Dedication

We dedicate this book in memory of Bert
Carron. His spirit, vitality, and passion for his
profession were contagious and inspirational.

Brief Contents

SECTION 1 Introduction to the Psychology of Exercise and Sedentary Behavior   **1**

Chapter 1   Introduction to the Psychology of Physical Activity   3
Chapter 2   Introduction to the Psychology of Sedentary Behavior   35

SECTION 2 Theoretical Models for Exercise and Sedentary Behavior   **61**

Chapter 3   Social Cognitive Theory   63
Chapter 4   Motivational Theories   85
Chapter 5   Theory of Planned Behavior   109
Chapter 6   Transtheoretical Model   137

SECTION 3 Psychological Health Effects of Exercise and Sedentary Behavior   **157**

Chapter 7   Cognition   159
Chapter 8   Anxiety and Depression   187
Chapter 9   Personality Traits   213
Chapter 10   Self-Esteem and Body Image   231
Chapter 11   Stress and Pain   257
Chapter 12   Sleep   285
Chapter 13   Health-Related Quality of Life and Positive Psychology   307
Chapter 14   Exercise-Related Disorders   335

SECTION 4 Environmental Effects of Exercise and Sedentary Behavior   **369**

Chapter 15   Social Environment   371
Chapter 16   Physical Environment   399

Contents

Foreword XIII

Preface XIV

About the Authors XVIII

Reviewers XIX

Section 1 Introduction to the Psychology of Exercise and Sedentary Behavior   1

Chapter 1   Introduction to the Psychology of Physical Activity   3
Vignette: Henry. 3
Introduction 5
    Physical Activity and the Tomato Effect .6
What Is a Meta-Analysis? 13
    Research Integration Through a Meta-Analysis 13
    Interpretation of Effect Sizes 15
Exercise Psychology 16
Individual Correlates of Exercise 16
Guidelines for Physical Activity. 19
    Upper Limit to Physical Activity Guidelines? 22
Historical Developments 25
Topics of Interest 26
Related Terms 26
Summary 30
    Key Terms. 30
    Review Questions. 31
    Applying the Concepts 31
    References 32

Chapter 2   Introduction to the Psychology of Sedentary Behavior   35
Vignette: Sarah. 35
Introduction 36
Defining Sedentary Behavior 38
Health Significance of Sedentary Behavior. 42
Guidelines for Sedentary Behavior. 43
Prevalence of Sedentary Behavior 45
Individual Correlates of Sedentary Behavior 50
Measures of Sedentary Behavior 53
Summary 56
    Key Terms. 56
    Review Questions. 57
    Applying the Concepts 57
    References 57

Section 2 Theoretical Models for Exercise and Sedentary Behavior   61

Chapter 3   Social Cognitive Theory   63
Vignette: Jennifer 63
Introduction 65
Self-Efficacy in Social Cognitive Theory 66
Sources of Self-Efficacy Beliefs 68
Nature and Measurement of Self-Efficacy 70
    Self-Efficacy in Physical Activity Contexts 72
Self-Efficacy and Physical Activity Behavior. 73
    Initiation and Maintenance of Physical Activity 73
    Effort Expended in Physical Activity 74
Self-Efficacy and Mental States 74
Enhancing Self-Efficacy: Experimental Evidence 75
    Social Cognitive Theory Applied to Sedentary Behavior 78
Summary 79
    Key Terms 80
    Review Questions 80
    Applying the Concepts 81
    References 81

Chapter 4   Motivational Theories   85
Vignette: Bryan 85
Introduction 87
Health Belief Model 88
    Health Belief Model Constructs 89
    Application of the Health Belief Model to Physical Activity. 93
Protection Motivation Theory 94
    Application of the Protection Motivation Theory
        to Physical Activity 96
    Protection Motivation Theory and Physical Activity Intervention. . . .97
    Limitations of the Health Belief Model and Protection
        Motivation Theory 98
Self-Determination Theory. 99
    Sources of Motivation. 100
    The Antecedents of Intrinsic and Extrinsic Motivation 101
    Research on Self-Determination Theory in Physical
        Activity Settings 102
    Self-Determination Theory in Physical Activity Intervention 103
Summary 104
    Key Terms 105
    Review Questions. 105
    Applying the Concepts 106
    References 106

Chapter 5 **Theory of Planned Behavior**   **109**
Vignette: Rachel. 109
Introduction 111
Theory of Planned Behavior Variables 112
    Intention. 112
    Attitude. 113
    Subjective Norm 113
    Perceived Behavioral Control. 113
Theory of Planned Behavior Research. 115
    Physical Activity Research 115
    Sedentary Behavior Research. 118
Elicitation Studies 119
Using Theory for Practice. 121
Limitations of the Theory of Planned Behavior 125
    Other Variables. 125
    Perceived Behavioral Control Issues. 126
    Intention–Behavior Gap. 127
    Habit and Planning. 128
    Subjective Norm Issues. 129
Summary 131
    Key Terms. 131
    Review Questions. 132
    Applying the Concepts 132
    References 132

Chapter 6 **Transtheoretical Model**   **137**
Vignette: Gina 137
Introduction 139
Constructs of the Transtheoretical Model. 140
    Stages of Change 140
    Decisional Balance 144
    Processes of Change 145
    Self-Efficacy 145
    Temptation 146
Advantages and Limitations of the Transtheoretical Model. 146
    Advantages. 146
    Limitations 148
Physical Activity Research Examining the Transtheoretical Model. 149
    Observational Studies. 150
    Intervention Research 151
Summary 152
    Key Terms. 153
    Review Questions. 153
    Applying the Concepts 153
    References 154

Section 3 Psychological Health Effects of Exercise and Sedentary Behavior   157

Chapter 7	**Cognition**	**159**
	Vignette: Mike	159
	Introduction	162
	The Brain	162
	What Is Cognition?	163
	Cognition, Physical Activity, and Sedentary Behavior	164
	Exercise and Cognition in Children and Adolescents	165
	Adult Populations	172
	Cognition and Sedentary Behavior	179
	Mechanism of Effect	179
	Summary	181
	Key Terms	181
	Review Questions	182
	Applying the Concepts	182
	References	182

Chapter 8	**Anxiety and Depression**	**187**
	Vignette: Laura	187
	Introduction	189
	Affect, Emotion, and Mood	189
	Depression, Physical Activity, and Sedentary Behavior	191
	Nonclinical Depression	192
	Clinical Depression	196
	Anxiety, Physical Activity, and Sedentary Behavior	200
	Anxiety Disorders	200
	State and Trait Anxiety	201
	Nonclinical Anxiety	203
	Clinical Anxiety	204
	Optimal Amount of Exercise Needed	205
	Potential Mechanisms	206
	Summary	206
	Key Terms	207
	Review Questions	207
	Applying the Concepts	208
	References	208

Chapter 9	**Personality Traits**	**213**
	Vignette: Lauren	213
	Introduction	215
	Structure of Personality	216
	Personality and Physical Activity	219
	Moderators of Personality and Physical Activity	221
	Lower-Order Traits	222

How Does Personality Affect Physical Activity?. 223
Personality and Intervention 224
Personality and Sedentary Behavior. **225**
Summary. **226**
Key Terms. 227
Review Questions. 227
Applying the Concepts 227
References 228

Chapter 10   Self-Esteem and Body Image   231
Vignette: Divya 231
Introduction 234
Self-Esteem 234
Physical Self-Esteem. 236
Effects of Exercise and Sedentary Behavior on Self-Esteem 239
Body Image 241
Scope and Significance of Body Image. 243
Body Image and Physical Activity 245
Self-Presentational Anxiety 248
Summary. 251
Key Terms. 252
Review Questions. 252
Applying the Concepts 253
References 253

Chapter 11   Stress and Pain   257
Vignette: Carla. 257
Introduction 259
Stress. 259
Types of Stress. 262
Stress, Exercise, and Sedentary Behavior. 263
Mechanisms of Effect 267
Stress Disorders and Exercise 268
Pain 269
Components of Pain. 271
Pain, Exercise, and Sedentary Behavior. 272
Effects of Exercise and Sedentary Behavior on Endogenous Pain . . .273
Effects of Exercise on Experimentally Induced Pain 277
Summary. 280
Key Terms. 280
Review Questions. 280
Applying the Concepts 281
References 281

Chapter 12   Sleep   285
Vignette: Omar 285
Introduction 287

What Is Sleep?. 287
How Much Sleep Do We Need?. 288
Sleep, Exercise, and Sedentary Behavior. 291
    Affects of Acute and Chronic Exercise on Sleep. 294
    Evening Exercise and Sleep 295
    Exercise and Clinical Sleep Disorders. 296
Mechanisms of How Exercise Affects Sleep 301
    Anxiety Reduction 301
    Antidepressant Effects 302
    Thermoregulation. 302
    Circadian Rhythms 302
Summary. 303
    Key Terms. 303
    Review Questions. 304
    Applying the Concepts 304
    References 304

Chapter 13   **Health-Related Quality of Life and Positive Psychology**   **307**
Vignette: Beverly 307
Introduction 309
Health-Related Quality of Life 309
    Measurement of Health-Related Quality of Life. 312
Health-Related Quality of Life, Exercise, and Sedentary Behavior. 316
    General Population. 316
    Health-Related Quality of Life and Exercise in
        Special Populations 317
Positive Psychology. 321
    Positive Psychology, Exercise, and Sedentary Behavior. 322
    Happiness 324
    Exercise-Induced Feelings 326
Summary. 328
    Key Terms. 328
    Review Questions. 329
    Applying the Concepts 329
    References 329

Chapter 14   **Exercise-Related Disorders**   **335**
Vignette: Katie. 335
Introduction 338
Exercise Dependence 338
    Does Exercise Have Negative Health Effects?. 338
    Exercise Dependence Defined 341
    Origins of Research on Exercise Dependence. 344
    Prevalence of Exercise Dependence 345
    Correlates of Exercise Dependence 348
    Exercise Deprivation. 351
    Explanations of Exercise Dependence 353

Eating Disorders 355
   Anorexia Nervosa 356
   Bulimia Nervosa 356
   Eating Disorders and Exercise 357
Muscle Dysmorphia 359
   Correlates of Muscle Dsymorphia 361
   Muscle Dysmorphia Measures 362
Summary 362
   Key Terms 363
   Review Questions 363
   Applying the Concepts 364
   References 364

Section 4 Environmental Effects of Exercise and Sedentary Behavior   369

Chapter 15 Social Environment   371

Vignette: Madeline 371
Introduction 372
Social Support 373
   Taxonomies for Social Support 374
   Negative Aspects of Social Support 375
   Social Support as a Personality Trait 376
   Measurement of Social Support 377
   Social Support, Physical Activity, and Sedentary Behavior 380
Group Dynamics 388
   Cohesion 388
   Leadership 390
Summary 393
   Key Terms 394
   Review Questions 394
   Applying the Concepts 394
   References 395

Chapter 16 Physical Environment   399

Vignette: Clayton 399
Introduction 401
Influences of the Physical Environment on Delayed Gratification 402
Modernization of the Physical Environment: A Comparison
  of Two Cultures 404
   The Case of the Inuit 405
   The Case of the Old Order Amish 407
Travel Patterns 410
   Youth Travel Patterns 410
   Travel in Different Countries 412
   The Case of the Dutch 413

Seasonal Variation 414
Point-of-Choice Environmental Prompts 416
Physical Environment Correlates 419
    Home Environment Correlates. 422
Summary 423
    Key Terms. 424
    Review Questions. 424
    Applying the Concepts 424
    References 425

Glossary 429
Index 443

Foreword

Two of my well-regarded colleagues, Heather Hausenblas and Ryan Rhodes, have undertaken a formidable task in putting together this book. Each of them brings a wealth of knowledge, expertise, and experience in the psychology of physical activity area to the table. Having met both at conferences as emerging young scholars (many years ago), I was impressed at that time with their ability to grasp the bigger picture, synthesize information, articulate concepts, and come up with important and meaningful research questions. As evidenced by their achievements and this book, clearly this has not changed. They both are established and well-respected leaders in our field. Just as important, we have collaborated on many projects and papers, and I have rarely come across two more positive, productive, and thoughtful individuals whom I am proud to call my colleagues.

This book will undoubtedly serve as an excellent resource to researchers, practitioners, and students. The book is set up in a logical manner—which will help you, the reader, build the foundation of knowledge in this area. This should enable you to become informed on what is known about physical activity and sedentary behaviors, why physical activity and sedentary behaviors are important, why and how to change physical activity and sedentary behaviors, and how to use this knowledge in research and application.

I would like to point out some highlights. Introducing the concept of sedentary behavior is timely and much needed as physical activity is further engineered out of our lives and with the rapid increase of screen technology (tablets/iPads, smartphones, web TV, etc.). The theories presented are the major theories in our field, thus providing a description of our current understanding of behavior and why people would change. The consequences and outcomes presented include psychological and physiological aspects, and, importantly, also address negative outcomes of physical activity. The book concludes with looking at the environment, both social and physical, to complete the picture.

Heather and Ryan have taken a very conversational approach to this book, which makes it easy to read and facilitates understanding. This includes providing learning objectives, asking questions, providing examples, defining terms as you read along, and presenting figures and tables. Such interactive and engaging writing makes it easy for the reader to continue and see what else there is to learn. I am confident that this text will be very valuable to our field and motivate practitioners, researchers, professors, and students to push their contributions to the next level. In so doing, the book will be a catalyst to our field.

Claudio R. Nigg, PhD, FSBM
Professor and Director, HBCR Workgroup and Editor, ACSM's Behavioral Aspects of Physical Activity and Exercise
Department of Public Health Sciences
University of Hawaii
Honolulu, Hawaii

Preface

What contributes to our overall health? What might surprise you is that our behavior—that is, what we are actually doing (or not doing)—has the most significant impact on our overall health. According to the U.S. Department of Health and Human Services (2014), our behavior has more of an impact on our health than our genetics, our environment, and our access to medical care.

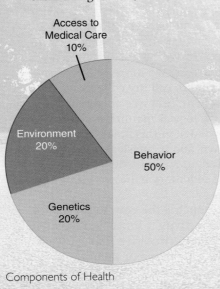

Components of Health

Data from U. S. Department of Health and Human Services. (2010). Physical activity for everyone: Recommendations. Retrieved March 27, 2010, from http://www.cdc.gov /physicalactivity/everyone/guidelines/adults.html.

If we break our behavior down even further, physical activity has one of the biggest impacts on our overall health. The science is clear—every system of the body benefits when a person exercises. Regular exercise is likely the single best prescription that people of all ages could take to reap a huge host of health benefits. Physical activity is highly effective for preventing and treating many of our most prevalent chronic diseases, including coronary heart disease, hypertension, heart failure, obesity, depression, and diabetes. The bottom line is that physical activity is very (very) good for our health. In fact, people who are regular exercisers can expect to have a mean life expectancy that is 7 years longer than that of their physically inactive friends (Chakravarty, Hubert, Lingala, & Fries, 2008).

Physical activity by itself, however, isn't enough to achieve overall health because it needs to be paired with a reduction in sedentary behavior. Sedentary behavior includes activities undertaken in either a sitting or reclined position, such as watching TV, reading, and engaging in activities on the computer. Too much sitting appears to be a health risk that is additional to, and distinct from, too little exercise. The consequence is that even if people are meeting the physical activity guidelines, if they spend most of their remaining waking hours in sedentary activities, they will experience a distinct negative impact on their overall health. We need to not only move more at a moderate and/or vigorous pace, but we also need to stand up more during the day.

The editor of *The Lancet* concluded in the July 2012 issue that was dedicated to physical activity and health: "In view of the prevalence, global reach, and health effect of physical inactivity, the issue should be appropriately described as pandemic, with far-reaching health, economic, environmental, and social consequences" (July 2012). This powerful conclusion reveals that more than ever the field of exercise and sedentary behavior psychology is of great importance.

How can we get people to move more and sit less? We have tackled this question in this book by exploring the research, summarizing the key areas in this increasingly significant area of scientific inquiry in order to shed light on possible answers to this question. Our main goal in writing this book was to produce the first targeted book to bring the research examining the psychology of both exercise and sedentary behavior together in a comprehensive, educational, and informative format with a socioecological scope.

This book is intended for health professionals, researchers, professors, and students who are interested in learning more about the psychological basis of exercise and sedentary behavior. It is our hope that it will stimulate continued interest and research in these important aspects of human behavior.

ORGANIZATION OF THE BOOK

All areas of science proceed through four general stages. The first stage is *description*. The descriptive stage is essential because it informs us about "what is." A large proportion of the research in the psychology of exercise and sedentary behavior has been descriptive in nature. Section 1 is devoted to the introductory material describing exercise psychology (Chapter 1) and the psychology of sedentary behavior (Chapter 2).

The second and third stages of science, *explanation* and *prediction*, involve theory development and testing. In Section 2, various theoretical models that have been advanced to explain and predict involvement in exercise and sedentary behavior are discussed. Chapter 3 deals with one of the most extensively used theoretical models used to understand human behavior—social cognitive theory. In Chapter 4, motivational theories are examined, including the health belief model, self-determination theory, and protection motivation theory. The theory of planned behavior is described in Chapter 5. A popular approach to the study of involvement in exercise, the transtheoretical model, is discussed in Chapter 6.

Section 3 of the book provides an overview of research that has centered on the relationships between exercise and sedentary behavior and various health outcomes. Considerable research has identified a number of psychological benefits of being physically active, including reduced anxiety and depression, improved stress reactivity, enhanced self-esteem, increased body satisfaction, and improved cognitive functioning. In Chapter 7, we examine the mind–body connection between physical activity and sedentary behavior and cognition. In Chapter 8, we explore how physical activity and sedentary behavior affect both depression and anxiety. In Chapter 9, we examine how our personality, in particular the Big Five personality traits of extraversion, openness to experience, neuroticism, agreeableness, and conscientiousness, affect our exercise and sedentary behaviors. In Chapter 10, we discuss the effect of exercise and sedentary behavior on self-esteem and the related construct of body image. The effects of exercise and sedentary behavior on our stress levels and our ability to handle pain are discussed in Chapter 11. Chapter 12 explores how exercise and sedentary behavior affect our sleep habits. In Chapter 13, we examine how exercise affects overall health-related quality of life and positive mood states such as vigor and happiness in the general population as well as special populations, such as cancer patients, pregnant women,

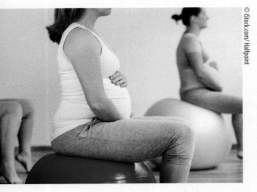

and obese individuals. Finally, a number of potential exercise-related disorders and negative behaviors have been associated with exercise, such as exercise dependence, steroid use, muscle dysmorphia, and eating disorders. The final chapter in this section (Chapter 14) focuses on the potential dark side of exercise behavior.

An important characteristic that helps to define the psychology of exercise and sedentary behavior as a discipline is its focus on the environmental factors that influence individual behavior. Section 4 provides an overview of research that has centered on an individual's social and physical environments. Chapter 15 focuses on the social environment (i.e., family, friends, and teammates), whereas Chapter 16 outlines aspects of the physical environment (e.g., neighborhoods, parks, green spaces) that have been found to be important influences on physical activity and sedentary behavior.

The fourth stage of science is *intervention*. Essentially, the description stage provides a basis for the explanation stage (theory), the prediction stage involves a test of theory, and the intervention stage involves the application of what has been learned from the other three stages. Because the benefits of exercise are so important for the individual and society in general, numerous attempts have been made to develop effective intervention strategies to not only increase exercise behavior but also reduce sedentary behavior. Strategies on how to promote exercise involvement and reduce sedentary behavior, including those that have focused on the individual level, social level, policy level, and environment, are integrated within each of the chapters.

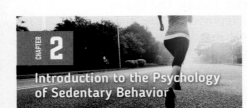

KEY FEATURES

- **Learning Objectives.** Each chapter begins with a list of goals to focus the reader in their learning and engagement with the content.
- **Vignettes.** A fictional vignette is presented to depict how a person might encounter that chapter's topic in real life and its impact on that person's health.
- **Applying the Concepts.** At the end of each chapter, readers are asked questions that tie the knowledge gained in the chapter to real-world scenarios.

- **Critical Thinking Activities.** Short questions and activities are included throughout each chapter to present opportunities for the reader to challenge and delve deeper in the theories, concepts, and research presented.

CRITICAL THINKING ACTIVITY 7-2

© ecco/Shutterstock, Inc.

Do you think that moderate and/or mild physical activity can improve the attention and concentration of children with ADHD? Explain why or why not.

- **Review Questions.** At the end of each chapter, Review Questions allow readers to evaluate the achievement of the objectives outlined at the start of the chapter.

INSTRUCTOR RESOURCES

The following resources are available to instructors to aid in teaching the content:
- **Test Bank** of more than 750 questions for assessment and practice.
- **Slides in lecture format** to support course lectures for each chapter.
- **Sample answers and Tips & Tricks** are provided to instructors for the Review Questions and Applying the Concepts questions at the end of each chapter.
- **Projects** that feature in-class activities are included for each chapter.
- **Instructor's Manuals** for selected chapters provide tips and grading rubrics for the additional projects provided.
- **Sample Syllabus** depicts an example of how to teach the topics in this book in a typical course.
- **Image Bank** slide deck includes the key images from the text.

REFERENCES

Chakravarty, E. F., Hubert H. B., Lingala V. B., & Fries J. F. (2008). Reduced disability and mortality among aging runners: A 21-year longitudinal study. *Archives of Internal Medicine, 168*, 1638–1646.

U.S. Department of Health and Human Services. (2014). Determinants of health. Healthy People 2020. Retrieved November 10, 2015, from http://www.healthypeople.gov/2020/about/foundation-health-measures/Determinants-of-Health.

Kohl, H. W., Craig, C. L., Lambert, E. V., et al. (2012). The pandemic of physical inactivity: global action for public health. *The Lancet.* doi:10.1016/S0140-6736(12)60898-8.

About the Authors

Heather Hausenblas, PhD is a physical activity and healthy aging expert, researcher, and author. She obtained her doctorate from the University of Western Ontario, Canada. She was a faculty member and the director of the Exercise Psychology Laboratory at the University of Florida from 1998 to 2012. She is currently a professor in the Brooks Rehabilitation College of Healthcare Sciences at Jacksonville University. Her research focuses on the psychological effects of health behaviors, in particular physical activity and diet, across the lifespan. She examines the effects of physical activity and diet on body image, mood, adherence, quality of life, and excessive exercise. Dr. Hausenblas is the co-author of five scientific books, and she has published over 90 scientific journal articles on these topics. In 1996, she was awarded the Canadian Association for Psychomotor Learning and Sport Psychology Young Scientist Award for Scholarly Research. In 2003, Heather was the recipient of the Dorothy V. Harris Memorial Award for outstanding early career development in health and exercise psychology from the Association of Applied Sport Psychology. In 2005, she was the recipient of the early career distinguished scholars award by the North American Society for the Psychology of Sport and Physical Activity. In 1998, she received the Sport Science Award of the International Olympic Committee. She is a mom to three young boys, and she enjoys exercising outdoors, spending time with her family and friends, and coaching and watching her sons play sports. She resides in Jacksonville, Florida, with her husband and boys.

Ryan E. Rhodes, PhD is the director of the Behavioural Medicine Laboratory and a professor at the School of Exercise Science, University of Victoria, Victoria, British Columbia. His primary research and teaching areas are focused on the psychology of physical activity and sedentary behavior, with applied interests in early family development of physical activity and special populations. Dr. Rhodes has written over 250 peer-reviewed publications on these topics and has taught annual courses in the psychology of physical activity and sedentary behavior since 2002. He has held research chairs from the Michael Smith Foundation for Health Research (Population Health Scholar, 2003–2008), the Canadian Institutes of Health Research (Gender and Health Investigator, 2006–2011), and the Canadian Cancer Society (Prevention Scientist, 2011–2016). He received the Early Career Scholar award from the North American Society for the Psychology of Sport and Physical Activity in 2008 and was awarded fellowship in the Society of Behavioral Medicine in 2014. When not working, he spends time with his two daughters, Lauren and Rachel, and his golden retriever named Cooper, who always manages to keep him active.

Reviewers

Heather R. Adams–Blair, PhD
Professor
Exercise and Sport Science
  Department
Eastern Kentucky University
Richmond, Kentucky

Brandon L. Alderman, PhD
Assistant Professor
Department of Exercise Science
  and Sport Studies
Rutgers University
Brunswick, New Jersey

Alison Castellano
Adjunct Professor
Psychology Department
Western New England University
Springfield, Massachusetts

Joseph B. Hazzard, Jr., PhD, LAT, ATC
Assistant Professor and Program
  Director
Clinical Athletic Training Program
Bloomsburg University
Bloomsburg, Pennsylvania

Dorothy Hyman, PhD
Lecturer
Exercise Science and Physical
  Education Department
McDaniel College
Westminster, Maryland

John Koshuta, MA, CHES
Senior Lecturer
Health Sciences Department
Carroll University
Greendale, Wisconsin

Beverly B. Palmer, PhD
Emeritus Professor
Psychology Department
California State University,
  Dominguez Hills
Carson, California

Kelley J. Reno, MS
Lecturer
Health & Kinesiology Department
University of Texas–San Antonio
San Antonio, Texas

Douglas Sanders, MS Ed
Senior Lecturer
Department of Kinesiology
Southern Illinois University
Carbondale, Illinois

Donna J. Terbizan, PhD
Professor and Coordinator
Exercise Science Department
North Dakota State University
Fargo, North Dakota

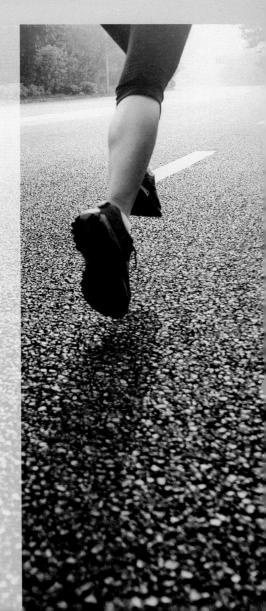

SECTION 1

Introduction to the Psychology of Exercise and Sedentary Behavior

This text is subdivided into four sections. The general purpose of Section 1 is to introduce you to the research area of the psychology of exercise and sedentary behavior. The scientific inquiry into exercise psychology is also referred to as *physical activity psychology*, *behavioral medicine*, or *fitness psychology*. In Chapter 1, we discuss physical activity from the perspective of why it is important, the degree to which people are involved in physical activity, and some of the physical activity guidelines (i.e., minimum levels) that have been developed for general as well as special populations. Also, a hallmark of effective communication is definitional clarity—it is important for you to understand some of the terms that are used throughout the text. So, in Chapter 1, definitions are provided for *exercise*, *physical activity*, and related terms such as *health*. A brief history of exercise psychology also is provided.

In Chapter 2, we discuss the psychology of sedentary behavior as a related, yet distinct, area from the psychology of physical activity. We will describe the health significance of sitting too much. We also take a closer look at the science behind the question: "Is sitting the new smoking?" In other words, is our current sedentary lifestyle more dangerous to our health than smoking? We will examine the science behind the health effects of prolonged sitting as well as the prevalence of sedentary behavior, correlates of sedentary behavior, and the emerging sedentary behavior guidelines. So let's get moving!

Introduction to the Psychology of Physical Activity

Runner: © lzf/Shutterstock

Vignette: Henry

My parents were by no means paragons of health. I was in elementary school the day mom came back from the doctor with a diagnosis of type 2 diabetes. The doc said it was because of all the weight she'd put on after pregnancy, as well as her diet. (Her favorite activity was watching daytime television on the couch, and if she ever did eat a vegetable it was soaked in butter and salt.) Since giving birth to me she'd developed back problems and found it painful to walk for more than 5- to 10-minute stretches at a time, so implementing the doc's recommended 30 minutes of movement a day struck her as impossible. (Needless to say, she didn't follow his advice.)

Dad had also been slapped with a diagnosis while I was still a kid. I can't remember a time where he wasn't bemoaning the blood pressure pills he had to take for his hypertension. He'd injured his ACL in college playing sports and was too afraid to get back into exercise, lest he hurt himself again. Plus, he barely had the time. He worked a demanding job as a truck driver and often went days without enough sleep.

Suffice it to say that exercise just wasn't something you went out of your way to do where I came from. Sure, some of my classmates did outdoorsy types of activities that got their blood pumping—biking, hiking, kayaking in the

LEARNING OBJECTIVES

After completing this chapter, you will be able to:

- Outline the importance of physical activity from a health perspective.
- Provide estimates of the number of people who are physically active.
- Describe the guidelines for a physically active lifestyle.
- Differentiate among the key terms used in the area known as the psychology of physical activity.
- Identify individual correlates and determinants of physical activity.
- Understand research integration via meta-analysis.

summers—but since I didn't have as much money to afford all the gear, and since I also worked at the local gas station to save up for college, I usually met up with those pals after they'd finished huffing and puffing so we could play video games at my house or drive into town for a movie.

I'll admit, too, that my more athletic peers intimidated me. I wasn't ever picked first in PE class and I never played sports because I didn't think I had it in me. I tried to stand out, instead, as someone who built up his brain instead of his body. The time I might have spent attending practice for a soccer, baseball, or basketball team I preferred to devote to studying. (If I wasn't hunched over my books, I'd just try to pick up an extra shift at the gas station.)

I got into engineering college early decision. I was thrilled to start on the path toward my degree. It's something I'd wanted to do since third grade. But once I got to campus and started classes the stress of having to work part time and meet all my academic deadlines was purely overwhelming. I didn't have an outlet to burn off the stress. It just kept mounting.

My roommate, an avid exerciser who woke up at an unfathomably early hour to squeeze in his morning runs, suggested I give jogging a try. "It'll help you relax," he kept trying to convince me, each time I turned down his invitations to drag me along. Then, one Friday afternoon, when neither of us had any plans and midterms were mostly finished, he asked if I wouldn't mind taking a walk with him to the college's fitness center. Not having anything better to do with my time, I (reluctantly) agreed.

To be honest, I was humiliated to walk into a gym not looking like anyone in there. I was already sweating at the thought of other students looking at my protruding midsection and rolling their eyes. I wasn't even sure that my shoes qualified as appropriate for the venue. I tiptoed from one machine to the other in high-top Converses with holes in the heels. Catching glimpses in the mirrors of students who could have very well been professional weightlifters for all I knew, I felt completely out of place. But my roommate urged me to just try a few machines. "You'll be better able to focus on your work," he reassured me.

So I gave the treadmill a go. He plugged in a few numbers and forward I went, walking at an incline (and trying not to fall over). The first 5 minutes were rough, but once I got into the swing of things the movement actually felt pretty good. At the 10-minute mark my roommate chided me: "Is that a smile I see?" (I couldn't deny, this wasn't so bad after all.)

After about 15 minutes of walking, he brought me over to the weight rack to show me how to do some basic bicep curls and overhead presses. ("Don't compare yourself to the other people in here," he kept telling me, when I'd look in shame at the other exercisers who were so much stronger than I was. "Everyone has to start somewhere.")

I didn't tell him then but part of why I stuck our first gym session out was the fear of becoming my parents. They'd always encouraged me to be better than them. And though it hurt me to hear in their voices a certain sense of self-defeat—of giving up on taking care of their health—I gathered that by giving exercise a shot I'd be making them proud. (While at the same time avoiding the health issues they'd faced throughout their adulthood.)

I've been regularly active ever since this date—I'm about to graduate, and I'm not sure I would have been able to make it this far without the added health boosts from my newfound love of movement.

No, I'll never be a bodybuilder. Or a marathon runner. Or even someone who can flaunt six-pack abs at the beach. But had you told me fitness didn't require any of the above—that it could be a lot simpler, entailing a 30-minute walk once or twice a day or a light jog a few times a week with some basic weight training sprinkled throughout, I probably would have started a lot sooner.

Being active isn't as hard as I thought it would be. I just never had a healthy amount of physical activity modeled for me by my parents, and the athletes in my high school, as well as the exercisers I saw in workout videos on TV, seemed to be doing things that were just way out of my range of possibility.

But I've found what works for me. It isn't an exorbitant amount of activity. Rather, it's just enough. And I think it's pretty incredible that a few weekly trips to the gym, a stroll or two around campus each day, and the occasional bike ride I now try to accomplish on weekends has improved my ability to focus on schoolwork while making me feel stronger, more energetic, and even less stressed. Even better? It's also been a boon to my confidence in approaching girls!

■ Introduction

Lao Tzu was a famous ancient Chinese philosopher who is quoted as saying that "the journey of a thousand miles begins with a single step." This proverb means that even the longest and most difficult ventures or journeys have a starting point. From the perspective of personal fitness, we know that the road to physical fitness and a healthy lifestyle is a lifetime journey with many obstacles. This is highlighted in Henry's personal story of becoming physically active. Unfortunately, like Henry's parents, most people are not on a physical fitness journey. In fact, it seems that participation in physical activity shows signs of a "**tomato effect**," an interesting term indeed. You might rightly ask, "What's a tomato effect?" Moreover, because it sounds mysterious, and possibly a bit dangerous, you might also be tempted to ask, "And how can this so-called tomato effect be eradicated?"

The tomato effect is a term James and Jean Goodwin (1984) used to describe a phenomenon whereby highly efficacious therapies are either ignored or rejected. Generally, the reason for this is that the therapies do not seem to make sense in light of popular beliefs or common understandings. A tomato effect, however, can also occur if people simply ignore the evidence available.

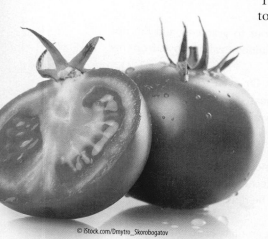

© iStock.com/Dmytro_Skorobogatov

The term *tomato effect* is derived from the history of the tomato in North America. The tomato was discovered in Peru and then transported to Spain, from where it made its way to Italy, France, and most of the rest of Europe. By 1560, the tomato played a major role in the diet of most Europeans. In North America, however, tomatoes were avoided because they were considered to be poisonous. The basis for this belief was that they belong to the nightshade family of plants, and some fruits from plants in the nightshade family can cause death if eaten in sufficient quantities. Thus, throughout the 18th century, tomatoes were not grown in North America. In fact, the turning point did not occur until 1820. Apparently, in a dramatic gesture, Robert Gibbon Johnson ate a tomato on the courthouse steps in Salem, New Jersey, and survived! According to legend, he stood on the courthouse steps and ate tomatoes in front of a large, amazed crowd that had assembled to watch him do so. When he neither dropped dead nor suffered any apparent ill effects, witnesses of his "experiment" slowly began to open their minds. By the end of the decade, American gardeners were growing tomatoes for food. Subsequently, tomatoes began to be accepted as a nutritious food source. It was not until the 20th century, however, that commercial marketing of the tomato began in earnest. Today, it represents one of the largest commercial crops in North America (Goodwin & Goodwin, 1984).

So, to answer the question "Does physical activity show a tomato effect?" we need to address the following three issues:

1. Is physical activity an efficacious therapy?
2. Do people either ignore or reject physical activity?
3. Do people know the benefits of physical activity?

Physical Activity and the Tomato Effect

1. Is Physical Activity an Efficacious Therapy?

According to Goodwin and Goodwin (1984), the use of aspirin for the alleviation of pain, swelling, and stiffness of rheumatoid arthritis also is characterized by a tomato effect. They noted that high doses of aspirin only became an accepted treatment about 70 years after initial studies demonstrated that aspirin is effective in treating some of the symptoms of arthritis. What about physical activity? Is a tomato effect toward physical activity prevalent in our society?

One part of the answer to this question, of course, pertains to whether physical activity is an efficacious activity. Scientists spent a large portion of the previous century conducting research on the physiological benefits of both **acute** and **chronic physical activity**. What their research has shown is that every system of the body benefits when a person engages in physical activity. In fact, regular physical activity is likely the single best prescription that people of all ages can take for a host of health benefits (Church & Blair, 2009). Regular exercise is one of the cornerstones of a therapeutic lifestyle change for producing optimal cardiovascular and overall health. Physical exercise, although not a drug, possesses many traits of a powerful pharmacological agent. Indeed, the saying "exercise is

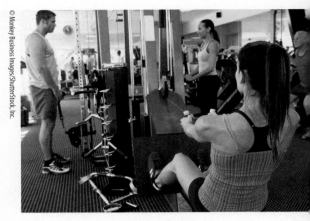

medicine" is supported by science. A routine of daily physical activity stimulates a number of beneficial physiological changes in the body and it can be highly effective for the prevention and treatment of many of our most prevalent chronic diseases, including coronary heart disease, hypertension, heart failure, obesity, depression, and type 2 diabetes. The bottom line is that physical activity is very good for our health.

But just how good is physical activity for our health? In terms of the skeletal system, for example, frequent physical activity leads to increased bone density in youth and an increased likelihood that bone mineral density will be retained in older adulthood (Marques, Mota, & Carvalho, 2012). How about the muscle system? Frequent physical activity results in hypertrophy, increased strength and endurance, as well as capillarization, maximization of blood flow, and enhanced metabolic capacity (e.g., Ferreira et al., 2012). How about the cardiovascular system? Along with increased cardiac mass, frequent physical activity contributes to increased stroke volume and cardiac output at rest and during physical activity and lower heart rate and blood pressure at rest and during submaximal physical activity (e.g., Cornelissen, Fagard, Cockelberghs, & Vanhees, 2011). How about the respiratory system? There is increased ventilatory-diffusion efficiency during physical activity and possible decreased work of breathing. How about the body's metabolism? Being physically active is associated with decreased triglycerides and increased high-density cholesterol, increased insulin-mediated glucose uptake, and decreased adiposity (Ekelund et al., 2012). What about psychological health? Physical activity is related to improved mood, sleep, stress reactivity, and body image, as well as a reduced likelihood of suicide later in life (Aberg et al., 2013). The end result is that people who exercise regularly have markedly lower rates of morbidity and mortality. In fact, people who are regular exercisers can expect to have a mean life expectancy that is 7 years longer than that of their physically inactive contemporaries (Chakravarty, Hubert, Lingala, & Fries, 2008). See **TABLE 1-1** for a summary of some of the health benefits of regular physical activity by age.

TABLE 1-1   Benefits of Physical Activity by Age Group

Early Years (0–4 years)	Children (5–11 years)	Youth (12–17 years)	Adults (18–64 years)	Older Adults (65+ years)
Maintain a healthy body weight.	Improve health.	Improve health.	Reduce premature death.	Less chronic disease (such as heart disease).
Improve movement skills.	Do better in school.	Do better in school.	Reduce heart disease and stroke.	Less premature death.
Increase fitness.	Improve fitness.	Improve fitness.	Reduce certain types of cancer.	Help maintain functional independence.
Build healthy hearts.	Have fun playing with friends.	Have fun playing with friends.	Reduce type 2 diabetes, osteoporosis.	Help improve mobility.
Feel happy, have fun.	Feel happier.	Feel happier.	Reduce high blood pressure.	Help improve fitness.
Develop self-confidence.	Maintain healthy body weight.	Maintain healthy body weight.	Improve strength and fitness.	Help improve/ maintain body weight.
Improve learning and attention.	Improve self-confidence.	Improve self-confidence.	Improve mental health.	Help maintain mental health and feel better.

Adapted from http://www.participaction.com/get-moving/benefits-of-physical-activity/.

These substantial physiological benefits of physical activity are no secret. Within the past 30 years, there has been an almost global endorsement of the value of physical activity. For example, the **World Health Organization (WHO)** (2009) has cited physical inactivity as one of the five leading global risk factors for mortality. The five leading global risks for mortality are high blood pressure (responsible for 13% of deaths globally), tobacco use (9%), high blood glucose (6%), physical inactivity (6%), and overweight and obesity (5%). These risks increase a person's chances of developing chronic diseases such as heart disease, diabetes, and some cancers.

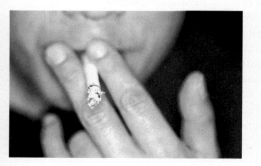

In an attempt to quantify the effect of physical inactivity on coronary heart disease, type 2 diabetes, breast cancer, and colon cancer, Lee and colleagues (2012) calculated the **population-attributable fraction** to estimate risks by country as well as globally.

They found that 9.4% of deaths from any cause are attributed to physical inactivity. More specifically, physical inactivity is responsible for 5.8% of the burden of coronary heart disease worldwide, ranging from 3.2% in Southeast Asia to 11.4% in Swaziland and Saudi Arabia. The burden of type 2 diabetes attributable to physical inactivity is 7.2% worldwide, ranging from 3.9% in Southeast Asia to 9.6% in the Eastern Mediterranean. Worldwide, 10.1% of breast cancers and 10.4% of colon cancers are attributable to a lack of physical exercise. These researchers concluded that if all of the inactive people in the world were to suddenly get off the couch and become engaged in just a modest level of physical activity, the estimated gain in life expectancy would be 0.68 years.

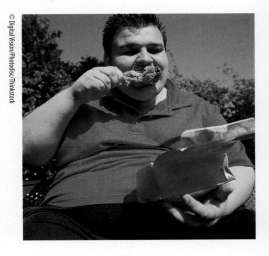

© Digital Vision/Photodisc/Thinkstock

A recent large-scale study highlights the role of physical inactivity in the rise in obesity in the United States. Ladabaum, Mannalithara, Myer, and Singh (2014) found that increases in obesity in the United States over the past 20 years may be due to sedentary lifestyles, not high caloric intake. They found that the average calorie intake of American adults has remained the same over the last two decades. However, American adults' physical activity levels have decreased significantly over the last two decades.

The study was conducted using data from the National Health and Nutrition Examination Survey (NHANES) to examine trends in obesity, physical activity, and calorie intake from 1988 to 2010 in adults. The researchers considered survey results from 17,430 participants from 1988 through 1994 and from about 5,000 participants each year from 1995 through 2010. The study results support previous findings on the growing prevalence of obesity, showing substantial increases in **body mass index (BMI)**, waist circumference, and abdominal adiposity in American adults. In fact, obesity increased, climbing from 25% to 35% in women and from 20% to 35% in men, during the study period. The study also found that Americans, on average, are consuming about the same number of calories per day as they were in 1988. However, they found a significant increase in the percentage of Americans reporting no leisure-time physical activity during this same time period.

CRITICAL THINKING ACTIVITY 1-1

© ecco/Shutterstock, Inc.

What is the difference between body mass index (BMI), waist circumference, and abdominal adiposity? Which of these three measures of body composition is considered the most significant for understanding the health impact of overweight or obesity?

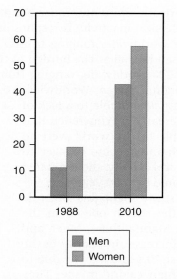

FIGURE 1-1   Percentage of American Adults Reporting No Leisure-Time Physical Activity from 1988 to 2010

Data from Ladabaum, U., Mannalithara, A., Myer, P. A., & Singh, G. (2014). Obesity, abdominal obesity, physical activity, and caloric intake in U.S. adults: 1988 to 2010. *The American Journal of Medicine, 127*, 717–727.

More specifically, the percentage of women reporting no leisure-time physical activity more than doubled from 1988 to 2010, increasing from 19.1% to 51.7%. Similarly, the percentage of men reporting no leisure-time physical activity nearly quadrupled, from 11.4% to 43.2% (see **FIGURE 1-1**). Although they were not able to see an association between daily caloric intake and increases in BMI or waist circumference, the researchers did find a relationship between decreased physical activity levels and increased BMI. The researchers concluded that the nationwide drop in exercise may be responsible for the upward trend in obesity rates.

Note that this study highlights the correlation between obesity and sedentary lifestyles, but because it is an observational study it does not address the possible causal link between inactivity and weight gain. The bottom line, however, is that physical inactivity rather than higher calorie intake could be driving the dramatic increase in obesity over the past few decades.

2. Do People Either Ignore or Reject Physical Activity?

The second part of the tomato-effect question pertains to whether people tend to ignore or reject exercise. Are people eating the tomatoes? Or, stated another way, is physical activity being embraced by a large portion of the world's population? Unfortunately, the answer is a qualified *no*. Despite the negative impact of physical inactivity, studies suggest that getting active is simply not happening (Dumith, Hallal, Reis, & Kohl, 2011).

TABLE 1-2 Adult Physical Inactivity Rates by Region	
Region	**Physically Inactive (%)**
Southeast Asia	17.0%
Africa	27.5%
Western Pacific	33.7%
Europe	34.8%
Eastern Mediterranean	43.3%
North America	43.3%
South America	43.3%
Central America	43.3%

For example, Pedro Hallal and his colleagues (2012) examined physical activity levels for adults aged 15 years or older from 122 countries. They found that, worldwide, 31% of adults failed to meet the public health guidelines for physical activity, defined as 150 minutes of moderate physical activity per week, but that the frequency of inactivity varied across regions, with proportions ranging from 17% in Southeast Asia to about 43% in North, South, and Central America and the Eastern Mediterranean. See **TABLE 1-2** for the physical inactivity rates by region.

CRITICAL THINKING ACTIVITY 1-2

© ecco/Shutterstock, Inc.

What are some possible explanations for why physical activity levels vary from country to country?

Hallal and his colleagues (2012) also found that inactivity increases with age and it is higher in women than in men. They also examined worldwide data for adolescents aged 13 to 15 years from 105 countries. They found that the proportion of 13- to 15-year-olds doing fewer than 60 minutes of moderate to vigorous physical activity intensity per day is about 80%. Similar to adult populations, boys are more active than girls.

The take-home message is that relatively few individuals are physically active on a regular basis, and this situation seems to generalize across a number of nations. Dr. Harold Kohl and his colleagues (2012) have called the current worldwide low activity levels a "**pandemic** of physical inactivity." Worldwide there has been a shift from concerns about infectious diseases (e.g., tuberculosis,

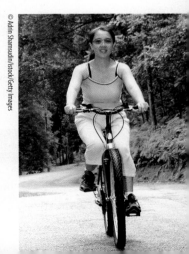

© Azim Shamsudin/istock/Getty Images

measles, and influenza) undermining public health to risks posed by chronic diseases, such as coronary heart disease, obesity, and type 2 diabetes. Even in countries such as China and India and those in Latin America and Africa the burden of chronic disease has outpaced the risk of infectious diseases, and physical inactivity is a contributing factor.

3. Do People Know the Benefits of Physical Activity?

As discussed earlier, scientists, healthcare professionals, and politicians are aware of the physical, biological, and physiological benefits of physical activity. A third part of the question pertaining to whether a tomato effect toward physical activity exists in society is whether the portion of the population who are not physically active (i.e., the non-tomato-eaters) have a full understanding of the benefits of a physically active lifestyle.

Jim Morrow and his colleagues (2004) attempted to answer this question by asking American adults whether they knew which types of physical activities affect their health and how much physical activity they should be doing to achieve a health benefit. Using a national random telephone survey of 2,002 American households, they found that 94% of adults were aware of traditional physical activities that provide a health benefit, and 68% were aware of specific exercise guidelines for health. Because most adults are physically inactive, the authors concluded that physical activity knowledge alone is not sufficient to cause people to become physically active.

So, the answer to the first question of this chapter—"Does participation in physical activity show evidence of a tomato effect?"—seems to be a qualified *yes* because we have answered yes to the following three issues:

1. *Yes*, physical activity is an efficacious therapy.
2. *Yes*, people either ignore or reject physical activity.
3. *Yes*, people know the benefits of physical activity.

The second question was how we overcome the tomato effect toward physical activity (i.e., "How can this so-called tomato effect be eradicated?"). One useful approach is through science—science that focuses on the psychology of physical activity and sedentary behavior. Before we examine what exercise psychology is, we must describe an important statistical technique that is often used to review this research.

CRITICAL THINKING ACTIVITY 1-3

© ecco/Shutterstock, Inc.

What other types of treatments or interventions have shown signs of a tomato effect?

■ What Is a Meta-Analysis?

Given the impressive list of the benefits of exercise, a strong case can be (and often is) made for increased physical activity on the basis of physical benefits alone. Historically, however, there has also been a long-standing belief that being physically active has consequences far beyond the physical. One illustration of that long-standing belief can be traced back to the following famous ancient Latin quotation *mens sana in corpore sano*, which is often translated as "a sound mind in a sound body." As another example, Hippocrates, who is acknowledged to be the Father of Medicine, strongly urged individuals thousands of years ago suffering from mental illness to exercise. However, only recently have scientists begun to evaluate systematically the association between exercise, sedentary behavior, and mental health in empirical studies.

The implicit belief that a link exists between physical health and mental health has led many social scientists to empirically test various relationships over the past 100 years. Not all of the research has been scientifically sound. Furthermore, not all of that research showed the same pattern of results. Thus, it was difficult to draw conclusions. This point was emphasized several years ago by Christian North, Penny McCullagh, and Zung Vu Tran (1990) when they attempted to summarize the literature on the impact of physical activity on depression. In their commentary, they pointed out "given the discrepant findings ... it is likely that a narrative review of literature would conclude that there is no consistent findings" (p. 383).

North and colleagues (1990) offered the solution of conducting a meta-analysis in an attempt to provide a firm conclusion from all the discrepant results. A **meta-analysis** is a statistical method of reviewing a body of research evidence that is both *systematic* and *quantitative*. A **systematic review** is a literature review focused on a particular research question that tries to identify, appraise, select, and synthesize all high-quality research evidence relevant to that question. **Quantitative research** refers to the systematic empirical investigation of a phenomena via statistical, mathematical, or numerical data or computational techniques. Fortunately, much of the research on the impact of exercise on psychological variables has been summarized through the use of meta-analysis. Thus, continually in our book we make reference to the findings of meta-analyses to illustrate the effects of exercise and sedentary behavior on various psychological outcomes. But before discussing the conclusions from these meta-analyses, an understanding of what exactly a meta-analysis is and why it is used by researchers is needed.

Research Integration Through a Meta-Analysis

Consider the following question: Is physical fitness related to anxiety? Across different studies, the operational definition of anxiety could vary markedly. For example, participants' level of anxiety might be tested with a single self-report question such as "I feel very anxious." Responses could then be obtained on a nine-point scale containing anchor statements such as "Strongly Disagree" and "Strongly Agree." Or, it might be tested with a psychometrically sound inventory containing 20 anxiety-relevant questions to which the individual responds "True" or "False." Or, it might even be assessed using a physiological measure such as heart rate with responses indicated in beats per minute.

Across that same cross-section of studies, the **operational definition** of fitness also could vary. For example, fitness might be assessed through the self-reported amount of time spent running per week. Then, responses could be obtained in minutes and/or hours per week. Or, fitness might be defined through measures of muscular strength and responses expressed in grams or kilograms (or ounces or pounds) lifted. Finally, fitness might even be assessed using a physiological measure such as maximal oxygen uptake with responses stated in milliliter per kilogram of body weight.

Imagine carrying out a literature review focusing on the question of the relationship between fitness and anxiety. If 50 studies were located, they might vary in the operational definitions used for anxiety, the operational definitions used for fitness, the size of the samples tested, and the nature of the samples tested by, for example, age, gender, physical health status, and mental health status. Also, the 50 studies might vary in their findings relative to the question. That is, 35 studies might show that fitness is associated with reduced anxiety, 10 studies might find that fitness is unrelated to anxiety, and 5 studies might conclude that fitness is associated with increased anxiety. Any scholar attempting to summarize this body of research with a narrative review would be forced to conclude that the results were either *mixed* or *unclear*.

In 1976, Gene Glass introduced a protocol for conducting a meta-analysis whereby the magnitude of the treatment effects in individual studies were quantified and the results of several studies were averaged. As Glass, McGaw, and Smith (1981) stated, the essential characteristic of a meta-analysis is that it "is the statistical analysis of the summary findings of many empirical studies" (p. 21). In other words, in statistics a meta-analysis refers to methods focused on contrasting and combining results from different studies in the hope of identifying patterns among study results, sources of disagreement among those results, or other interesting relationships that may come to light.

In essence, the result from an individual study is converted to a standard score, which is called an **effect size**. Because effect sizes are **standard scores**, the measures (and the units used to express those measures) in the various studies are not relevant. (A percentile is another example of a standard score.) Moreover, standard scores can be added and then averaged to draw conclusions about the overall impact of a particular treatment.

Finally, and this is also important, the possible influence of what are called moderator variables should be examined. **Moderator variables** directly influence the relationship of an independent variable to a dependent variable. So, returning to our example, it would be possible to assess statistically through a meta-analysis whether age is a moderator variable in the fitness–anxiety relationship. If increased fitness is associated with reduced anxiety, does that relationship hold across the age spectrum from adolescents to older adulthood?

Meta-analysis is particularly useful in areas of research where a large number of studies are available, not all the studies are of uniform quality, there is wide variability in the operational definition of the variables, there are differences in the nature of the subjects or differences in designs, and the results have not been completely consistent. Meta-analysis offers the opportunity to statistically average the effects from various studies in order to come to some conclusion for the population as a whole. It is also possible, of course, to subdivide the pool of studies and examine conditions that might serve to moderate the basic relationship.

Interpretation of Effect Sizes

Most of us can easily interpret quantities or amounts when commonly used measures such as inches, feet, seconds, and kilograms are used. Most of us also have a common understanding of the meaning of standard statistical scores such as a percentile (e.g., you scored in the 85th percentile on your SAT). However, interpretation of an effect size is not as intuitively obvious. Fortunately, Jacob Cohen (1992) has provided some guidelines that are useful for understanding the results from a meta-analysis. Thus, the descriptive term *small* can be used for any effect size within the range of 0.10 to 0.30. Also, the descriptive term *moderate* can be used for effect sizes in the range of 0.40 to 0.70. Finally, the descriptive term *large* can be used for any effect size that is greater than 0.80.

Another statistical way to interpret an effect size is available. Consider, for example, the differences in anxiety scores in an experimental group exposed to 16 weeks of exercise versus the improvement in anxiety scores in a control group that simply met and talked for the 16 weeks. An effect size of 0.33 for the improvement (i.e., reduction) in anxiety scores in the experimental group over that in the control group would mean that the average experimental person improved in (showed a reduction for) anxiety one-third of a standard deviation more than was the case for the average control person.

Most students find it easier to use the descriptive terms *small*, *medium*, and *large* for effect sizes of 0.20, 0.50, and 0.80, respectively. However, they sometimes ask, "Well, what about effect sizes of 0.35 or 0.75? How are these effect sizes described? They are not included in the ranges above." In response, we remind students that the descriptive terms are intended to be guidelines, not fixed criteria. So, to a large extent, the verbal descriptors used for effect sizes that are outside the ranges we have presented are a matter of personal choice. There is a parallel in academia. Universally, we might agree that someone in the 30th percentile is a poor student, someone in the 50th percentile is a good student, and someone in the 85th percentile is an excellent student. Where is the boundary between a poor and a good student and a good and an excellent student? It seems likely that there would be wide variability in the answers given by different groups. Now let's turn our focus to introducing exercise psychology.

Exercise Psychology

If physical activity is efficacious, one important challenge facing scientists, health professionals, and governments is to help large segments of the population become more physically active. How this will be achieved is not likely to come

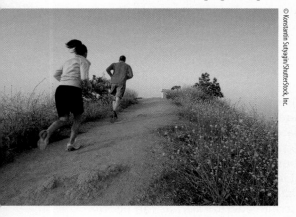

© Konstantin Sutyagin/ShutterStock, Inc.

through additional research in exercise physiology, although that discipline will undoubtedly provide answers to important questions such as how much activity is necessary to obtain the physiological benefits described earlier. As a science, exercise physiology does not concern itself with general issues associated with understanding and modifying behavior, influencing public opinion, motivating people, and changing people's attitudes. Nor is it a concern of the biomechanics, historians, or sociologists of sport and physical activity. Questions concerning human attitudes, moods, cognitions, and behavior fall directly under the mandate of psychology.

Psychology is a science devoted to gaining an understanding of human behavior. In turn, the area of science we refer to in this text as **exercise psychology** (also called *physical activity psychology* or *fitness psychology*) is devoted to gaining an understanding of (1) individual attitudes, moods, cognitions, and behaviors in the context of exercise and (2) the social and physical factors that influence those attitudes, moods, cognitions, and behaviors. In other words, exercise psychology is defined as the study of psychological issues and theories related to physical activity. Exercise psychology is a subdiscipline within the field of psychology, as well as a subdiscipline within the field of kinesiology.

Individual Correlates of Exercise

To understand, promote, and maintain exercise and decrease sedentary behavior, we need to examine determinants and correlates of these behaviors. In the case of exercise, a **correlate** is a variable that is associated with either an increase or decrease of physical activity. Correlates research assesses only statistical associations, rather than providing evidence of a causal relationship between a factor and physical activity (Bauman, Sallis, Dzewaltowski, & Owen, 2002). In comparison, when a variable has been assessed in a longitudinal observational study or an experimental design it is called a **determinant**. Thus, a determinant is a variable that has a strong causal association with physical activity. Given that the research examining physical activity determinants has largely been generated in either cross-sectional or retrospective studies, the implicit suggestion of causation often is not appropriate (Bauman et al., 2012).

For ease of interpretation, we will use the term *correlate* in this section because most often this is the more accurate term for physical activity adherence. For example, it is well documented that as we get older we tend to be less active. It is not true, however, that advancing age causes people to be less active. All of us know older people who are very physically active and younger individuals who are sedentary. Also, there is no single variable that explains all physical activity behavior. Different variables exert different degrees of influence on different people. For example, spousal support may be important for some people to exercise, but not others. Also, the strength of spousal influence for each person may vary during different stages of their married life. Spousal support for physical activity may be relatively unimportant in early adulthood but important in older adulthood.

Another way to look at individual correlates is to ask the question "Why do some people exercise and others don't?" This is a difficult question to answer. Because physical activity is affected by diverse factors, behavioral theories and models (such as the theory of planned behavior and the transtheoretical model) are used to guide the selection of variables to study. Integration of ideas from several theories into an ecological model (including inter-relations between individuals and their social and physical environments) is now common (Sallis, Owen, & Fisher, 2008). An ecological approach uses a comprehensive framework to explain physical activity, proposing that determinants at all levels (i.e., individual, social, environmental, and policy) contribute to or influence whether someone engages in exercise. A key principle is that knowledge about all types of influence can inform development of multilevel interventions to offer the best chance of success.

FIGURE 1-2 presents a social ecological framework for physical activity (see Nigg, Rhodes, & Amato, 2013). This ecological framework highlights people's interactions with their physical and social/interpersonal environments, with individuals shaping their environments, as well as being shaped by their environments (McLeroy, Bibeau, Steckler, & Ganz, 1998). The focus of this section is on

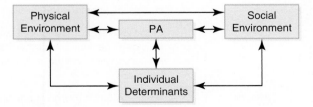

FIGURE 1-2   A Conceptualization of the Social Ecological Framework for Physical Activity (PA)

Reproduced from Nigg, C. R., Rhodes, R., & Amato, K. R. (2013). Determinants of physical activity: Research to application. In J. M. Rippe (Ed.), *Lifestyle medicine* (pp. 1435–1446). Taylor & Francis Group.

the individual correlates of physical activity. The list of physical activity correlates is long, and individual-level factors such as age, sex, health status, self-efficacy, and previous physical activity are correlated with physical activity levels (Bauman et al., 2012). **TABLE 1-3** summarizes some of the main individual correlates of

TABLE 1-3 Summary of the Individual Correlates of Physical Activity		
Correlate Category	**Specific Correlate**	**Relationship with Physical Activity (PA)**
Demographic	Age	Negative: PA levels continually decline as we get older.
	Ethnicity	Whites exercise more than minorities.
	Socioeconomic status	Positive: Higher socioeconomic status associated with higher PA levels.
	Gender	Male populations exercise more than female populations.
	Health status	Healthy people are more active than persons with medical and psychological conditions.
	Education level	Positive: Higher education level correlated with higher PA levels.
	Weight	Negative: Obese and overweight people exercise less than normal weight people.
	Marital status	Unrelated. No relationship with marital status and PA levels.
Behavioral	Previous PA	Positive: Previous PA is positively related to future/current PA behavior.
	Smoking	Negative: Negative relationship between cigarette smoking and PA.
Psychological	Self-efficacy	Positive: Higher self-efficacy (confidence in the ability to be physically active in specific situations) correlated with higher PA levels.
	Barriers	Negative: Negative relationship between an individual's perception that there are barriers to PA participation and that individual's actual PA behavior.
	Attitude	Positive: Attitude (overall appraisal or evaluation of PA) positively related with PA intention and behavior.
	Enjoyment	Positive: Enjoyment positively related to PA.

physical activity into categories of demographic, psychological, and behavioral (Bauman et al., 2012; Nigg et al., 2013).

Of importance, few researchers have examined the correlates of physical activity in low- and middle-income countries (Bauman et al., 2012).

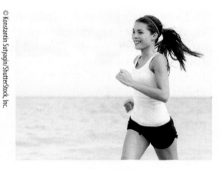

© Konstantin Sutyagin/ShutterStock, Inc.

Guidelines for Physical Activity

A possible reason for the high rate of physical inactivity may be a misperception that exercise-mediated health benefits can only be achieved by strenuous sustained aerobic activity such as a vigorous 45-minute run. Such perceptions were fostered by the original exercise guidelines established by the American College of Sports Medicine in 1978 (see TABLE 1-4 for a description of these 1978 guidelines). These guidelines were based on the improvement of cardiovascular fitness; however, they were often applied to general health (Haskell, 1994). These original guidelines were very specific and led to somewhat regimented thinking about how much exercise should be recommended. This caused many people to think that exercise amounts that did not meet these specific criteria would be of either limited or no value (Blair, LaMonte, & Nichaman, 2004). More recently, however, recommendations by leading authorities have significantly influenced the traditional beliefs about the amount, intensity, and frequency of exercise that is necessary to elicit physical and psychological benefits.

TABLE 1-4 Former Adult Guidelines for Physical Activity		
Activity Characteristics	**American College of Sports Medicine (1978)**	**U.S. Department of Health and Human Services (1996)**
Frequency	3–5 times per week	Most (preferably all) days of the week
Intensity	Vigorous	Moderate
Duration	20–45 minutes	Accumulation of ≥ 30 minutes of daily activity in bouts of at least 10 minutes
Type	Aerobic activity	Any activity that can be performed at an intensity similar to that of brisk walking

How much physical activity do we need to achieve its health-related benefits? The next guidelines established by the American College of Sports Medicine and the Centers for Disease Control in 1996 stated that adults should accumulate a minimum of 30 minutes of moderate-intensity physical activity on most, if not all, days of the week (U.S. Department of Health and Human Services, 1996; see Table 1-4). Moderate-intensity physical activity, for example, could include brisk walking at a pace of 3 to 4 miles per hour, climbing stairs, and doing heavy housework. The accumulation of physical activity indicates that people can engage in shorter bouts of activity spread out over the course of the day. For example, a person could go for a 10-minute brisk walk in the morning, afternoon, and evening to reach the daily goal of 30 minutes. The suggestion that physical activity can be accumulated over the course of the day, rather than performed continuously in a single session, was motivated by the difficulties reported by numerous individuals in trying to find a block of 30 minutes per day for physical activity. A main goal of these guidelines was to show people that they do indeed have the time to exercise.

These U.S. Department of Health and Human Services (USDHHS, 1996) physical activity guidelines emphasize moderate-intensity levels for a duration of 30 minutes. Does this mean that people do not need to engage in physical activity at vigorous-intensity levels or for durations greater than 30 minutes to achieve the health-related benefits? The answer to this question is an emphatic *no*! It is important to note that the benefits of physical activity are related to the effort that one devotes (USDHHS, 1996). Thus, additional health and fitness advantages are gained from physical activities that are undertaken for longer durations or at more strenuous intensity levels, or both (USDHHS, 1996).

In 2012, the WHO developed the "Global Recommendations on Physical Activity for Health," with the overall goal of providing guidance on the dose–response relationship between the frequency, duration, intensity, type, and total amount of physical activity needed for the prevention of **noncommunicable diseases** (e.g., cardiovascular diseases, cancers, respiratory diseases). Many countries have adopted similar physical activity recommendations and guidelines (e.g., Canadian Society for Exercise Physiology, 2011; USDHHS, 2010).

The WHO guidelines for the general adult population (18 to 64 years) recommend at least 150 minutes of moderate-intensity aerobic physical activity throughout the week or at least 75 minutes of vigorous-intensity aerobic physical activity throughout the week or an equivalent combination of moderate- and vigorous-intensity activity. The aerobic activity bouts must be at least 10 minutes in duration to count toward the weekly total. For additional health benefits, adults should increase their moderate-intensity aerobic physical activity to 300 minutes per week, or engage in 150 minutes of vigorous-intensity aerobic physical activity per week, or an equivalent combination of moderate- and vigorous-intensity activity.

These guidelines also suggest that larger doses of exercise may be necessary in some groups. Those with or at risk for coronary heart disease are recommended to do 30 to 60 minutes of exercise daily. Adults trying to prevent the transition to either overweight or obesity are encouraged to exercise 45 to 60 minutes per day.

And it is recommended that formerly obese individuals trying to prevent weight regain should exercise 60 to 90 minutes per day.

For older adults (aged 65 years and older), the guidelines are identical to adults but with the following two caveats. First, when older adults cannot do the recommended amounts of physical activity due to health conditions, they should be as physically active as their abilities and conditions allow. Second, older adults with poor mobility should perform physical activity to improve their balance and prevent falls on three or more days per week. See **TABLE 1-5** for an outline of the physical activity guidelines for youth, adults, and older adults.

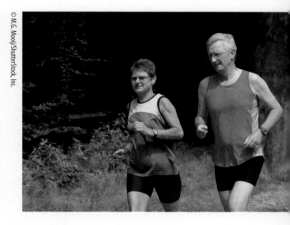

Most recently, Australia developed new guidelines on physical activity that double the levels previously recommended as a "wake-up call" for Australians (Australian Government Department of Health, 2014). The new Australian physical activity guidelines recommend that adults complete between 150 and 300 minutes of physical activity per week, twice the amount of the previous government

TABLE 1-5   World Health Organization Physical Activity (PA) Guidelines

Activity Characteristics	Children (5–17 years)	Adults (18–64 years)	Older adults (65+ years)
Frequency	Daily	Weekly accumulation of minutes as opposed to a frequency per week	Weekly accumulation of minutes as opposed to a frequency per week
Intensity	Moderate to vigorous	Moderate and/or vigorous	Moderate and/or vigorous
Duration	60 minutes per day. Most PA should be aerobic	150 minutes of moderate PA a week *or* 75 minutes of vigorous PA *or* a combination of moderate and vigorous PA. Aerobic activity bouts at least 10 minutes	150 minutes of moderate PA a week *or* 75 minutes of vigorous PA *or* a combination of moderate and vigorous PA. Aerobic activity bouts at least 10 minutes
Muscle training	Three or more times per week	Two or more days a week	Two or more days a week

Data from: World Health Organization. (2012). *Recommended levels of physical activity for adults aged 18–64 years* [Electronic Version]. Retrieved December 20, 2012, from http://www.who.int/dietphysicalactivity/factsheet_adults/en/index.html.

TABLE 1-6 **The 2012 Australian Physical Activity Guidelines**
Criteria
Doing any physical activity is better than doing none. If you currently do no physical activity, start by doing some, and gradually build up to the recommended amount.
Be active on most, preferably all, days every week.
Accumulate 150 to 300 minutes (2.5 to 5 hours) of moderate-intensity physical activity or 75 to 150 minutes (1.25 to 2.5 hours) of vigorous-intensity physical activity, or an equivalent combination of both moderate and vigorous activities, each week.
Do muscle strengthening activities on at least two days each week.

Data from: Australian Government Department of Health. (2014). Physical activity and sedentary behavior guidelines. Retrieved March 2014 from http://www.health.gov.au/internet/main/publishing.nsf/Content/health-pubhlth-strateg-phys-act-guidelines/%24File/Brochures_PAG_Adults18-64yrs.PDF.

recommendations. The guidelines draw on research that suggests while the previous recommendation of 150 minutes per week of moderate activity was sufficient for general health benefits, a higher level is needed to prevent weight gain and some cancers. To successfully limit weight gain, Australian adults need to aim for that upper recommendation of 300 minutes per week. For those who are currently inactive, one of the main messages of the new Australian guidelines is that some activity is always better than none. See **TABLE 1-6** for more information on the Australian physical activity guidelines.

Recent research findings are challenging the guidelines that physical activity bouts must be at least 10 minutes in duration to achieve health benefits—or at least weight loss benefits. Jessie Fan and colleagues (2013) examined if moderate to vigorous physical activity in less than the recommended 10-minute bouts was related to weight loss in a random national sample of 4,511 American adults between the ages 18 to 64 years. The adults had clinically measured BMI and accelerometer data that measured their minute-by-minute physical activity. The researchers found that higher-intensity physical activity of both short bouts (less than 10 minutes) and high bouts (longer than 10 minutes) were related to lower BMI and risk of being either overweight or obese. In comparison, neither lower-intensity short bouts nor lower-intensity long bouts were related to BMI or risk of overweight or obesity. The researchers concluded that for weight gain prevention, accumulated higher-intensity physical activity bouts of fewer than 10 minutes are highly beneficial, supporting the public health promotion message "every minute counts."

Upper Limit to Physical Activity Guidelines?

The physical activity guidelines state the minimal amount of exercise needed to achieve health-related benefits; however, they offer no information regarding the maximal amount of exercise needed. In other words, when is exercise too much of a good thing? Is it possible for people to exercise too much, resulting in negative health effects? Preliminary research suggests that high amounts of exercise may have some negative physical and mental health outcomes.

British researchers examined the heart health of a group of very fit older men (Wilson et al., 2011). They recruited men who had been part of a British national or Olympic team in either distance running or rowing, as well as members of the **100 Marathon Club**, which admits runners who, not surprisingly, have completed at least 100 marathons. All of the men had trained and competed through-out their adult lives and continued to engage in strenuous exercise. For comparison purposes, the researchers also recruited 20 healthy older men who were not endurance athletes. All the men underwent a type of magnetic resonance imaging of their hearts that identifies early signs of fibrosis, or scarring, within the heart muscle. Fibrosis, if it becomes severe, can lead to either stiffening or thickening of portions of the heart, which can eventually contribute to irregular heart function and heart failure.

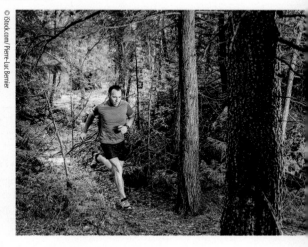

The researchers found that none of the younger athletes or the older nonath-letes had fibrosis in their hearts. However, half of the older athletes showed some heart muscle scarring. The affected men were those who had trained the longest and hardest. In other words, spending more years exercising strenuously or run-ning more marathons was associated with a greater likelihood of heart damage.

Another study quantified the amount of weekly exercise that promotes men-tal health and found that, while too little is not healthy, neither is too much (Kim et al., 2012). The researchers used self-reported data on physical activity and men-tal health symptoms from 7,674 American adults. They measured participants' mental health using a self-report questionnaire that assessed their psychological distress, depression, and anxiety levels over the past 30 days. The participants also answered questions about the frequency and duration of physical activities that caused an increase in breathing. Not surprisingly, mental health was better in peo-ple who reported some physical activity compared to sedentary people. Moreover, as shown in **FIGURE 1-3**, there were improvements in mental health with just a lit-tle physical activity, supporting the fact that the biggest gains from exercise often come from going from a couch potato to slightly active.

After about 2 hours per week of physical activity, however, there was no significant continued gain in mental health for the adults. And then, after about 7.5 hours of physical activity, the gains in mental health plateaued, and then started to reverse. That reversal in health benefits was ever so slight at first, as weekly physical activity climbed to 10 hours. But with more and more activity,

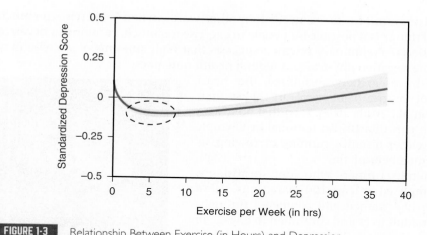

FIGURE 1-3   Relationship Between Exercise (in Hours) and Depression

According to one study, the optimal range for the best mental health is between 2.5 and 7.5 hours of exercise per week, which is illustrated in the oval area.

Reprinted from Kim, Y. S. et al. (2012). Relationship between physical activity and general mental health. *Preventive Medicine*, 55, 458–463. With permission from Elsevier.

the mental-health benefits of exercise declined significantly. Nearing 25 hours a week, reported mental health was no better than in slightly active people.

The researchers concluded that the optimal amount of exercise for improved mental health might be between 2.5 to 7.5 hours per week, because people who exercised beyond 7.5 hours per week had poorer mental health. While excess exercise is related with diminished mental health, without further evidence, it is not clear from this study that excessive exercise is the cause. People who have a propensity to poor mental health may be inclined to exercise excessively. Furthermore, excessive exercise may also be at the expense of other activities that

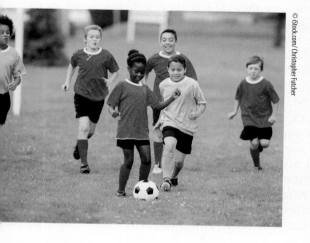

contribute to psychological well-being, such as relationships, sleep, proper nutrition, and rest.

Similar results have been found in an adolescent population. Arnaud Merglen and his colleagues (2014) examined weekly sport practice on 1,245 Swiss adolescents (aged 16 to 20 years). Weekly sport practice was categorized into four groups: low (less than 3.5 hours), average (about the recommended 7 hours), high (about 14 hours), and very high (greater than 17.5 hours). They found that compared with adolescents in the average group, those in the very high group and the low group had a higher risk of poor well-being. In contrast, those in the high group had a lower risk of poor well-being than those in the average group. In other words, the best well-being was found with the adolescents who participated in about 14 hours of sport training. In contrast, the lowest well-being was found with adolescents who engaged in less than 2.5 hours or more than 17.5 hours per week of training. The researchers concluded that there was an inverted, U-shaped relationship between weekly sport practice duration and well-being among adolescents.

In summary, the science is clear that exercise in general is very good for your overall health. But the emerging science does suggest that there may be a threshold of distance, intensity, or duration beyond which exercise can have undesirable physical and mental health effects. Unfortunately, it remains impossible, at the moment, to predict just what that threshold is for any given person, and which people might be most vulnerable as a result of excessive exercise.

■ Historical Developments

The first exercise psychology (as well as first social psychology and sport psychology) research study was conducted by Norman Triplett in 1898. Triplett noticed that cyclists tended to have faster times when riding against another person compared to when cyclists rode alone. He then demonstrated this effect in a controlled, laboratory experiment, and he concluded that people perform a simple lab task faster in pairs than when performing it alone.

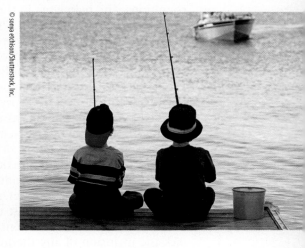

For example, in one research design, Triplett had children play a game that involved turning a small fishing reel as quickly as possible. He found that the children who played the game in pairs turned the reel faster than those who were alone. These findings were termed **social facilitation**, which is the tendency for people to do better on simple tasks when in the presence of other people. This implies that whenever people are being watched by others they will do well on things that they are already good at doing.

Rejeski and Thompson (1993) noted that although interest has been directed toward the psychology of physical activity since Triplett's (1898) social facilitation studies, most of the research has appeared since the early 1970s. Several reasons were advanced by Rejeski and Thompson for the relatively slow development of the psychology of physical activity as a science. First, the popularity of sport preceded the popularity of exercise within the general population. Thus, scientists inevitably gravitated toward sport to ask and attempt to answer sport-related research questions. Second, the importance of physical activity for disease prevention and the maintenance of general health has long been suspected but not fully known until relatively recently. Consequently, understanding the psychological dimensions of involvement in physical activity was not perceived to be a pressing priority. Finally, throughout history, the use of a **biomedical model** has been the traditional approach to understanding health and disease. The biomedical model of illness excludes psychological and social factors and includes only biological factors in an attempt to understand a person's medical illness or disease. The dominant concern of the biomedical model is with the treatment of disease as opposed to its prevention. It has only been relatively recent that the importance of a biopsychosocial approach to disease prevention has been acknowledged. The **biopsychosocial model** acknowledges that the mind and the body together determine health and illness. As its name implies, the biopsychosocial model's fundamental assumption is that health and illness are the consequences of the interplay of biological, psychological, and social factors.

Topics of Interest

When research into the psychological aspects of involvement in physical activity increased in the 1970s, it tended to focus on the first portion of the definition outlined above; namely, gaining an understanding of human attitudes, moods, cognitions, and behaviors in the context of physical activity. More recently, Ryan Rhodes and Gabriella Nasuti (2011) examined trends and changes in psychology of physical activity research across 20 years (i.e., 1990–2008) by auditing leading journals where exercise psychology research is often published. They found that the volume of exercise psychology research tripled between the 1990s and 2000s. While these results clearly support a growth in research volume, a critical question for the evolution of exercise psychology is whether the quality of the research has evolved over time. For this assessment, the researchers considered the methods employed, the stage of research, and the use of various theoretical approaches to guide exercise interventions. They found evidence that the domain has shifted from measurement studies to descriptive research, but experimental intervention research is still relatively scant. Further, methodological characteristics such as physical activity measurement, sampling, designs, and intervention characteristics have changed little in the last two decades. By contrast, there has been a major theoretical shift to environmental models of physical activity, but many studies still lack the inclusion of any theoretical frame. The most common exercise psychology research topics investigated are outlined in **TABLE 1-7** (Rejeski & Thompson, 1993; Rhodes & Nasuti, 2011).

Related Terms

A variety of related terms have been the focus of research under the umbrella term *exercise psychology*. Researchers and practitioners, operating under the assumption that definitional clarity is essential for effective communication, have taken care to draw a distinction among terms. Though people often use physical activity and

TABLE 1-7	Common Exercise Psychology Research Topics
Topic	**Description**
Mental health	Influence of acute and chronic physical activity on mental health parameters such as anxiety and depression
Body image and self-esteem	Influence of acute and chronic physical activity on self-perceptions and self-esteem
Psychophysiological reactivity	Influence of acute and chronic physical activity on modulating psychological and physiological responses to social stressors
Perceived exertion	Subjective perceptions of physical functioning during acute bouts of physical activity
Adherence	Identifying correlates and determinants of involvement in chronic physical activity
Sleep	Impact of acute and chronic physical activity on quantity and quality of sleep
Cognition	Influence of acute and chronic physical activity on mental acuity
Interventions	Interventions to increase physical activity behavior
Exercise dependence	Nature and consequences of obsessive involvement in physical activity
Social support	Comparing the influence of peers versus parents for children's physical activity
Leadership and cohesion	Role played by the exercise leader in sustaining involvement in physical activity programs
Environment	Identifying aspects of the environment (aesthetics, structural characteristics, safety) related to physical activity
Theories of behavior change	Developing and testing theory-based physical activity interventions

exercise interchangeably, the terms have different definitions. **Physical activity** is an umbrella term used to describe any body movement produced by skeletal muscles that requires energy expenditure. In other words, physical activity refers to any body movement that burns calories, whether it is for work or play, daily chores, engaging in a competitive sport, or a daily commute. **Exercise**, a subcategory of physical activity, refers to planned, structured, and repetitive activities aimed at improving physical fitness and health (Caspersen, Powell, & Christenson, 1985). A characteristic that helps to define exercise is that the person must

TABLE 1-8	The FITT Principle Defined	
Principle	**Definition**	**Example**
Frequency	How often you exercise	Five times per week
Intensity	How hard you work during exercise	Moderate intensity
Type	The type of activity you're doing	Brisk walk
Time	How long you exercise	30 minutes

conform to a recommended frequency, intensity, type, and time (often called the FITT principle; see TABLE 1-8 for a description) to achieve the specific purpose desired. Researchers sometimes use the terms *leisure-time physical activity* or *recreational physical activity* as synonyms for exercise. Other subcategories of physical activity include sport, occupational physical activity, household physical activity, self-care physical activity, and transportation physical activity (see FIGURE 1-4).

Exercise psychology has also been referred to as a component of **behavioral medicine**. Behavioral medicine is an interdisciplinary field of medicine concerned with the development and integration of knowledge in the biological, behavioral,

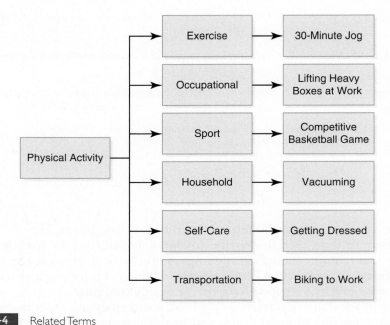

FIGURE 1-4   Related Terms

psychological, and social sciences relevant to health and illness. The practice of behavioral medicine also includes applied psychophysiological therapies such as biofeedback, hypnosis, and biobehavioral therapy of physical disorders, aspects of occupational therapy, rehabilitation medicine, and psychiatry, as well as preventive medicine.

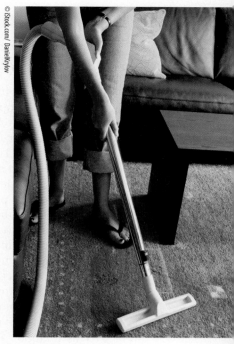

© iStock.com/ DanielKrylov

Health may be viewed as a human condition with physical, social, and psychological dimensions, each characterized by a continuum varying from positive to negative poles. As defined by the WHO over a half century ago (1946), health is a state of complete physical, mental, and social well-being and not merely the absence of disease or infirmity. Both physical activity and exercise, along with a number of other activities, such as maintaining a proper diet and refraining from smoking, contribute to the development and maintenance of health on the positive end of the continuum. Although every health behavior is important in its own right, this textbook concentrates on physical activity, exercise, and sedentary behavior.

Health psychology is the study of the psychological and behavioral processes in health, illness, and health care (Johnston, 1994). It is concerned with understanding how psychological, behavioral, and cultural factors are involved in physical health and illness, in addition to the biological causes that are well understood by medical science. Health psychologists take a biopsychosocial approach; that is, they understand health to be the product not only of biological processes (e.g., a virus, tumor), but also of psychological processes (e.g., stress, thoughts and beliefs, behaviors such as smoking and exercise) and social processes (e.g., socioeconomic status, culture, and ethnicity). The term *health psychology* is often used interchangeably, and incorrectly, with *exercise psychology*.

CRITICAL THINKING ACTIVITY 1-4

© ecco/Shutterstock, Inc.

How has the biopsychosocial model shaped the field of exercise psychology?

Finally, *sport psychology* is the study of the how psychological factors affect athletes' performance and well-being. Some sport psychologists work with professional athletes and coaches to improve the performance and increase the motivation of athletes. Although sport psychology is commonly referred to as *sport and exercise psychology*, it is important to understand the important distinction between these two related fields.

■ Summary

Is there a tomato effect—a tendency for people to avoid efficacious activities—insofar as physical activity is concerned? A large number of benefits are associated with involvement in physical activity. Furthermore, it is reasonable to suggest that physical activity is considered to be health producing and beneficial by large portions of the population. Physical inactivity has been identified as the fourth leading risk factor for global mortality, causing an estimated 3.2 million deaths globally each year. Despite the known risks of inactivity, in general, throughout the world physical inactivity levels are still unacceptably high. Changes in exercise behaviors and attitudes are necessary. Both of these fall within the domain of psychology as a science. This textbook focuses on the area of science referred to as the psychology of physical activity and sedentary behavior.

A variety of diverse behaviors have been the focus of research under the umbrella term *psychology of physical activity*. These were defined. Physical activity represents bodily movements produced by skeletal muscles that lead to substantial increases in energy expenditure. Exercise is considered to be a specific form of physical activity that the individual engages in to improve fitness, physical performance, and/or health. Health is a condition that is composed of physical, social, and psychological dimensions, each of which exists along a continuum that ranges from positive to negative.

This textbook centers on physical activity, not other areas, such as rehabilitation psychology, sport psychology, or health psychology. What this means, essentially, is that this text incorporates information from research where physical activity or sedentary behavior was the dependent (outcome) variable.

KEY TERMS

acute physical activity
behavioral medicine
biomedical model
biopsychosocial model
body mass index (BMI)
chronic physical activity
correlate
determinant
effect size
exercise
exercise psychology
health
health psychology
meta-analysis

mens sana in corpore sano
moderator variables
noncommunicable diseases
100 Marathon Club
operational definition
pandemic
physical activity
population-attributable fraction
quantitative research
social facilitation
standard score
systematic review
tomato effect
World Health Organization (WHO)

REVIEW QUESTIONS

1. Does physical activity show a tomato effect? (Hint: Use the three issues to justify your answer.)

2. What is the difference between a correlate and a determinant of physical activity? List five individual demographic correlates of physical activity, and describe how these correlates are related to physical activity.

3. What are the current physical activity guidelines for adults?

4. Describe what social facilitation is and how it is historically linked to the psychology of physical activity.

5. List six topics of interest for the psychology of physical activity.

6. How do the American College of Sports Medicine's (1978) physical activity guidelines differ from the U.S. Department of Health and Human Services's (1996) physical activity guidelines?

7. Define *meta-analysis*. How can a meta-analysis help us understand a body of literature?

8. What is a moderator variable? Provide an example.

APPLYING THE CONCEPTS

1. How did the lifestyle of Henry's parents illustrate the tomato effect?

2. What factors help explain why Henry was able to change into a more active individual?

3. How do Henry's new exercise habits measure up to the current guidelines for physical activity?

REFERENCES

Aberg, M. A., Nyberg, J., Toren, K., Sorberg, A., Kuhn, H. G., & Waern, M. (2013). Cadiovascular fitness in early adulthood and future suicidal behaviour in men followed for up to 42 years. *Psychological Medicine, 6,* 1–10.

American College of Sports Medicine. (1978). American College of Sports Medicine position statement on the recommended quantity and quality of exercise for developing and maintaining fitness in healthy adults. *Medicine and Science in Sports, 10,* vii–x.

Australian Government Department of Health. (2014). Physical activity and sedentary behavior guidelines. Retrieved March 2014 from http://www.health.gov.au/internet/main/publishing.nsf/Content/health-pubhlth-strateg-phys-act-guidelines/%24File/Brochures_PAG_Adults18-64yrs.pdf

Bauman, A. E., Reis, R. S., Sallis J. F., Wells, J. C., Loos, R. J., & Martin, B. W. (2012). Correlates of physical activity: Why are some people physically active and others not? *Lancet, 380,* 258–271.

Bauman, A. E., Sallis, J. F., Dzewaltowski, D. A., & Owen, N. (2002). Toward a better understanding of the influences on physical activity: The role of determinants, correlates, causal variables, mediators, moderators, and confounders. *American Journal of Preventive Medicine, 23,* 5–14.

Blair, S. N., LaMonte, M. J., & Nichaman, M. Z. (2004). The evolution of physical activity recommendations: How much is enough? *American Journal of Clinical Nutrition, 79,* 9135–9205.

Canadian Society for Exercise Physiology. (2011). Canadian physical activity guidelines for adults 18–64 years [Electronic Version]. Retrieved February 1, 2013, from http://www.csep.ca/english/view.asp?x=804

Caspersen, C. J., Powell, K. E., & Christenson, G. M. (1985). Physical activity, exercise, and physical fitness: Definitions and distinctions for health-related research. *Public Health Reports, 100,* 126–131.

Chakravarty, E. F., Hubert H. B., Lingala, V. B., & Fries, J. F. (2008). Reduced disability and mortality among aging runners: A 21-year longitudinal study. *Archives of Internal Medicine, 168,* 1638–1646.

Church, T. S., & Blair, S. N. (2009). When will we treat physical activity as a legitimate medical therapy ... even though it does not come in a pill? *British Journal of Sports Medicine, 42,* 80–81.

Cohen, J. (1992). A power primer. *Psychological Bulletin, 112,* 155–159.

Cornelissen, V. A., Fagard, R. H., Coeckelberghs, E., & Vanhes, L. (2011). Impact of resistance training on blood pressure and other cardiovascular risk factors: A meta-analysis or randomized, controlled trials. *Hypertension, 58,* 950–958.

Dumith, S. C., Hallal, P. C., Reis, R. S., & Kohl, H. W 3rd. (2011). Worldwide prevalence of physical inactivity and its association with human development index in 76 countries. *Preventive Medicine, 53,* 24–28.

Ekelund, U., Luan, J., Sherar, L. B., Esliger, D. W., Griew, P., & Cooper, A. (2012). Moderate to vigorous physical activity and sedentary time and cardiometabolic risk factors in children and adolescents. *JAMA, 307,* 704–712.

Fan, J. X., Brown, B. B., Hanson, H., Kowaleski-Jones, L., Smith, K. R., & Zick, C. D. (2013). Moderate to vigorous physical activity and weight outcomes: Does every minute count? *American Journal of Health Promotion, 28,* 41–49.

Ferreira, M. L., Sherrington, C., Smith, K., Carswell, P., Bell, R., Bell, M., ... Vardon, P. (2012). Physical activity improves strength, balance, and endurance in adults aged 40–65 years: A systematic review. *Journal of Physiotherapy, 58,* 145–156.

Glass G. V. (1976). Primary, secondary, and meta-analysis of research. *Educational Researcher, 5*, 3–8.

Glass, G. V., McGaw, B., & Smith, M. L. (1981). *Meta-analysis in social research*. Beverly Hills, CA: Sage.

Goodwin, J. S., & Goodwin, J. M. (1984). The tomato effect: Rejection of highly efficacious therapies. *JAMA, 251*, 2387–2390.

Hallal, P. C., Andersen, L. B., Bull, F. C., Guthold, R., Haskell, W., & Ekelund, U. (2012). Global physical activity levels: Surveillance progress, pitfalls, and prospects. *Lancet, 21*, 247–257.

Haskell, W. L. (1994). J. B. Wolffe Memorial Lecture. Health consequences of physical activity: Understanding and challenges regarding dose-response. *Medicine and Science in Sports and Exercise, 26*, 649–660.

Johnston, M. (1994). Current trends in health psychology. *The Psychologist, 7*, 114–118.

Kim, Y. S., Park, Y. S., Allegrante, J. P., Marks, R., Ok, H., Cho, K. O., & Garber, C. E. (2012). Relationship between physical activity and general mental health. *Preventive Medicine, 55*, 458–463.

Kohl, H. W., Craig, C. L., Lambert, E. V., Inoue, S., Alkandari, J. R., Leetongin, G., & Kahlmeier, S. (2012). The pandemic of physical inactivity: Global action for public health. *Lancet, 380*, 294–305.

Ladabaum, U., Mannalithara, A., Myer, P. A., & Singh, G. (2014). Obesity, abdominal obesity, physical activity, and caloric intake in U.S. adults: 1988 to 2010. *American Journal of Medicine, 127*, 717–727.

Lee, I. M., Shiroma, E. J., Lobela, F., Puska, P., Blair, S. N., & Katzmarzyk, P. T. (2012). Effect of physical inactivity on major noncommunicable diseases worldwide: An analysis of burden of disease and life expectancy. *Lancet, 380*, 219–229.

Marques, E. A., Mota, J., & Carvalho, J. (2012). Exercise effects on bone mineral density in older adults: A meta-analysis of randomized controlled trials. *Age, 34*, 1493–1515.

McLeroy, K. R., Bibeau, D., Steckler, A., & Glanz, K. (1988). An ecological perspective on health promotion programs. *Health Education Quarterly, 15*, 351–377.

Merglen, A., Flatz, A., Belanger, R. E., Michaud, P. A., & Suris, J. C. (2014). Weekly sport practice and adolescent well-being. *Archives of Disease in Children, 99*, 208 – 210.

Morrow, J. R., Krzewinski-Malone, J. A., Jackson, A. W., Bungum, T. J., & FitzGerald, S. J. (2004). American adults' knowledge of exercise recommendations. *Research Quarterly in Exercise and Sport, 75*, 231–237.

Nigg, C. R., Rhodes, R., & Amato, K. R. (2013). Determinants of physical activity: Research to application. In J. M. Rippe (Ed.), *Lifestyle medicine* (pp. 1435–1446). New York, NY: Taylor & Francis Group.

North, T. C., McCullagh, P., & Tran, Z. V. (1990). Effect of exercise on depression. *Exercise and Sport Sciences Reviews, 18*, 379–415.

Rejeski, W. J., & Thompson, A. (1993). Historical and conceptual roots of exercise psychology. In P. Seraganian (Ed.), *Exercise psychology: The influence of physical exercise on psychological processes* (pp. 3–38). New York, NY: Wiley.

Rhodes, R. E., & Nasuti, G. (2011). Trends and changes in research on the psychology of physical activity across 20 years: A quantitative analysis of 10 journals. *Preventive Medicine, 53*, 17–13.

Sallis, J. F., Owen, N., & Fisher, E. B. (2008). Ecological models of health behavior. In K. Glanz, B. K. Rimer, and K. Viswanath (Eds.), *Health behavior and health education: Theory, research, and practice* (pp. 465–486). San Francisco, CA: Jossey-Bass.

Triplett, N. (1898). The dynamogenic factors in pacemaking and competition. *American Journal of Psychology, 9*, 507–533.

U.S. Department of Health and Human Services. (1996). *Physical activity and health: A report of the Surgeon General*. Atlanta, GA: U.S. Department of Health and Human Services, Centers for Disease Control and Prevention, National Center for Chronic Disease Prevention and Health Promotion.

U.S. Department of Health and Human Services. (2010). *Physical activity for everyone: Recommendations*. Retrieved March 27, 2010, from http://www.cdc.gov/physicalactivity/everyone/guidelines/adults.html

Wilson, M., O'Hanlon, R., Prasad, S., Deighan, A., Macmillan, P., Oxborough, D., & Whyte, G. (2011). Diverse patterns of myocardial fibrosis in lifelong, veteran endurance athletes. *Journal of Applied Physiology, 110,* 1622–1626.

World Health Organization. (1946). Preamble to the Constitution of the World Health Organization as adopted by the International Health Conference, New York, 19-22 June 1946, and entered into force on 7 April 1948.

World Health Organization. (2009). *Global health risks: Mortality and burden of disease attributable to selected major risks.* Retrieved from http://www.who.int/healthinfo/global_burden_disease/GlobalHealthRisks_report_full.pdf

World Health Organization. (2012). *Recommended levels of physical activity for adults aged 18–64 years* [Electronic Version]. Retrieved December 20, 2012, from http://www.who.int/dietphysicalactivity/factsheet_adults/en/index.html

CHAPTER 2

Introduction to the Psychology of Sedentary Behavior

Runner: © lzf/Shutterstock

Vignette: Sarah

I wake up around 6:30 a.m. each morning to give myself enough time to shower and get dressed and dab some makeup on before starting my hour commute via car to work. Most mornings I'm lucky if I grab a muffin to eat while I drive. It's rare that I have time to sit down for a full breakfast.

I arrive at the office around 8:45, sometimes a bit after 9:00 if traffic is bad. As an executive assistant to the CEO of a small insurance company, the majority of my day is spent fielding phone calls and emails from clients, scheduling the boss's meetings and travel plans, coordinating with our account director to manage billing inquiries, and organizing reports from the focus groups my company conducts on a monthly basis.

Needless to say, most of this requires me to stay seated. I'd say the most exercise I get during normal business hours depends on how many times I walk to the copy machine down the hallway and how often I make trips to the restroom throughout the day.

I know that I'm supposed to get more exercise. And the need's especially strong considering my cholesterol levels were higher than normal on my most recent blood test. I try

LEARNING OBJECTIVES

After completing this chapter, you will be able to:

- Describe what sedentary behavior is and how it is distinct from physical inactivity.
- Estimate the numbers of people who are sedentary.
- Describe the guidelines for sedentary behavior.
- Differentiate among key terms such as *inactive*, *screen time*, and *sedentary*.
- Identify individual correlates of sedentary behavior.
- Understand the health effects of sedentary behavior.

to watch what I eat so as to control my weight, but I'm well aware health isn't just about being able to fit into a size 4.

I've tried joining a gym before but my commitment to training usually lasts only a few months—often around New Year's or during the first few weeks of spring, when I'm getting ready to be seen in less clothing come summer. The trouble with me is that I just don't feel like I have the energy or the time to commit to working out. Going to the gym adds time to my already lengthy commute to and from work. And, honestly, by the time I leave the office I'm completely exhausted. On particularly stressful days, I'm more likely to come home, order takeout, and watch Netflix for the few hours I have to myself before bedtime rather than hoofing it to my local fitness center.

I'm single now and I don't have kids, so I am at an advantage in terms of being able to squeeze a few sessions of exercise in during a week. I've tried recently to commit to doing a few at-home yoga and Pilates routines that I learned from a fitness DVD set. But it's frustrating to me that physical activity simply isn't built into the typical workday—and also that my commute saps the time and energy I'd have to really put more effort into a legitimate workout.

I've considered getting a treadmill or elliptical machine for my home. But I rent a small apartment and worry about the noise it would make for the neighbors below as well as how much space it would take up. (Not to mention the machine's cost.) I want to imagine there's an easier way to fit it all in. But while I'm working to repay my student loans, make rent each month, and put money into a savings account, the prospect of keeping in shape just seems completely out of reach. Sometimes I wonder: Would I need to go part time just to make room in my life for the gym?

■ Introduction

The health benefits of regular moderate- to vigorous-intensity exercise are well established and our knowledge of these benefits continues to increase. The science clearly shows that regular physical activity is associated with the reduction of more than 25 chronic diseases. Today, however, a new trend is the rapid rise in research examining how sedentary behavior, as opposed to physical activity, affects our health (Biddle, 2011). Sedentary behavior includes waking activities undertaken in a sitting or reclined position, such as watching television, reading, playing video games, and engaging in computer activities. Because sedentary behavior is so prevalent, and has so many negative health effects, experts are now beginning to ask the question: "Is sitting the new smoking of our generation?" An interesting question indeed.

CRITICAL THINKING ACTIVITY 2-1

© ecco/Shutterstock, Inc.

What is meant by the statement: "Is sitting the new smoking of our generation?" Do you think that this is true?

The inquiry into the scientific study of sedentary behavior is very recent. It is only within the last 15 years that an explosion of research into the science of sedentary behavior has occurred despite the fact that we have known since the 1950s that sitting too much is hazardous to our health (Morris et al., 1953). In a landmark series of studies, Jeremy Morris and his colleagues (1953) examined the activity levels among different occupations. Their seminal study revealed that the sedentary drivers of London's double-decker buses had higher rates of cardiovascular disease than the conductors who climbed the stairs and walked around the bus taking people's tickets. The data were so compelling because the bus drivers and the conductors were similar demographically; that is, the bus drivers and the conductors were the same age and social class. There was only one obvious difference between these two groups—the drivers were sedentary and the conductors were unavoidably active. In fact, the conductors ascended and descended 500 to 750 steps per working day. And they were half as likely as the drivers to die of a sudden heart attack.

Morris and his colleagues extended their study findings to other populations, and they noticed that postmen who delivered the mail by either bike or on foot had fewer heart attacks than the sedentary postal men who either served behind the counters or as the telephone switchboard operators. Although, collectively these early studies provided evidence for the role of physical activity in averting premature mortality, it has only recently been hypothesized that some of these observed associations may be explained by differences in time spent sitting rather than the time spent being physically active; that is,

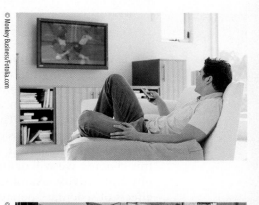

© Monkey Business/Fotolia.com

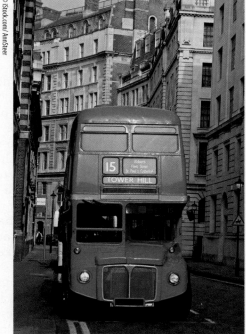

© iStock.com/ AmiSteer

the bus drivers sat more than the conductors, and the telephone switchboard operators and clerks sat more than the postmen. Unfortunately, the independent roles of sitting versus physical activity cannot be determined from these early studies. However, they do provide an intriguing look into the potential health effects of sitting too much.

CRITICAL THINKING ACTIVITY 2-2

© ecco/Shutterstock, Inc.

Why were the independent roles of sitting versus physical activity not examined in these landmark studies?

Exercise studies traditionally have focused on physical activities performed at moderate to high intensities, rather than sedentary behavior or mild physical activity. In health guidelines, physical activity of at least moderate intensity has been imposed, and often the exercise treatment has been vigorous in intensity and prolonged in duration. Thus, there is a dearth of research on sedentary behavior, in general, and even less on the psychology of sedentary behavior. The main purposes of this chapter are to examine this emerging field of scientific inquiry. In this chapter, we will define and describe how sedentary behavior is distinct from physical activity, examine the sedentary behavior guidelines, discuss the health effects of sedentary behavior, outline individual correlates of sedentary behavior, and determine how sedentary behavior is measured.

■ Defining Sedentary Behavior

Too much sitting (or being sedentary) appears to be a health risk that is additional to, and distinct from, too little exercise. What exactly does this mean? Even if people are meeting the physical activity guidelines of, for example, exercising at a moderate intensity for 150 minutes per week, yet spend most of the remaining waking hours left in sedentary activities, this has a negative impact on their health. Thus, not only should people be meeting the physical activity guidelines, but people should also reduce the time that they spend sitting during the day. This is an emerging area of inquiry, with most research findings illustrating that sedentary behavior has negative health effects independent of physical activity (Maher, Olds, Mire, & Katzmarzyk, 2014). In other words, we need to not only move more at a moderate and/or vigorous pace, but we also need to stand up more during the day. Like Sarah, most people struggle to both exercise and stand more during the day.

But how does sedentary behavior differ from light activity? **Sedentary behavior** refers to any waking activity characterized by little physical movement and an energy expenditure of less than or equal to 1.5 **metabolic equivalents (METs)** in either a sitting or reclining position (Tremblay et al., 2012). This means that any time a person is either sitting or lying down, that person is engaging in sedentary behavior. Sleeping does not count as sedentary behavior—remember, you must be awake. Sedentary behavior encompasses activities based on technology (TV, computer use, video games), socializing (sitting, talking, texting), travel (car, train), work/school (desk job, studying), and leisure activities (reading, listening to music). The collective term of **screen time** is often used to refer to television watching, playing passive video games, and using mobile devices and computers. In comparison, **recreational screen time** refers specifically to television watching, passive video game playing, using the computer, or use of other screens during leisure time that are practiced while sedentary.

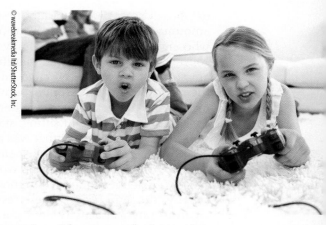

Light or mild physical activity, which often is incorrectly grouped with sedentary behavior, involves energy expenditure at the level of 1.6 to 2.9 METs. Mild physical activities include, for example, slow walking, cooking food, and washing dishes. For clarification, **TABLE 2-1** provides the categories and descriptions of the various physical activity intensities.

Is **sedentarism** different from just not getting enough exercise? Yes! Sitting is not the behavioral equivalent of exercising too little. The term **inactive behavior**

TABLE 2-1   Categories of Physical Activity Intensity

Intensity	METs	Description	Examples
Sedentary	< 1.6	Sitting or lying down. Little additional movement, low energy requirement.	Watching TV, riding in car, reading, sitting, and texting.
Light	1.6 to < 3	Aerobic activity that does not cause noticeable changes in breathing rate.	Standing, light walking, washing dishes, folding laundry.
Moderate	3 to 6	Aerobic activity that is able to be conducted while having an uninterrupted conversation.	Brisk walking, mopping, water aerobics, easy biking riding, doubles tennis.
Vigorous	6 to < 9	Aerobic activity in which a conversation generally cannot be maintained uninterrupted.	Singles tennis, running, high impact aerobics, biking uphill.

METs = metabolic equivalents.
Data from Norton, K., Norton, L., & Sadgrove, D. (2010). Position statement of physical activity and exercise intensity terminology. *Journal of Science and Medicine in Sport, 13,* 496–502.

or **physical inactivity** typically describes those who are performing insufficient amounts of moderate to vigorous physical activity. In other words, those people who are not meeting specified physical activity guidelines. Lynette Craft and her colleagues (2012) illustrated that the time we spend sitting is independent of the amount of time we spend engaged in moderate to vigorous physical activity. In their study, 91 healthy women between the ages of 40 to 75 years wore an activity monitor for 1 week. The researchers then determined the time (i.e., minutes per day) these women spent sitting, standing, stepping, and in bouts of moderate to vigorous physical activity that was at least 10 minutes in duration.

They found that the time spent sitting, standing, and in **incidental physical activities** did not differ between women who either met or exceeded the physical activity guidelines compared to those with either no or minimal levels of physical activity (see **FIGURE 2-1**). These results show that our time spent in moderate to vigorous physical activity does not replace significant periods of sitting time. In other words, exercise and sedentary behaviors are independent classes of behavior. In fact, some people who meet the physical activity guidelines may spend a great deal of their remaining waking time sitting. This is an excellent example of what is meant by "the active couch potato" (Owen, Healey, & Dunstan, 2010). In other words, sitting may be the new smoking—even for regular exercisers.

CRITICAL THINKING ACTIVITY 2-3

© ecco/Shutterstock, Inc.

Describe what is meant by "the active couch potato." Do you know anyone who is an active couch potato? How does this affect that person's health?

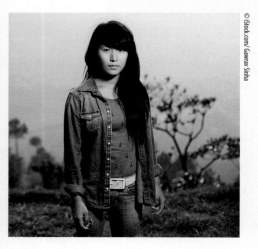
© iStock.com/Gawrav Sinha

Thus, there is a need to examine not only how to make a physically inactive public more active, but how to also make a sedentary public stand more. Most of society sits for prolonged periods almost every day. The healthy and relatively very active women in the aforementioned study sat about 9 hours a day, which is more than the average adult sleeps. As Craft and colleagues (2012) noted, sitting is now more abundant than sleeping, which is likely an important milestone in human history. Public health recommendations and interventions aimed at increasing exercise behavior are unlikely to impact how much time people spend sitting because they are independent behaviors. As seen in **TABLE 2-2** , sedentary behavior operates in a different way from physical activity; thus, sedentary behavior is in need of its own guidelines, basic research inquiry, and interventions (Biddle, 2011).

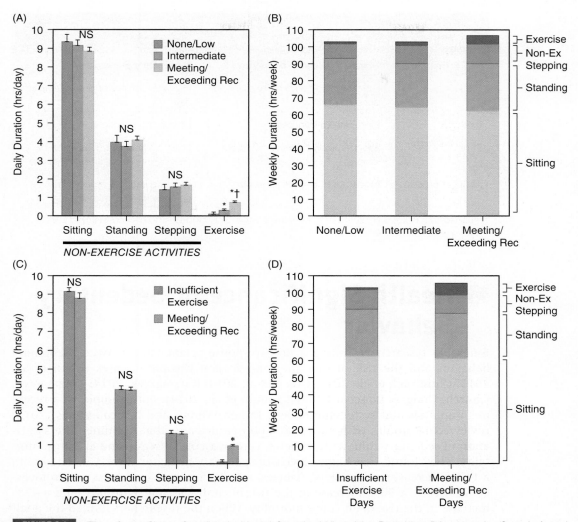

FIGURE 2-1   Time Spent Sitting, Standing, Incidental Stepping When Not Exercising (Non-exercise Stepping), and Exercising as Defined by the Federal Physical Activity Guidelines

Panels A and B illustrate the results for a cross-sectional comparison between subjects for the mean daily duration of each behavior (A) and the sum of all behaviors accumulated over an entire week (B) for the three groups stratified by time spent exercising. Panels C and D illustrate the within subject analysis results comparing the days that subjects had insufficient exercise (< 30 minutes) compared to days where they perform at least 30 minutes of aerobic exercise. Values are expressed as means with SEM bars.

* $p < 0.001$ vs. None/Low Exercise or Insufficient Exercise; † $p < 0.001$ vs. Intermediate.

Reproduced from Craft, L. L., Zderic, T. W., Gapstur, S. M., VanIterson, E. H., Thomas, D. M., Siddique, J., & Hamilton, M.T. (2012). Evidence that women meeting physical activity guidelines do not sit less: An observational inclinometry study. *International Journal of Behavioral Nutrition and Physical Activity, 9*, 122. doi:10.1186/1479-5868-9-122

TABLE 2-2   FITT (Frequency, Intensity, Time, and Thought Process) Principles Applied to Physical Activity and Sedentary Behavior

FITT Principle	Physical Activity Behavior	Sedentary Behavior
Frequency	Low: Likely to be no more than once per day.	High: Regular, prolonged bouts every day.
Intensity	Moderate to vigorous.	Little to no exertion.
Time	Short: Typically between 10 to 30 minutes.	Long: Such as 2 to 3 hours of TV viewing or prolonged sitting at work.
Thought process	Moderate to high; requires planning.	Low and habitual; requires little or no conscious decision making.

Modified from Biddle, S. H. (2011). Fit or sit? Is there a psychology of sedentary behavior? *Sport and Exercise Psychology Review, 7,* 5–10.

Health Significance of Sedentary Behavior

Emerging research is finding a dose–response relationship between sedentary behavior and the risk of mortality and several chronic diseases (Chau et al., 2013; Chomistek et al., 2013; Green et al. 2014; Katzmarzyk, 2014; Katzmarzyk, Church, Craig, & Bouchard, 2009; Sequin et al., 2014). For example, in a recent meta-analysis and systematic review, Emma Wilmot and her colleagues (2012) reviewed 18 studies with almost 800,000 participants that examined the association of sedentary time with diabetes, cardiovascular disease, and all-cause mortality. They found that higher levels of sedentary behavior were associated with a 112% increase in the risk of diabetes, a 147% increase in the risk of cardiovascular disease, a 90% increase in the risk of cardiovascular mortality, and a 47% increase in the risk of all-cause mortality. When the researchers limited the analysis to studies that controlled for physical activity as a covariate, they still found that sedentary time was related, although to a lesser extent, to increased risk for the aforementioned conditions. The researchers concluded the existence of a strong and consistent association between sedentary time and diabetes, cardiovascular disease, and all-cause mortality. These reported associations were largely independent of physical activity, revealing that sedentary behavior and moderate to vigorous physical activity are distinct behaviors.

Other systematic and meta-analytic reviews have confirmed that prolonged sedentary behavior is independently associated with negative health outcomes regardless of physical activity (Biswas et al., 2015). For example, researchers found that sedentary time is related to increased risk of all-cause mortality in older adults, and that a positive relationship exists between sedentary behavior and metabolic syndrome, waist circumference, and overweight/obesity (Rezende, Rey-Lopez, Matsudo, & Luiz, 2014).

As well, evidence suggests that having a high level of sedentary behavior negatively impacts health independent of other factors, including body weight, diet, and physical activity. For example, a 12-year prospective study of about 17,000 Canadian adults found that those who spent most of their time sitting were 50% more likely to die during the follow-up than those who sat the least, even after controlling for age, smoking, and physical activity levels (Katzmarzyk et al., 2009). These data demonstrate a dose–response association between sitting time and mortality from all causes and cardiovascular disease, independent of exercise. The bottom line (no pun intended) is that prolonged sitting time is associated with increased morbidity and mortality, independent of leisure-time physical activity.

■ Guidelines for Sedentary Behavior

The current model of physical activity and health is well supported by over 70 years of scientific inquiry, and the beneficial effects of moderate to vigorous physical activity have been more clearly defined in recent years. As Peter Katzmarzyk (2010) noted, if we are complacent with the existing paradigm—that increasing levels of moderate to vigorous physical activity will result in the greatest improvements in public health—then we may not obtain the full return on investment with respect to improving quality of life and life expectancy through human movement.

Researchers, healthcare professionals, and government agencies have realized the health importance of limiting people's sedentary behavior in addition to trying to increase their physical activity levels. Some countries, such as Australia and Canada, have been leaders in advancing guidelines on how to reduce sedentary behavior and screen time (Australia Department of Health and Aging, 2012). Because the research is still in its infancy, the current sedentary behavior guidelines are considered consensus "sensible" guidelines. This means that as more science emerges on the health effects of sedentary behavior the guidelines will be updated to reflect the new knowledge.

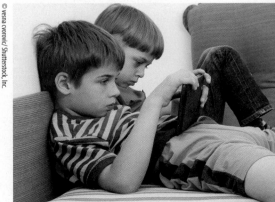

In 2011, the Canadian Society for Exercise Physiology released sedentary behavior guidelines for children and youth. These sedentary behavior guidelines were developed with the goal of getting the well-known, yet undervalued, statement across: "Move more and sit less every day." These guidelines recommend that, for health benefits, children and youth should minimize the time that they spend being sedentary each day. This may be achieved by the following two general categories of (1) limiting recreational screen time to no more than 2 hours per day (with lower levels of screen time being associated

TABLE 2-3 Sedentary Behavior Guidelines for Children		
Infants and Young Children 0–4 Years	**Children 5–11 Years**	**Children 12–17 Years**
Minimize time spent being sedentary.	Minimize time spent being sedentary.	Minimize time spent being sedentary.
For children under 2, screen time is not recommended.	Limit screen time to less than 2 hours a day; lower levels are associated with additional health benefits.	Limit recreational screen time to no more than 2 hours per day; lower levels are associated with additional health benefits.
For children 2–4 years, screen time should be limited to under 1 hour per day; less is better.	Limit sedentary (motorized) transport, extended sitting, and time spent indoors throughout the day.	Limit sedentary (motorized) transport, extended sitting, and time spent indoors throughout the day.

Data from Salmon, J., Tremblay, M. S., Marshall, S. J., & Hume, C. (2011). Health risks, correlates, and interventions to reduce sedentary behavior in young people. *American Journal of Preventive Medicine, 41*, 197–206.

with additional health benefits) and (2) limiting sedentary (motorized) transport, extended sitting time, and time spent indoors throughout the day. **TABLE 2-3** provides a more detailed description of the sedentary guidelines for children. See **TABLE 2-4** for recommendations on how young people should limit their involvement in sedentary pursuits to reduce health risks (Tremblay et al., 2011; Tremblay et al., 2012).

TABLE 2-4 Ways to Reduce Children's Sedentary Behavior Time	
Early Years (0–4 years)	**Children (5–17 years)**
Limit the use of playpens and infant seats when baby is awake.	Turn the TV off.
Explore and play with your child.	Hide the remote.
Stop during long car trips for playtime.	Reduce the number of TVs in the home. Take TVs out of kitchens and bedrooms.
Set limits and have rules about screen time.	Plan outdoor family time.
Keep TVs and computers out of bedrooms.	Create a TV watching and computer schedule.
Take children outside every day.	

Data from Salmon, J., Tremblay, M. S., Marshall, S. J., & Hume, C. (2011). Health risks, correlates, and interventions to reduce sedentary behavior in young people. *American Journal of Preventive Medicine, 41*, 197–206.

TABLE 2-5   Adults (18 to 65 years) Sedentary Behavior Guidelines
Guidelines
Minimize the amount of time spent in prolonged sitting.
Break up long periods of sitting as often as possible.

Data from Australian Government Department of Health. (2014). Physical activity and sedentary behavior guidelines. Retrieved March 2014 from http://www.health.gov.au/internet/main/publishing.nsf/Content/health-pubhlth-strateg-phys-act-guidelines/%24File/Brochures_PAG_Adults18-64yrs.pdf.

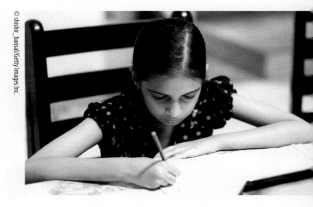
© shishir_bansal/Getty Images Inc.

Data from more than 23,000 Canadian students in grades 9 through 12 revealed that youth spend almost 500 minutes per day in sedentary behavior (Leatherdale & Harvey, 2015). In other words, high school students are spending over 8 hours a day in sedentary pursuits. Furthermore, 97% of these students exceeded the sedentary guidelines of no more than 2 hours per day of recreational screen time. The researchers concluded that most youth are highly sedentary and there is a need to develop effective interventions to reduce their sedentary time.

More recently, Australia developed the first sedentary guidelines for adults ages 18 to 65 years (Australian Government Department of Health, 2014). These guidelines, although brief, are designed to encourage adults to sit less and move more (see **TABLE 2-5**). Prolonged sitting is often quantified as sitting without a break for 1 hour. In other words, if you have been sitting for an hour, you have been sitting for too long. The ultimate goal for people should be to break up sitting times with light-intensity activity one to two times per hour.

CRITICAL THINKING ACTIVITY 2-4

© ecco/Shutterstock, Inc.

How would you expand on the sedentary guidelines to other populations, including pregnant women, disabled adults, and older adults?

■ Prevalence of Sedentary Behavior

In addition to the promotion of moderate to vigorous physical activity, people should not sit for extended periods of time. Unfortunately, people, regardless of their age, spend too much time in sedentary activities. Based on the following quote it is likely that the former American educator Robert Maynard Hutchins (1899–1977) also spent a large portion of his day being inactive: "The secret of my abundant health is that whenever the impulse to exercise comes over me, I lie down until it passes away" (McEvoy, 1938, p. 482). How many people today hold his same view of physical activity and sedentary behavior? In other words, just how sedentary are we? To answer this question, let's take a closer look at the prevalence of sedentary behavior in a variety of populations.

Both children and adults spend a large portion of their day being sedentary. The average child spends about 5 to 10 hours a day being sedentary. Of this sedentary time, young people typically spend 2 to 4 hours a day in screen-based behaviors

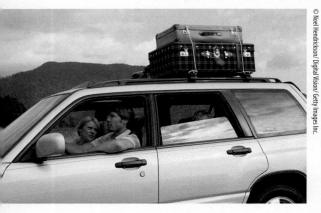

such as watching television, playing video games, and using the computer (Salmon, Tremblay, Marshall, & Hume, 2011). And the average adult spends more than 9 hours a day in sedentary behaviors (Gennuso et al., 2013; Healy, Matthews, Dunstan, Winkler, & Owen, 2011). **FIGURE 2-2** illustrates the typical adult pattern of daily activities when categorized in terms of intensity level (based on the percentage of a 24-hour day; Norton, Norton, & Sadgrove, 2010). This figure reveals graphically that most of our time during the day is spent engaged in sedentary types of activities.

Based on the quote from Robert Hutchins, it is likely that if he were alive today he would not be meeting either the physical activity or sedentary behaviors guidelines. How many people actually meet both the sedentary and physical

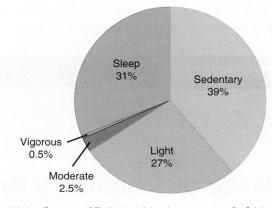

FIGURE 2-2 Typical Adult Pattern of Daily Activities (percentage of a 24-hour day)

Adapted from Norton, K., Norton, L., & Sadgrove, D. (2010). Position statement of physical activity and exercise intensity terminology. *Journal of Science and Medicine in Sport, 13*, 496–502.

activity guidelines? Research is revealing that very few people are meeting both health guidelines. Canadian researchers found that only 15% of 3- to 4-year-olds and 5% of 5-year-olds are meeting both the physical activity and sedentary behavior guidelines (Colley et al., 2013). These findings are a wake-up call that we need to stand up and get moving.

What about college students? Often, newly found independence allows college students to make decisions and choices that were previously made for them by their parents. An important decision a college student may make is how to incorporate physical activity into a busy lifestyle. The U.S. Department of Labor publishes the American Time Use Survey, which is a nationally representative estimate on how people living in America spend their time. Data equated from the 2008 to 2012 surveys showed that on an average weekday, full-time university and college students spend most of their waking hours in leisure and sport activities (3.8 hours), followed by educational activities (3.4 hours) and working activities (2.7 hours) (see **FIGURE 2-3**). When leisure time was categorized, television viewing comprised the largest percentage, at 1.84 hours per day (U.S. Department of Labor, 2009). Thus, when college students have free time they are most likely being sedentary by watching television.

Charles Fountaine and his colleagues (Fountaine, Liguori, Mozumdar, & Schuna, 2011) further examined sedentary behavior and physical activity by

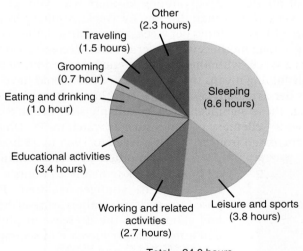

Total = 24.0 hours

NOTE: Data include individuals, ages 15 to 49, who were enrolled full time at a university or college. Data include non-holiday weekdays and are averages for 2008–2012.

FIGURE 2-3   Time Use on an Average Weekday for Full-Time University and College Students

U.S. Department of Labor, Bureau of Labor Statistics. American time use survey. Retrieved May 10, 2013, from http://www.bls.gov/tus/datafiles_2008.htm.

gender in a large sample of college students (*N* = 746). Consistent with previous studies, they found that male students reported higher levels of physical activity than did female students, as represented by days per week of aerobic exercise (3.37 vs. 3.04) and strength training activities (1.90 vs. 1.13). In regard to sedentary behavior, they found that college students spent 144 minutes per day dedicated to screen time, with 60 minutes spent watching television. Male students reported higher levels of overall screen time and television viewing compared to female students, whereas female students spent more time engaged in homework than male students. When the researchers categorized the data by activity level, they found that physically active students reported fewer minutes of total screen time than inactive students.

As another example, sedentary behavior and physical inactivity have increased significantly among American mothers over the last four decades. Edward Archer and his colleagues (2013) analyzed 45 years of national data (from 1965 to 2010) on the following two groups of mothers: (1) those with children 5 years or younger and (2) those with children aged 6 to 18 years. Physical activity was determined by the amount of time allocated to housework, childcare, laundry, food preparation, postmeal cleanup, and exercise. Sedentary behavior was the sum of time spent in a vehicle and using screen-based media.

The researchers found that with each passing generation, mothers have become more physically inactive, sedentary, and obese. From 1965 to 2010, the average amount of physical activity among mothers with younger children fell from 44 hours a week to less than 30 hours a week, resulting in a decrease in energy expenditure of 1,573 calories per week. In comparison, the average amount of physical activity among mothers with older children decreased from 32 hours to less than 21 hours a week, with a reduction in energy expenditure of 1,238 calories per week. This finding means that mothers in 2010 would have to eat 175 to 225 fewer calories per day to prevent weight gain than mothers in 1965.

Not surprising, these significant declines in physical activity corresponded with large increases in sedentary pastimes such as watching TV. On average, sedentary behaviors increased from 18 hours a week in 1965 to 25 hours a week in

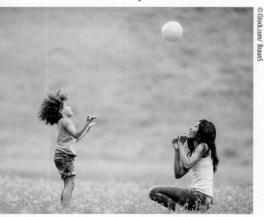

©iStock.com/ Braun5

2010 among mothers with older children, and from 17 hours a week to nearly 23 hours a week among mothers with younger children. Finally, compared to working mothers, stay-at-home mothers had about twice the decrease in physical activity and a much larger increase in sedentary behavior (see **FIGURES 2-4** and **2-5**).

Juliet Harvey and her colleagues (Harvey, Chastin, & Skeleton, 2013) found that with regard to older adults aged 65 and older, 67% of this population is sedentary for more than 8.5 hours a day. TV viewing encompassed a large portion of this population's sedentary time. Computer use is likely to increase with time as older adults become more

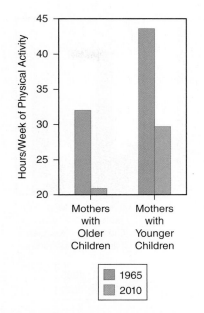

FIGURE 2-4   Time Allocated to Physical Activity in Mothers by Year

Note: From 1965 to 2010, the time allocated to physical activity decreased in mothers. Specifically, the time allocated to physical activity decreased by 11.1 hours/week (from 32.0 to 20.9 hours/week) in MOC and by 13.9 hours/week (from 43.6 to 29.7 hours/week) in MYC.

Reprinted from Archer, E., Lavie, C. J., McDonald, S. M., et al. (2013). Maternal inactivity: 45-year trends in mothers' use of time. *Mayo Clinic Proceedings, 88*, 1368–1377. With permission from Elsevier.

familiar with computer technology. These researchers also found a slight increase in sedentary behavior in people over the age of 75 compared to those aged 65 to 74 years. Thus, in general, as we get older we become more sedentary.

In short, the prevalence of sedentary behavior is rapidly increasing across the globe in all age demographics. The increased prevalence in sedentary time is largely driven by reductions in movement at work, at home, and in travel. In particular, the rapid and dramatic changes in the workforce over the last century have resulted in increased sedentary behavior at work (Kirk & Rhodes, 2011). Current estimates reveal that people today spend about 80% of their working day sitting (Thorp et al., 2009). Because people spend a large portion of their waking hours at work, it provides an ideal environment to intervene to get people to stand and move more. Emerging research is revealing that

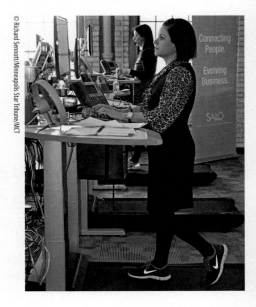

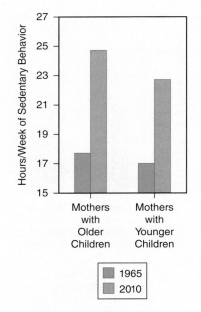

FIGURE 2-5   Time Allocated to Sedentary Behavior in Mothers by Year

Note: From 1965 to 2010, the time allocated to physical activity decreased in mothers. Specifically, the time allocated to physical activity decreased by 11.1 hours/week (from 32.0 to 20.9 hours/week) in mothers with older children (between the ages of 6 and 18 years) and by 13.9 hours/week (from 43.6 to 29.7 hours/week) in mothers with younger children (i.e., children 5 years of age or younger).

Reprinted from Archer, E., Lavie, C. J., McDonald, S. M., et al. (2013). Maternal inactivity: 45-year trends in mothers' use of time. *Mayo Clinic Proceedings, 88,* 1368–1377. With permission from Elsevier.

active workstations such as treadmill desks and pedal deskscan increase energy expenditure without affecting work performance (Koepp et al., 2013; Thompson, Koepp, & Levine, 2013; Tudor-Locke, Schuna, Frensham, & Proenca, 2013). In other words, replacing traditional office chair and desktop computer workstations with active workstations may be a strategy for mitigating the low energy expenditure inherent to contemporary office workstations.

■ Individual Correlates of Sedentary Behavior

While the health benefits of meeting the physical activity guidelines are well established, the health risks of sedentary behavior, independent of meeting the physical activity guidelines, are evolving. Studies have shown that prolonged sedentary behavior, independent of physical activity level, is associated with various negative health conditions, such as cardiovascular disease, obesity, type 2 diabetes, cancer, metabolic syndrome, and psychological distress. From this evidence, it is essential to identify correlates of sedentary behavior so that interventions can target those individuals at a higher likelihood for engaging in sedentary behaviors.

Several studies have examined correlates of sedentary behavior (e.g., Al-Hazzaa, Abahussain, Al-Sobayel, Qahwaji, & Musaiger, 2011; Dogra & Stathokostas, 2014; Dunlop et al., 2014; Harrington, Barreira, Staiano, & Katzmarzyk, 2013; Mielke, da Silva, Owen, & Hallal, 2014; Pearson & Biddle, 2011; Rhodes, Mark, & Temmel, 2012; Salmon et al., 2011; Thorp, Owen, Neuhaus, & Dunstan, 2011; Uijdewilligen et al., 2011). In many cases, these studies operationalized sedentary behavior as the amount of time spent watching TV. Most of the research examining the correlates of sedentary behavior has focused on demographic factors. Thus, we know little about personal motives or environmental and social correlates of sedentary behavior. A summary of emerging findings on the correlates of sedentary behavior is presented in **TABLE 2-6**. This is a developing area of research, and further study is needed to substantiate these correlates in high-quality studies with standardized and objective measures of sedentary behavior.

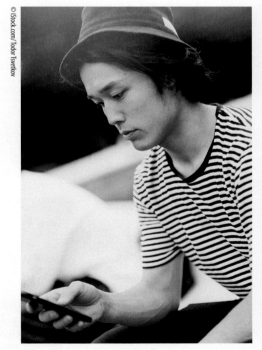

Of interest is the use of technology and how it affects sedentary behavior. In other words, is technology a correlate of sedentary behavior? Today's college students are a unique population to examine the effects of technology on activity levels because they are the first cohort of young people raised entirely in the **digital age** (also known as the *new media* or *information age*). These **digital natives** have interacted with technology from an early age and are often described as "hyperconnected" to their cell phones and other electronic devices (Anderson & Rainie, 2012). Because cell phone use is so pervasive among college students, this population makes a logical starting point for investigating the relationship between cell phone use and how it affects physical activity and sedentary behavior levels.

In a recent study, Andrew Lepp and his colleagues (Lepp, Barkley, Sanders, Rebold, & Gates, 2013) examined the relationship between cell phone use and college students' levels of sedentary behavior and physical activity. In the first part of their study, 305 college students completed a self-report questionnaire measuring cell phone use in the following three ways: (1) total cell phone use per day, (2) total number of text messages sent per day, and (3) total number of calls made per day. In the second part of their study, 49 students were interviewed regarding their cell phone use and physical activity behavior; they also completed a progressive treadmill exercise test to exhaustion to assess cardiorespiratory fitness (i.e., VO_2 max test).

TABLE 2-6 Individual Correlates of Sedentary Behavior		
Correlate Category	**Specific Correlate**	**Relationship with Sedentary Behavior**
Demographic	Age	Positive: Sedentary behavior increases as we get older.
	Ethnicity	Caucasians are less sedentary than ethnic minorities.
	Socioeconomic status	Negative: Higher socioeconomic status is associated with less sedentary behavior.
	Gender	Sedentary time is higher in women.
	Health status	People with chronic diseases, disabilities, and mood disorders are more sedentary than healthy persons.
	Education level	Negative: Higher education level is correlated with less sedentary behavior.
	Weight	Positive: Obese and overweight people sit more than normal weight people.
	Retirement status	People who are retired sit more than people who are not retired.
	Employment status	Unemployed are more sedentary than employed.
Behavioral	Physical activity behavior	People who are physically active tend to be less sedentary.
	Smoking	Smokers are more sedentary than nonsmokers.
	Diet	Those who eat a less healthy diet (e.g., high consumption of energy-dense snacks and fast food) are more sedentary.
	Alcohol consumption	No relationship.
	Cell phone use	Positive: Cell phone use positively related to sedentary behavior.
	TV viewing	Positive: TV viewing positively related to sedentary behavior.

The researchers found that students averaged just over 300 minutes (5 hours) of cell phone use per day. In addition, 88.2% of participants reported using the cell phone primarily for leisure. No significant gender differences were found for cell phone use (see **TABLE 2-7**). The researchers, however, found that cell phone use was negatively related with cardiorespiratory fitness; that is, high-frequency cell phone users tended to be less physically fit than low-frequency cell phone users.

The researchers concluded that cell phone use is associated with physical activity and fitness in a manner similar to other types of sedentary behaviors such as watching television and using a computer. Although cell phones provide many

TABLE 2-7 Self-Reported Cell Phone Use by Gender		
Cell Phone Use	**Men (*n* = 134)**	**Women (*n* = 168)**
Total use per day (minutes)	299	313
Text messages sent per day	214	158
Calls made per day	6.7	5.0

Data from Lepp, A., Barkley, J. E., Sanders, G. J., Rebold, M., & Gates, P. (2013). The relationship between cell phone use, physical and sedentary activity, and cardiorespiratory fitness in a sample of U.S. college students. *International Journal of Behavioral Nutrition and Physical Activity, 21*. doi:10.1186/1479-5868-10-79

of the same temptations as television and Internet-connected computers, the main difference is that cell phones fit in our pockets and purses and are with us wherever we go. Thus, they provide an ever-present invitation to "sit and play." It appears that compared to low-frequency cell phone users, high-frequency cell phone users are more likely to forgo being physically active to use their cell phones for more sedentary activities such as using Facebook and Twitter, playing video games, and surfing the Internet.

CRITICAL THINKING ACTIVITY 2-5

© ecco/Shutterstock, Inc.

Compare and contrast the correlates for sedentary behavior and physical activity. What are the main differences? What are the main similarities?

Measures of Sedentary Behavior

To date, few self-report instruments have been developed to detect sedentary behavior and light-intensity physical activity, and even fewer measures have been validated. Recent advances in **accelerometers** have made it possible to measure the full range of physical activity levels, from sedentary to vigorous, with a single instrument. Although accelerometers can accurately classify participants' behavior as sedentary, they do not provide information about either the type of sedentary behavior or the context (Lubans et al., 2011). In other words, an accelerometer, for example, can tell us if someone is sedentary, but we do not know if the person is sitting and watching TV at home or sitting at a computer at work. Thus, it is recommended that objective measures of sedentary behavior such as accelerometers be used in conjunction with subjective measures (e.g., self-reports) to assess both the type and context of the sedentary behavior (Lubans et al., 2011).

Several self-report measures have recently been developed in an attempt to measure various aspects of sedentary behavior in a variety of populations. For example, the Sedentary Behavior Questionnaire is a brief, yet comprehensive, assessment of sedentary behavior in adults. The questionnaire assesses the time that people spend in the following nine sedentary behaviors: watching television, playing computer/video games, sitting while listening to music, sitting and talking on the phone, doing paperwork or office work, sitting and reading, playing a musical instrument, doing arts and crafts, and sitting and driving/riding in a car, bus, or train (see **TABLE 2-8**).

When participants are completing the Sedentary Behavior Questionnaire they are asked to report their sedentary time separately for weekdays versus weekend days. Wording for weekday reporting is: "On a typical weekday, how much time do you spend (from when you wake up until you go to bed) doing the following?" In comparison, the wording for weekend day reporting is: "On a typical weekend day, how much time do you spend (from when you wake up until you go to bed) doing the following?"

Researchers using the Sedentary Behavior Questionnaire have found that demographic variables are related to sedentary behavior. For example, body mass

TABLE 2-8   Sedentary Behavior Questionnaire

SEDENTARY BEHAVIOR: Weekday

On a typical WEEKDAY, how much time do you spend (from when you wake up until you go to bed) doing the following?

	None	15 min. or less	30 min.	1 hr	2 hrs	3 hrs	4 hrs	5 hrs	6 hrs or more
1. Watching television (including videos on VCR/DVD).	O	O	O	O	O	O	O	O	O
2. Playing computer or video games.	O	O	O	O	O	O	O	O	O
3. Sitting listening to music on the radio, tapes, or CDs.	O	O	O	O	O	O	O	O	O
4. Sitting and talking on the phone.	O	O	O	O	O	O	O	O	O
5. Doing paperwork or computer work (office work, emails, paying bills, etc.)	O	O	O	O	O	O	O	O	O
6. Sitting reading a book or magazine.	O	O	O	O	O	O	O	O	O
7. Playing a musical instrument.	O	O	O	O	O	O	O	O	O
8. Doing artwork or crafts.	O	O	O	O	O	O	O	O	O
9. Sitting and driving in a car, bus, or train.	O	O	O	O	O	O	O	O	O

Reproduced from Rosenberg, D. E., Norman, G. J., Wagner, N., Patrick, K., Calfas, K. J., & Sallis, J. F. (2010). Reliability and validity of the Sedentary Behavior Questionnaire (SBQ) for adults. *Journal of Physical Activity and Health, 7*, 697–705.

index (BMI) has a negative relationship with sedentary time (Rosenberg et al., 2010); that is, overweight and obese people sit more than those who are normal weight. And gender differences have been found with regard to specific sedentary activities. For example, men spend more time watching television, playing computer games, playing musical instruments, and doing office work or paperwork. In comparison, women spend more time sitting and talking on phone and doing arts and crafts than men.

In another study, researchers examined the amount of time **bariatric surgery** candidates spent in different forms of sedentary behavior (Bond et al., 2013). Participants included 52 bariatric surgery candidates with an average BMI in the morbidly obese range (median BMI = 45.3) who completed the Sedentary Behavior Questionnaire and also wore an accelerometer for one week.

The researchers found that bariatric surgery candidates reported engaging in many different types of sedentary behavior, although, on average, they spent almost 30% of their sedentary time watching television (see **FIGURE 2-6**). Thus,

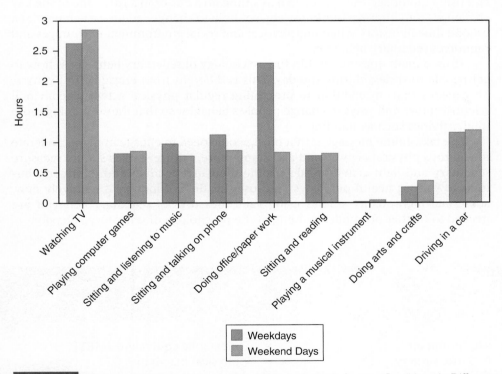

FIGURE 2-6   Reported Average Hours per Day Spent by Bariatric Surgery Candidates in Different Forms of Sedentary Behavior Assessed by the Sedentary Behavior Questionnaire

Adapted from Bond, D. S., Thomas, J. G., Unick, J. L., Raynor, H. A., Vithiananthan, S., & Wing, R. R. (2013). Self-reported and objectively measured sedentary behavior in bariatric surgery candidates. *Surgery for Obesity and Related Diseases, 9*, 123–128.

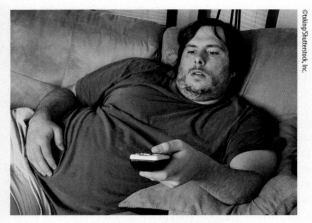
©txking/Shutterstock, Inc.

the researchers concluded that interventions that help these patients to substitute television watching with physical activity may help reduce sedentary time in this high-risk population.

■ Summary

Sedentary behavior has become a popular area of research in the psychology of physical activity, and for good reason. The prevalence of sedentary behavior is increasing rapidly across the globe, and it is negatively affecting our health (Nq & Popkin, 2012). Some examples of sedentary behavior are sitting for prolonged periods watching television, playing passive video games, and using motorized transport (such as sitting on a bus or in a car). One of the key challenges is to improve our knowledge of how to change sedentary behavior at a unique time in history when our physical and social environment encourages and reinforces sedentary behavior.

Thus, a main question within the psychology of sedentary behavior is how to get people to sit less during the day. This is different from engaging in exercise. This means that, in addition to promoting regular physical activity, behavioral scientists must find ways to change people's behavior so that they are doing more mild activities such as standing.

The take-home message is that most people need to engage in more moderate to vigorous physical activity and also stand more. Future studies should measure sedentary and light activity to determine their independent and joint contributions to various health outcomes. Because this field of inquiry is relatively new, additional high-quality studies using valid measures of sedentary behavior are needed to further our understanding of the psychology of sedentary behavior.

KEY TERMS

accelerometer
bariatric surgery
digital age
digital native
inactive behavior
incidental physical activity

metabolic equivalent (MET)
physical inactivity
recreational screen time
screen time
sedentarism
sedentary behavior

REVIEW QUESTIONS

1. What are the sedentary guidelines for children aged 0 to 4 years?

2. What is the difference between sedentary behavior and inactive behavior?

3. What are some of the health implications of sedentary behavior?

4. Describe the prevalence of sedentary behavior in children, adults, and older adults.

5. How much time do college students spend on cell phone use daily? How does this affect their levels of physical activity and sedentary behavior?

6. Describe two correlates of sedentary behavior.

7. How has sedentary behavior and physical inactivity changed among American mothers over the last four decades? What role do children play?

8. Is sitting the new smoking of our generation? Describe your answer in detail using information provided in this chapter.

APPLYING THE CONCEPTS

1. How has Sarah's sedentary lifestyle affected her health?

2. Why is Sarah so sedentary? What factors in Sarah's life contribute to her sedentary lifestyle?

REFERENCES

Al-Hazzaa, H. M., Abahussain, N. A., Al-Sobayel, H. I., Qahwaji, D. M., & Musaiger, A. O. (2011). Physical activity, sedentary behaviors, and dietary habits among Saudi adolescents relative to age, gender, and region. *International Journal of Behavioral Nutritional and Physical Activity*, *8*, 140. doi:10.1186/1479-5868-8-140

Anderson, J., & Rainie, L. (2012). Millennials will benefit and suffer due to their hyperconnected lives. The Pew Research Center's Internet and American Life Project. Retrieved from http://www.pew-internet.org/Reports/2012/Hyperconnected-lives/Overview.aspx

Archer, E., Lavie, C. J., McDonald, S. M., Herbert, J. R., Taverno Ross, S. E., McIver, R. M., & Blair, S. N. (2013). Maternal inactivity: 45-year trends in mothers' use of time. *Mayo Clinic Proceedings, 88*, 1368–1377.

Australian Government Department of Health. (2014). Physical activity and sedentary behavior guidelines. Retrieved March 2014 from http://www.health.gov.au/internet/main/publishing.nsf/Content /health-pubhlth-strateg-phys-act-guidelines/%24File/Brochures_PAG_Adults18-64yrs.pdf

Biddle, S. H. (2011). Fit or sit? Is there a psychology of sedentary behavior? *Sport and Exercise Psychology Review, 7*, 5–10.

Biswas, A., Oh, P. I., Faulkner, G. E., Bajaj, R. R., Silver, M. A., Mitchelle, M. S., & Altern D. A. (2015). Sedentary time and its association with risk of disease incidence, mortality, and hospitalization in adults: A systematic review and meta-analysis. *Annals of Intern Medicine, 162*, 123–132.

Bond, D. S., Thomas, J. G., Unick, J. L., Raynor, H. A., Vithiananthan, S., & Wing, R. R. (2013). Self-reported and objectively measured sedentary behavior in bariatric surgery candidates. *Surgery for Obesity and Related Diseases, 9*, 123–128.

Canadian Society for Exercise Physiology. (2011). Canadian physical activity guidelines for adults 18–64 years [Electronic Version]. Retrieved from http://www.csep.ca/english/view.asp?x=804

Chau, J. Y., Grunseit, A. C., Chey, T., Stamatakis, E., Brown, W. J., Matthews, C. E., Bauman, A . E., & van der Ploeg, H. P. (2013). Daily sitting time and all-cause mortality: A meta-analysis. *PLoS One, 8*(11), e80000. doi:10.1371/journal.pone.0080000

Chomistek, A. K., Manson, J. E., Stefanick, M. L., Lu, B., Sands-Lincoln, M., Going, S. B., ... Eaton, C. B. (2013). Relationship of sedentary behavior and physical activity to incident cardiovascular disease: Results for the Women's Health Initiative. *Journal of the American College of Cardiology, 61*, 2346–2354.

Colley, R. C., Garriquet, D., Adamo, K. B., Carson, V., Janssen, I., Timmons, B. W., & Tremblay, M. S. (2013). Physical activity and sedentary behavior during the early years in Canada: A cross-sectional study. *International Journal of Behavioral Nutrition and Physical Activity, 10* (epub).

Craft, L. L., Zderic, T. W., Gapstur, S. M., Vanlterson, E. H., Thomas, D. M., Siddique, J., & Hamilton, M. T. (2012). Evidence that women meeting physical activity guidelines do not sit less: An observational inclinometry study. *International Journal of Behavioral Nutrition and Physical Activity, 9*, 122.

Dogra, S., & Stathokostas, L. (2014). Correlates of extended sitting time in older adults: An exploratory cross-sectional analysis of the Canadian Community Health Survey Healthy Aging Cycle. *International Journal of Public Health, 59*, 983–991.

Dunlop, D., Song, J., Arnston, E., Semanik, P., Lee, J., Chang, R., & Hootman, J. M. (2014). Sedentary time in U.S. older adults associated with disability in activities of daily living independent of physical activity. *Journal of Physical Activity and Health, 12*, 93–101.

Fountaine, C. J., Liguori, G. A., Mozumdar, A., & Schuna, J. R. (2011). Physical activity and screen time sedentary behaviors in college students. *International Journal of Exercise Science, 4*, 102–112.

Gennuso, K. P., Gangnon, R. E., Matthews, C. E., Thraen-Borowski, K. M., & Colbert, L. M. (2013). Sedentary behavior, physical activity, and markers of health in older adults. *Medicine and Science in Sports and Exercise, 45*, 1493–1500.

Green, A. N., McGrath, R., Martinez, V., Taylor, K., Paul, D. R., & Vella, C. A. (2014). Associations of objectively measured sedentary behavior, light activity, and markers of cardiometabolic health in young women. *European Journal of Applied Physiology, 114*, 907–919.

Harrington, D. M., Barreira, T. V., Staiano, A. E., & Katzmarzyk, P. T. (2013). The descriptive epidemiology of sitting among U.S. adults, NHANES 2009–2010. *Journal of Science in Sport.* doi:10.1016/j. jsams.2013.07.017

Harvey, J. A., Chastin, S. F., & Skelton, D. A. (2013). Prevalence of sedentary behavior in older adults: A systematic review. *International Journal of Environmental Research and Public Health, 10*, 6645–6661.

Healy, G. N., Matthews, C. E., Dunstan, D. W., Winkler, E. A. H., & Owen, N. (2011). Sedentary time and cardio-metabolic biomarkers in U.S. adults: NHANES 2003–06. *European Heart Journal, 32*, 590–597.

Katzmarzyk, P. T. (2010). Physical activity, sedentary behavior, and health: Paradigm paralysis or paradigm shift? *Diabetes*, *59*, 2717–2725.

Katzmarzyk, P. T. (2014). Standing and mortality in a prospective cohort of Canadian adults. *Medicine and Science in Sports and Exercise*, *46*, 940–946.

Katzmarzyk, P. T., Church, T. S., Craig, C. L., & Bouchard, C. (2009). Sitting time and mortality from all causes, cardiovascular disease, and cancer. *Medicine and Science in Sports and Exercise*, *41*, 998–1005.

Kirk, M. A., & Rhodes, R. E. (2011). Occupation correlates of adults' participation in leisure-time physical activity: A systematic review. *American Journal of Preventive Medicine*, *40*, 476–485.

Koepp, G. A., Manohar, C. U., McCrady-Spitzer, S. K., Ben-Ner, A., Hamann, D. J., Runge, C. F., & Levine, J. A. (2013). Treadmill desks: A 1-year prospective trial. *Obesity*, *21*, 705–711.

Leatherdale, S. T., & Harvey, A. (2015). Examining communication- and media-based recreational sedentary behaviors among Canadian youth: Results from the COMPASS study. *Preventive Medicine*, *74*, 74–80.

Lepp, A., Barkley, J. E., Sanders, G. J., Rebold, M., & Gates, P. (2013). The relationship between cell phone use, physical and sedentary activity, and cardiorespiratory fitness in a sample of U.S. college students. *International Journal of Behavioral Nutrition and Physical Activity*, *21*. doi:10.1186/1479-5868-10-79

Lubans, D. R., Hesketh, K., Cliff, D. P., Barnett, L. M., Salmon, J., Dollman, J., ... Hardy, L. L. (2011). A systematic review of the validity and reliability of sedentary behaviour measures used with children and adolescents. *Obesity Reviews*, *12*, 781–799.

Maher, C., Olds, T., Mire, E., & Katzmarzyk, P. T. (2014). Reconsidering the sedentary behavior paradigm. *PLOS One*. doi:10.1371/journal.pone.0086403

McEvoy, J. P. (1938, December). Garlands for the living: Young man looking backwards. *American Mercury*, 482.

Mielke, G. I., da Silva, I. C., Owen, N., & Hallal, P. C. (2014). Brazilian adults' sedentary behaviors by life domain: Population-based study. *PLoS One*, *9*(3): e91614. doi:10.1371/journal.pone.0091614

Morris, J. N., Heady, J. A., Raffle, P. A., Roberts, C. G., & Parks, J. W. (1953). Coronary heart disease and physical activity of work. *Lancet*, *265*, 1053 – 1057.

Norton, K., Norton, L., & Sadgrove, D. (2010). Position statement of physical activity and exercise intensity terminology. *Journal of Science and Medicine in Sport*, *13*, 496–502.

Nq, S. W., & Popkin, B. M. (2012). Time use and physical activity: A shift away from movement across the globe. *Obesity Reviews*, *13*, 659–680.

Owen, N., Healy, G. H., & Dunstan, D. W. (2010). Too much sitting: The population-health science of sedentary behavior. *Exercise and Sport Sciences Reviews*, *38*, 105–113.

Pearson, N., & Biddle, S. J. (2011). Sedentary behavior and dietary intake in children, adolescents, and adults. A systematic review. *American Journal of Preventive Medicine*, *41*, 178–188.

Rezende, L. F., Rey-Lopez, J. P., Matsudo, V. K., & Luiz, O. D. (2014). Sedentary behavior and health outcomes among older adults: A systematic review. *BMC Public Health*, *14*, 333. doi:10.1186/1471-2458-14-333

Rhodes, R. E., Mark, R. S., & Temmel, C. P. (2012). Adult sedentary behavior: A systematic review. *American Journal of Preventive Medicine*, *42*, e3–e28.

Rosenberg, D. E., Norman, G. J., Wagner, N., Patrick, K., Calfas, K. J., & Sallis, J. F. (2010). Reliability and validity of the Sedentary Behavior Questionnaire (SBQ) for adults. *Journal of Physical Activity and Health*, *7*, 697–705.

Salmon, J., Tremblay, M. S., Marshall, S. J., & Hume, C. (2011). Health risks, correlates, and interventions to reduce sedentary behavior in young people. *American Journal of Preventive Medicine*, *41*, 197–206.

Sequin, R., Buchner, D. M., Liu, J., Allison, M., Manini, T., Wang, C. Y., ... Lacroix, A. Z. (2014). Sedentary behavior and mortality in older women: The Women's Health Initiative. *American Journal of Preventive Medicine*, *46*, 122–135.

Thompson, W. G., Koepp, G. A., & Levine, J. A. (2013). Increasing physical activity with treadmill desks. *Work, 48,* 47–51.

Thorp, A., Dunstan, D., Clark, B., Gardiner, P., Healy, G., Keegel, T., ... Winkler, E. (2009, August). Stand up Australia. Sedentary behaviour in workers. Retrieved April 19, 2014, from http://www .medibank.com.au/Client/Documents/Pdfs/Stand_Up_Australia.pdf

Thorp, A. A., Owen, N., Neuhaus, M., & Dunstan, D. W. (2011). Sedentary behaviors and subsequent health outcomes in adults: A systematic review of longitudinal studies, 1996–2011. *American Journal of Preventive Medicine, 41,* 207–215.

Tremblay, M. (2012). Letter to the editor: Standardized use of the terms "sedentary" and "sedentary behaviours." *Applied Physiology Nutrition and Metabolism, 37,* 540–542.

Tremblay, M. S., Leblanc, A. G., Janssen, I., Kho, M. E., Hicks, A., Murumets, K., ... Duggan, M. (2011). Canadian sedentary behaviour guidelines for children and youth. *Applied Physiology, Nutrition, and Metabolism, 36,* 59–64.

Tremblay, M. S., Lablanc, A. G., Carson, V., Choquette, L., Connor Gorber, S., Dillman, C., ... Spence, J. C. (2012). Canadian sedentary behaviour guidelines for the early years (aged 0–4 years). *Applied Physiology, Nutrition, and Metabolism, 37,* 370–391.

Tudor-Locke, C., Schuna, J. M., Frensham, L. J., & Proenca, M. (2013). Changing the way we work: Elevating energy expenditure with workstation alternatives. *International Journal of Obesity.* doi:10.1038/ijo.2013.223

U.S. Department of Labor, Bureau of Labor Statistics. American time use survey. Retrieved May 10, 2013, from http://www.bls.gov/tus/datafiles_2008.htm

Uijtdewilligen, L., Nauta, J., Singh, A. S., van Mechelen, W., Twisk, J. W., van der Horst, K., & Chinapaw, M. J. (2011). Determinants of physical activity and sedentary behaviour in young people: A review and quality synthesis of prospective studies. *British Journal of Sports Medicine, 45,* 896–905.

Wilmot, E. G., Edwardson, C. L., Achana, F. A., Davies, M. J., Gorely, T., Gray, L. J., ... Biddle, S. J. H. (2012). Sedentary time in adults and the association with diabetes, cardiovascular disease, and death: Systematic review and meta-analysis. *Diabetologia, 55,* 2895–2905.

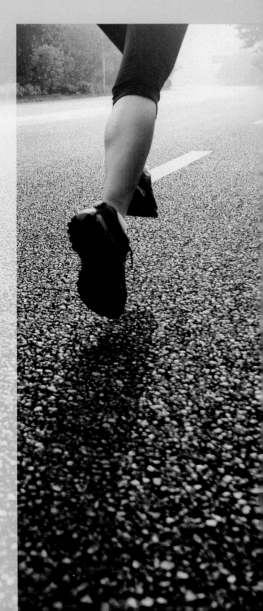

SECTION 2

Theoretical Models for Exercise and Sedentary Behavior

A story is told about a group of blind people who set out to describe an elephant. Each person is directed to a different area of the body, and after spending some time palpating the elephant each writes up a description. Each description is completely accurate in its own right, but none is entirely complete. This story serves as a metaphor for the various explanations that have been advanced to account for why people do or do not embrace a physically active lifestyle. Each of the theories is accurate in its own right, but none fully account for involvement in physical activity.

In Section 2 of this book, various theoretical models that have been advanced to explain and predict involvement in exercise and sedentary behavior are discussed. Chapter 3 deals with one of the most prominent theoretical models used to understand human behavior—social cognitive theory. In Chapter 4, motivational theories are examined, such as the health belief model, self-determination theory, and protection motivation theory. The theory of planned behavior is described in Chapter 5. A popular approach to the study of involvement in exercise, the transtheoretical model, is discussed in Chapter 6.

Social Cognitive Theory

Runner: © lzf/Shutterstock

Vignette: Jennifer

I was 42, going through an emotionally arduous divorce, and I hadn't been physically active in years. (After giving birth to my first baby at age 32, I cancelled my gym membership, tried to get back into fitness after my second child at 36, and then failed to maintain a regular exercise schedule under the pressures of motherhood and returning to full-time work.) Once my ex-husband moved out, I was determined to start afresh.

Workout DVDs in the basement of what used to be "our" house never did it for me—I'd commit to them for a few weeks only to find myself bored, if not more preoccupied with work obligations for the talent company at which I'm a senior project manager. (Let's not even mention childcare and housework.) So I committed to a morning boot camp program at a health club that was a short drive from my home and coordinated with a nanny to help take my 10- and 6-year-old kids to school on the mornings the boot camp met.

Throwing myself into a new physical activity routine was immensely taxing. The demands of the program were far beyond the limit of what my body could handle. But I wanted to be tough. I needed something to focus on that could distract me from the stressors at work, the toll (and

LEARNING OBJECTIVES

After completing this chapter, you will be able to

- Describe the main factors that have been proposed to influence self-efficacy.
- Explain how self-efficacy can be measured.
- Outline the relationship between social cognitive theory and physical activity behavior.
- Outline the relationship between social cognitive theory and sedentary behavior.
- Describe the current evidence for using social cognitive theory to change physical activity.

shame) of my recent divorce, and the satisfying, yet incessant, demands brought about by motherhood.

Two weeks into the boot camp I awoke in the middle of the night short of breath, bathed in sweat, and feeling as if a giant weight was pressing against my sternum. I didn't know it at the time—I chalked the sweats up to signs of impending menopause—but I was having a heart attack.

It didn't strike me as odd that I'd be experiencing physical manifestations of the stress I was under. Still, I placed a phone call to my primary care doctor the following morning. She demanded I come in immediately for a blood test and EKG—both of which confirmed a horrifying reality.

Needless to say, I immediately quit the boot camp program. This came as a blow to my self-esteem, in addition to my motivation to take care of my health. How could I get back into shape if the initial attempt to do so led me to a near-death situation?

Luckily, my doctor referred me to a cardiologist and a nutritionist. I also got the number of a psychologist with whom I could discuss my stress levels and strategize more effective coping skills. I took about 2 weeks off from all activity and, to the chagrin of my kids, threw out the junk food in my pantry for extra measure. (Though I never qualified as obese, I was disheartened to watch my dress size expand substantially over the years—especially after giving birth to my second child.)

Within a few weeks, after a stress test with the cardiologist during which I walked on a treadmill attached to a blood pressure cuff and several nodes stuck to my chest, I was cleared for regular, albeit "light," exercise.

It was at that point that I called the psychologist.

I needed to speak with someone about the dread I felt about approaching exercise, given the life-threatening outcome of my previous attempt to get fit. I didn't honestly believe I could do it without getting hurt. I assumed that, were I to attempt any type of exertion, I'd fail in the ultimate way—namely, by killing myself in the process.

It took me several months to even venture inside a gym again. And when I did, it was for a minimally exhausting yoga class. Gradually, I incorporated some weight training exercises I'd learned during and after college. A few months later, I bit the bullet and purchased an elliptical machine for my home.

I'm 44 now and I'm still terrified of doing anything that makes me too short of breath. It's unfortunate because many of my girlfriends have gotten into spin classes, and I just don't see myself as someone who is capable of joining them. But I have shed a few inches from my waistline, I've been incredibly fortunate to gain more flexible hours at the office, and I've stopped fearing the prospect of collaborating with my husband to help teach both of my kids to bike ride. (We've agreed, based on my heart attack episode and based on our own genetic histories—his father died of a heart attack and mine had a stent by age 60—that it's best they be as active as possible, so as to offset future health issues.)

I wish I could believe in myself enough to run. But I tend to be more cognizant of the risks associated with that level of exertion rather than its benefits. If it isn't my heart that could be a problem, it's the osteoporosis I'm at risk for. I've been told that doing some higher-impact exercises would strengthen my bones, but I just no longer see myself as someone who can do this without getting hurt.

I'm working on this with my psychologist, who I still see on a regular basis. Both she and my doctor keep affirming that I've done a wonderful turn around in terms of taking care of my health—from my diet to implementing a moderate and sustainable exercise regimen. I'm okay for now, but I still worry. I know I need to take care of my health in order to be a good mom and an efficient manager at work. I guess what keeps me going is resting assured that, at least when it comes to the latter two, I can definitely do a great job.

Introduction

A shift in thinking from a behaviorist (i.e., stimulus causes response) to a cognitive (i.e., stimulus causes thinking, which then causes a response) focus in the second half of the 20th century sparked the development of the social cognitive theory (SCT). Social cognitive theory, as currently conceptualized (Bandura, 2004), is a model that includes goals, sociostructural factors, and outcome expectations, but the central mediator of the model is the construct of self-efficacy. **Self-efficacy** "refers to beliefs in one's capabilities to organize and execute the courses of action required to produce given attainments" (Bandura, 1997, p. 2). It develops slowly, a fact reflected in the vignette used to introduce this chapter. However, in social cognitive theory, it is the foundation for human behavior. As Albert Bandura (1997) noted, "unless people believe they can produce desired effects by their actions, they have little incentive to act. Efficacy belief, therefore, is a major basis for action" (pp. 2–3).

Self-efficacy is thought to influence the course of action an individual chooses. Will you jog or cycle with friends or attend a box aerobics class? Or avoid all of these activities? A belief that you have the capability to successfully carry out any or all of these activities will influence your decision. Also, the amount of effort you expend in these activities will be influenced by your efficacy belief. With a weak belief in your personal capability

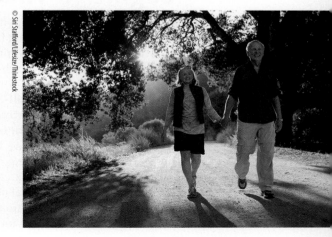

© Siri Stafford/Lifesize/Thinkstock

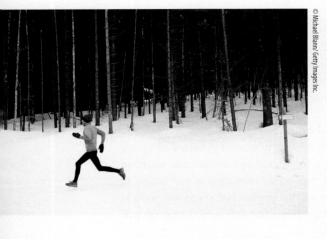

© Michael Blann/ Getty Images Inc.

to keep up or perform successfully, it is likely that you will be more tentative. Self-efficacy also will influence the degree of perseverance you demonstrate when obstacles and adversities arise. It will impact whether your thought patterns hinder or facilitate your performance. Expectations of failure generally serve as a self-fulfilling prophecy. Similarly, individuals with low self-efficacy are more likely to feel anxious, stressed, or depressed if environmental demands become high. Finally, as a result of all of the above, if your self-efficacy is low, social cognitive theory suggests your level of accomplishment will be detrimentally affected.

Given the important role that self-efficacy is thought to play in human behavior generally, it is hardly surprising that numerous researchers have studied its specific role in physical activity. Indeed, it is likely the most frequently applied construct in exercise psychology research (Rhodes & Nasuti, 2011). Issues that have been examined include whether self-efficacy is related to the intention to become active, the initiation of a more physically active lifestyle, the maintenance of a more physically active lifestyle, resisting a sedentary lifestyle, effort expended on physical activity, and thought patterns about physical activity. The results from that research are discussed in this chapter after the nature, structure, and sources of self-efficacy are introduced.

■ Self-Efficacy in Social Cognitive Theory

Self-efficacy is an integral component of social cognitive theory, a conceptual approach useful for understanding human behavior. Social cognitive theory combines aspects of operant conditioning, social learning theory, and cognitive psychology. **FIGURE 3-1** provides a schematic illustration of the main tenets of the theory, as proposed by Bandura (1998).

In social cognitive theory, self-efficacy affects behavior directly and through its impact on **outcome expectations**, the expectations an individual has about the outcomes of a behavior. These can be physical (e.g., performing exercise would be painful), social (e.g., my friends will be pleased if I go to aerobics class with them), or self-evaluative (e.g., I will feel proud of myself for sticking to my running schedule). The outcome expectation construct, in itself, has had mixed evidence as a correlate of physical activity (Williams, Anderson, & Winett, 2005). Self-efficacy is also thought to impact sociostructural factors (i.e., facilitators and barriers) that play a role in behavior change. A person must hold a strong enough

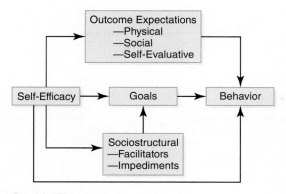

FIGURE 3-1   Social Cognitive Theory

Data from Bandura, A. (1998). Health promotion from the perspective of social cognitive theory. *Psychology and Health, 13,* 623–649.

level of self-efficacy to overcome these barriers. Finally, personal goals related to behavior can be formed through the combination of self-efficacy, outcome expectations, and sociostructural factors. Bandura (2004) suggests that short-term goals are the most manageable and are more linked to success.

CRITICAL THINKING ACTIVITY 3-1

Social cognitive theory is most famous for the self-efficacy construct, but outcome expectations also are considered to influence behavior. Consider the physical, social, and self-evaluative outcome expectations outlined in the theory. What outcomes make you physically active or inactive?

The basis of the social cognitive theory is the concept of triadic **reciprocal determinism** (Bandura, 1977). Specifically, three classes of determinants—behavior, internal personal factors, and external environment—are assumed to coexist. Behavior (i.e., its type, frequency, duration, and context) is influenced by and influences internal personal factors (i.e., individual cognitions such as self-efficacy, outcome expectations, and goals). An individual's outcome expectation and self-efficacy beliefs, for example, would influence dieting behavior. In turn, the effectiveness (or ineffectiveness) of dieting behavior would serve to shape the person's outcome expectations. As another example, an athlete's teammates (i.e., environment) might influence his or her self-efficacy about dieting behavior. Again, in turn, the athlete's own outcome expectations would have a reciprocal influence on his or her teammates (**FIGURE 3-2**).

What are some of the implications of accepting a triadic reciprocal causation perspective? One implication is relatively straightforward: cognitions such as self-efficacy are assumed to play a role in behavior. A cardiac rehabilitation patient may be physically capable of moderate physical activity. However, if he

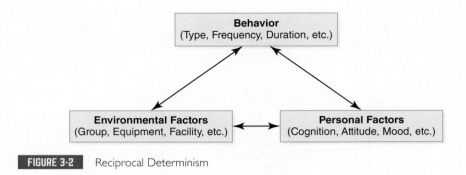

FIGURE 3-2 Reciprocal Determinism

or she does not possess the belief that this is the case, physical activity behavior is unlikely.

A patient also could learn through the consequences of his or her own actions. A cardiac rehabilitation patient who engages safely in physical activity would gain self-efficacy from the experience.

A third implication is that an individual's beliefs can be influenced by external environmental factors. A person does not have to engage directly in a behavior to develop the belief about personal capabilities. In short, self-efficacy can be influenced through social persuasion as well as the success of (similar) others. That same cardiac rehabilitation patient may gain efficacy by coming to a class and observing other patients with similar health problems engaging in physical activities.

CRITICAL THINKING ACTIVITY 3-2

© ecco/Shutterstock, Inc.

Triadic reciprocal determinism makes sense, but it definitely makes it difficult to understand what comes first in a "chicken-or-egg" type scenario because the environment, the individual, and behavior are all thought to cause each other. What do you think comes first in terms of physical activity? If you were asked to develop a physical activity intervention, what factor would you start with in your program?

◼ Sources of Self-Efficacy Beliefs

As **FIGURE 3-3** shows, self-efficacy can arise from a number of sources (Bandura, 1997). According to social cognitive theory, the most important, potent source of self-efficacy is personal **mastery experiences**. Carrying out a task successfully helps to cement the belief in the person that he or she has the capabilities necessary. In this regard, success is obviously important for self-efficacy to develop. However, Bandura has pointed out that an efficacy belief is more resilient if the individual has also had to overcome obstacles and adversity—and has done so

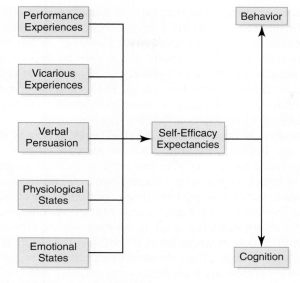

FIGURE 3-3   Proposed Sources of Self-Efficacy

Adapted from Bandura, A. (1997). *Self-efficacy, the exercise of control.* New York, NY: Freeman.

successfully. Similarly, of course, self-efficacy can be fragile; initial failure experiences can serve to undermine efficacy beliefs. The power of personal experiences can, therefore, shape self-efficacy for better or for worse.

Another source of efficacy is **vicarious experiences**, or observational learning. The behavior (and successes or failures) of others can be used as a comparative standard for the individual. Observing others who are similar achieve success increases self-efficacy, while observing them fail is thought to diminish it. Essentially, the individual is thought to be persuaded if a similar other has the capability and does as well.

Bandura also has pointed out that while vicarious experiences are generally a less powerful source of self-efficacy beliefs than mastery experiences, there are conditions under which this is not the case. For example, a woman may experience failure in her initial attempts to use a stair-climber and, as a result, lose self-efficacy. However, observing a friend who is perceived to be similar (or less fit) exercise successfully could serve as a catalyst to enhance self-efficacy.

A specialized form of vicarious experiences is cognitive self-modeling; that is, *imagery experiences*. Here, the individual uses visualization to repeatedly and successfully confront and master challenging situations.

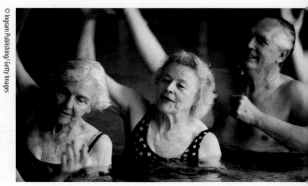

A third source of information that has an impact on self-efficacy is **verbal persuasion**. Its influence is generally thought to be weaker than observational vicarious experiences or personal experiences. However, as Bandura (1997) has pointed out, although "verbal persuasion alone may be limited in its power to create enduring increases in perceived efficacy … it can bolster self-change if the positive appraisal is within realistic bounds (p. 101). Generally, verbal persuasion has its greatest impact on self-efficacy on those individuals who have some reason to believe that they could be successful if they persist.

The fourth source of information for self-efficacy beliefs is the individual's **physiological state**. Bodily sensations such as increased heart rate, increased sweating, and increased respiratory rate can serve to provide a signal to the individual about his or her current level of efficacy. Bandura emphasized that the individual's physiological state—like performance experiences, vicarious experiences, and verbal persuasion—is not, by itself, an indicator of self-efficacy. The individual's appraisal of the information is crucial. If, for example, an elevated heart rate is interpreted as confirmation of suspected poor physical condition, it could serve to reduce self-efficacy. In contrast, if an elevated heart rate is interpreted as evidence of being adequately warmed-up, it could serve to enhance self-efficacy.

The final factor, **mood states**, can influence self-efficacy through either affective priming or cognitive priming. Affective priming occurs because previous successes and failures are stored in memory (and recalled) with associated mood states. Thus, when we are successful, we store that experience in memory along with the feelings of joy, elation, vigor, and so on that initially accompanied it. Similarly, when we fail, we store that experience in memory with the feelings of frustration, sorrow, depression, and so on that initially accompanied it. Therefore, the presence of a negative mood state prior to an effect serves to prime memories of failures, thereby serving to reduce self-efficacy.

The cognitive priming perspective is similar but with a subtle distinction. Memory of a failure might be stored with the negative mood state, but it is also stored with an accompanying cognition—an attribution for example. Consider the athlete who has just had a poor performance in a 10K race. The memory of that performance, the emotion associated with it (e.g., feeling depressed), and any accompanying attribution (e.g., "my failure to arrive 1 hour prior to the start was one reason for my poor performance") would be stored in memory together. Given similar or related experiences in a subsequent race, the cognition of the earlier causal event (arriving too close to the start time) would prime both the emotion (feeling depressed) and memory of the failure. The result would be diminished self-efficacy.

■ Nature and Measurement of Self-Efficacy

Theoreticians have stated that self-efficacy is a complex construct that can vary along three dimensions. One dimension, the *level* of self-efficacy, reflects a belief in personal ability to accomplish a particular task or component of a task. Generally, when people consider self-efficacy, this is the dimension that comes to mind. However, an individual's self-efficacy can also vary in *strength*; that is, the degree of conviction that a particular task or component of a task can be carried out successfully. Thus, for example, an individual might hold the belief that he or she can complete a 30-minute aerobics class (i.e., the level of self-efficacy). However, he or she also might only be 75% (not 100%) confident about this belief (i.e., the strength of self-efficacy). The third dimension, *generality*, reflects the degree to which efficacy beliefs transfer to related tasks. An individual who has high self-efficacy for an aerobics class may also have similarly high efficacy in all activities requiring aerobic fitness.

One of the measurement challenges in self-efficacy research is separating one's capability from one's motivation. Self-efficacy is an assessment of capability, but confidence can easily be misinterpreted or misconstrued from motivation independent of ability (Cahill, Gallo, Lisman, & Weinstein, 2006; Kirsch, 1982; Rhodes & Blanchard, 2007). For example, people could report that they are not confident that they can exercise regularly because they do not like to exercise, even if they feel they actually would have the ability to do so. This appraisal assesses an outcome expectation (I would enjoy/not enjoy exercise), rather than a judgment of efficacy (Bandura, 1977; Cahill et al., 2006). Williams and Rhodes (2014) suggest this often happens due to how people colloquialize the wording of "I can" in popular speech. For example, if someone asks you whether you can go to the movies tonight, you may answer that you can't. This likely has to do with other priorities or commitments and not a literal interpretation that you are physically or mentally unable to go to the movies! Indeed, when Rhodes and Blanchard (2007) asked college students why they were confident they could or could not exercise, almost half of the reasons were motivational in nature (enjoyment, health, motivation), while the other half were about capability (time, skill). To help reduce the chances of this mistaken meaning, Rhodes and colleagues have argued and demonstrated that "confidence" items with a motivational qualifier (e.g., "if I wanted to") help measure ability instead of outcome expectations (Rhodes & Blanchard, 2007; Rhodes & Courneya, 2003, 2004). Still, the challenge for physical activity scientists remains an attempt to separate motivation and outcome expectancies from self-efficacy expectations (Williams & Rhodes, 2014).

CRITICAL THINKING ACTIVITY 3-3

© ecco/Shutterstock, Inc.

Self-efficacy is one of the strongest correlates of physical activity in past research, but is that largely because of our colloquial use of "can" in speech, as Williams and Rhodes (2014) suggest? Think of the most common barriers to your physical activity. Do these barriers include factors such as time, fatigue, bad weather, or low social support? If so, do they really affect whether you can perform physical activity, or do they just affect your motivation and willingness to be active?

Self–Efficacy in Physical Activity Contexts

Because self-efficacy is a situation-specific construct, different manifestations (operational definitions of self-efficacy) have been assessed depending upon the

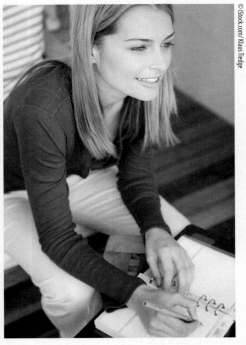

context and interest of the researcher. The best way to operationalize self-efficacy for physical activity has received research attention because it helps us understand where our promotion efforts should be focused. Several researchers have contributed to this area, and the three forms of efficacy highlighted in the following discussion do not represent a comprehensive list, but rather are among the most common in physical activity research.

One of the most common forms of self-efficacy is sometimes referred to as **barrier efficacy** (McAuley & Mihalko, 1998). It represents an individual's beliefs about possessing the capability to overcome obstacles to physical activity. These obstacles/barriers could be social, such as spousal lack of encouragement, or personal, such as limited time, or environmental, such as bad weather that might interfere with physical activity. Respondents indicate, for example, their confidence that they can attend exercise classes three times a week in spite of inclement weather. A special form of barrier efficacy is **scheduling efficacy**. It reflects the individual's confidence that physical activity can be scheduled into a daily or weekly routine.

McAuley and Mihalko (1998) also noted that many studies assess what they referred to as *disease-specific* or *health behavior efficacy*. Disease-specific efficacy is similar to barrier efficacy. However, it is directly aimed at assessing efficacy beliefs in specific populations engaged in the secondary prevention of disease through exercise rehabilitation (e.g., arthritis programs). Similarly, health behavior efficacy pertains to individuals' beliefs about their capability to engage in health-promoting behaviors.

Another form of self-efficacy used commonly in the literature is **task efficacy**. An early debate among self-efficacy theorists centered around self-efficacy and its role in repeated/complex behaviors such as regular exercise (Bandura, 1995; Kirsch, 1995; Maddux, 1995). The main debate focused on whether self-efficacy is about confidence to perform the act itself (walking involves putting one foot in front of the other) or the confidence to regulate the action. In physical activity, this has given rise to specific measurements of task efficacy (Blanchard et al., 2007). Task efficacy is the confidence to perform the specific physical activity act itself. As you could imagine, many people may feel that they have high task efficacy with simple activities (e.g., walking), but this would change as the difficulty of the activity increases (e.g., mountain climbing). In addition, task efficacy may be very important for clinical or physically compromised populations (Blanchard et al., 2007; Blanchard, Rodgers, Courneya, Daub, & Knapik, 2002). Finally, task self-efficacy may be more important for the initial adoption of physical activity, but barrier efficacy may become more important as one attempts to maintain a physically active lifestyle (Higgins, Middleton, Winner, & Janelle, 2014).

A student examining research on self-efficacy and physical activity behavior for the first time might wonder if all the ways of measuring efficacy are necessary; why can't one reliable and valid measure of self-efficacy be adopted and used? McAuley and Mihalko (1998) noted that the specificity of self-efficacy makes it unwise to adopt one general omnibus measure of self-efficacy. An individual might have extremely high self-efficacy for overcoming the barriers to distance running, but minimal or low efficacy for completing a 20K run. By assessing both task efficacy and barrier efficacy (or, if the research question dictates it, assessing one or the other), a better understanding of physical activity behavior is obtained. Continued research to decipher the most important efficacies associated with physical activity should improve our promotion success in interventions.

Self-Efficacy and Physical Activity Behavior

As Figure 3-3 shows, various factors contribute to self-efficacy. In turn, when self-efficacy is present, it is positively associated with behavior. Indeed, a meta-analysis by Spence and colleagues (2006) showed the effect size as $r = .35$, which makes it one of the largest and most reliable correlates of physical activity. In the physical activity domain, efficacy beliefs have been found to be associated with a wide cross section of behaviors.

Initiation and Maintenance of Physical Activity

Changes in behavior often unfold slowly. One reason is that people perceive the presence of a number of (real or perceived) barriers, and they are not confident about their ability to overcome those barriers. Not surprisingly, barrier efficacy plays a role insofar as initiating a lifestyle that involves being physically active. Early research showed that people who intend to become more active in the immediate future (but have not actually done so) have greater barrier efficacy than people who have no intention of adopting a physically active lifestyle (Armstrong, Sallis, Hovell, & Hofstetter, 1993). Oman and King (1998) conducted a 2-year randomized trial where 63 participants were randomly assigned to a condition for participation in an aerobic exercise program (higher-intensity home-based exercise, higher-intensity class-based exercise, or lower-intensity home-based exercise). Results from the study indicated that independent of treatment group, baseline self-efficacy was a significant predictor of exercise behavior during the adoption stage but not during the maintenance phase.

Still, exercise efficacy also plays a role insofar as maintaining a physically active lifestyle is concerned. In a review paper on self-efficacy and exercise, this positive, significant relationship has been illustrated among a variety of populations (clinical and nonclinical) and ages (ranging between adolescents and older adults) (McAuley & Blissmer, 2000). For example, a study of 174 older adults participating in an exercise program (randomized to an aerobic group or stretching and toning group) measured both exercise self-efficacy and physical efficacy levels across a 12-month trial (McAuley et al., 1999). Results showed that a curvilinear growth of self-efficacy occurred across the trial, with declines at the follow-up stage (postexercise program). Participants therefore had increases in self-efficacy throughout the program, but then declines occurred following. As a result of the interplay between physical activity participation and self-efficacy, it becomes essential for practitioners to develop physical activity opportunities that help to build personal self-efficacy levels.

Effort Expended in Physical Activity

It was pointed out earlier in the chapter that one expected consequence of self-efficacy pertains to the amount of effort expended; that is, efficacious individuals could be expected to try harder. Research has supported this expected relationship in regard to physical activity. A variety of indices of physical effort or exertion, such as perceived exertion, self-reports of activity intensity, peak heart rate, vital capacity, expiratory volume, and time to reach 70% of maximal heart rate, have been found to be related to exercise efficacy, as well as disease- and health-related efficacy (see McAuley and Mihalko, 1998, for an overview of this research).

It was pointed out earlier (see also Figure 3-2) that the strongest, most viable source of efficacy beliefs are expected to be mastery experiences. Thus, not surprisingly, the relationship between self-efficacy and involvement in physical activity is reciprocal. Efficacy beliefs are associated with the initiation and maintenance of physical activity. In turn, both acute and long-term involvement in a program of physical activity lead to significant gains in self-efficacy (McAuley & Blissmer, 2000).

The positive effects of physical activity on self-efficacy are not restricted to general populations only. Individuals involved in cardiac rehabilitation programs (Blanchard, Rodgers, Courneya, Daub, & Knapik, 2002) and other clinical populations have reported increased efficacy beliefs following a program of physical activity (McAuley & Blissmer, 2000).

■ Self-Efficacy and Mental States

Figure 3-3 is intended to illustrate schematically that when self-efficacy beliefs are stronger, cognitions about physical activity are greater, stronger, and more positive. Research on the role that efficacy beliefs play in physical activity has demonstrated this relationship.

It has been shown by Albert Bandura (1986) that individuals who possess greater self-efficacy also have lower depression and anxiety than those reporting lower self-efficacy. Similarly, efficacy beliefs are interrelated with *emotional responses* following acute sessions of physical activity. For example, individuals possessing greater exercise efficacy report more positive and less negative affect (McAuley, Shaffer, & Rudolph, 1995) following an acute bout of activity. Similarly, they also report enjoying the experience more (McAuley, Wraith, & Duncan, 1991).

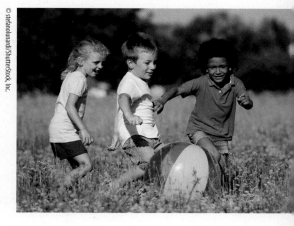

Efficacy beliefs also are associated with a number of positive intrapersonal characteristics. For example, Kavussanu and McAuley (1995) noted that individuals with greater self-efficacy tend to be more optimistic. As another example, exercise efficacy has been positively associated with self-esteem (Sonstroem, Harlow, & Josephs, 1994).

Enhancing Self-Efficacy: Experimental Evidence

The previous sections served to highlight the important role that efficacy beliefs play in involvement in physical activity—from initiation to maintenance, from effort to frequency and duration, and from attitudes to cognitions. Thus, an important question is, how can efficacy be enhanced in individuals uncertain about their capability to organize and execute the actions associated with a physically active lifestyle? Edward McAuley, an authority on the correlates of self-efficacy in physical activity, addressed this question in 1994. As he noted:

> It is vitally important for practitioners and programs to provide experiences that maximize individuals' beliefs in their sense of personal capabilities with respect to exercise and physical activity. If practitioners fail to organize, present, and develop their programs in such a way as to cultivate efficacy beliefs, participants are likely to perceive the activity negatively, become disenchanted and discouraged, and discontinue. On the other hand, adequately organizing exercise and physical activity sessions in a manner such that a strong sense of personal efficacy is promoted will result in individuals displaying more positive affect, evaluating their physical self-worth more positively, embracing more challenging activities, putting forth more effort, and persisting longer (p. 87).

McAuley then went on to propose a series of strategies within each of the main categories of antecedents for self-efficacy identified Figure 3-2: mastery

TABLE 3-1 Strategies for Strengthening Self-Efficacy Expectations	
Source	**Potential Strategy for Enhancing Self-Efficacy**
Mastery experiences	Exercises: Gradually increasing the (1) speed, grade, or duration of treadmills; (2) resistance or duration of stationary bicycles; and (3) load, repetitions, or sets in weightlifting Daily activities: Walking to work, school, or errands instead of using motor transportation; using stairs instead of elevators or escalators; walking around golf courses instead of riding
Vicarious learning	Showing videotapes of successful models similar in age, physical characteristics, and capabilities Providing frequent leader or expert demonstrations Encouraging attendance at orientation sessions at health and exercise facilities to observe others Employing participant modeling in which gradually diminished aid is provided to participants for more difficult activities Using cooperative activities in groups or with partners
Verbal persuasion	Providing information and orientation seminars for participants Providing videotape and multimedia health promotion information Providing articles, magazines, or information pamphlets and booklets Developing social support networks through the implementation of "buddy systems" and group social activities Providing a telephone hotline or telephone reminders for frequent absentees Providing a physical activity and health bulletin board and newsletter
Physiological states	Instructing participants how to accurately and positively interpret heart rate, perspiration, muscle soreness, weight changes, and general fatigue

McAuley, E. (1994). Enhancing psychological health through physical activity. In H. A. Quinney, L. Gauvin, & A. E. T. Wall (Eds.), *Toward active living: Proceedings of the International Conference on Physical Activity, Fitness, and Health* (pp. 83–90). Champaign, IL: Human Kinetics.

experiences, vicarious learning, verbal persuasion, and physiological states. A summary of that list of strategies is provided in **TABLE 3-1**.

Insofar as mastery experiences are concerned, the principle underlying strategy emphasized is gradual progression. Opportunities for initial success should be maximized. A way to ensure this is to gradually increase the physical challenge on equipment such as treadmills, Stairmasters, bicycles, and weights. Also, as Table 3-1 shows, gradual increases in activity should be promoted in daily endeavors (e.g., walking instead of riding). Finally, participants should be encouraged to chart their progress both in terms of physical accomplishments and physiological parameters such as heart rate.

The principle underlying approach emphasized to gain self-efficacy via *vicarious learning* is to ensure that participants see others successfully engaged in the target activity. This might be achieved through videotapes, demonstrations, or by having the participants themselves model the activity. Participant modeling, for example, could involve helping a prospective exerciser mount and stand without moving on a Stairmaster; begin stepping, but against large resistance; and, finally, begin stepping against appropriate resistance but for a limited duration.

The principle strategy that underlies the enhancement of self-efficacy through verbal persuasion is that participants are provided with considerable information about the "why," "what," and "where" of physical activity. This might be achieved through orientation sessions, pamphlets, articles, newsletters, and so on, or through media presentations (e.g., videotapes, television, newspapers).

Finally, the principle strategy underlying the enhancement of self-efficacy through physiological states is ensuring that participants understand the body's response to activity. Physical activity produces increases in heart rate and sweating, for example. The meaning the individual attaches to those physiological changes is important. Individuals who are frequently active expect and understand the body's response to a physical load. Participants new to physical activity may not. Therefore, they must be helped to interpret what the physiological changes mean and how those physiological responses to activity change with training.

Despite the clear, logical, and prescriptive grounds for how to change self-efficacy, the literature surrounding physical activity interventions is limited and also has mixed support (Baranowski, Anderson, & Carmack, 1998; Lubans, Foster, & Biddle, 2008; Rhodes & Pfaeffli, 2010). For example, in Rhodes and Pfaeffli's (2010) examination of whether self-efficacy interventions could account for changes in physical activity, only 1 of 19 studies supported a complete link between changes in self-efficacy and changes in physical activity. Thus, self-efficacy has considerably limited support for its role as a mediator of physical activity changes due to interventions at present.

The experimental evidence for the importance of various sources of self-efficacy to impart change also has relatively mixed evidence (Conn, Hafdahl, & Mehr, 2011; Prestwich et al., 2014). Ashford, Edmunds, and French (2010) reviewed 27 physical activity interventions that used sources of self-efficacy in order to change exercise self-efficacy. Overall, and similar to the findings of Rhodes and Pfaeffli (2010), the effectiveness to change self-efficacy was poor in a meta-analysis ($d = .16$). This was recently replicated in a meta-analysis separating barrier ($d = .13$) and task ($d = .21$) efficacy interventions (Higgins et al., 2014). Interestingly, mastery experiences were also not found to be the most effective way to change self-efficacy; positive feedback and vicarious experience were shown as more effective. The results of this review had relatively low numbers of studies with specific techniques (i.e., most studies employed a variety of sources, which could confound these results), yet it demonstrates the importance of testing theory. Recently, the same analysis was also performed in samples of older adults (French, Olander, Chisholm, & Mc Sharry, 2014). Overall, interventions were able to change self-efficacy ($d = .37$), but similar to past results, these changes did not link well to changes in behavior ($d = .16$). The results also showed no clear mechanism that was effective in changing self-efficacy, and positive feedback and vicarious experience were associated with less change! Again, these results were from a relatively small number of studies ($N = 24$), but the findings suggest that changing self-efficacy may represent only a small component of what is needed to promote and sustain changes in physical activity.

Social Cognitive Theory Applied to Sedentary Behavior

Unlike physical activity, the study of sedentary behavior is in its relatively early stages. Still, one cannot assume that the same principles and findings for social cognitive theory and physical activity can be used to understand sedentary behavior. The most obvious difference would be self-efficacy and its relationship with sedentary behavior. While physical activity is a complex behavior that often requires skill and control over various other temptations (i.e., high self-efficacy), sedentary behaviors are often known for their ease and tempting outcomes. Thus, low confidence to sit in a comfy chair and watch a screen hardly seems like a driving factor that would explain the variations in sedentary behavior! Indeed, research has generally demonstrated no relationship between control factors like self-efficacy and sedentary behavior (Rhodes, Temmel, & Mark, 2012), with the one caveat being video games, where skill is associated with play hours (Terlecki et al., 2011). Instead, social cognitive theory, when applied to sedentary behaviors, is often phrased in terms of limiting the behavior. For example, self-efficacy might be phrased as confidence to limit TV time or time spent online (Van Dyck et al., 2011).

Applications of social cognitive theory to sedentary behavior are too few at present to render any definitive judgment on how it applies to sedentary behavior, but early work does demonstrate that it may have utility. For example, Van Dyck and colleagues (2011) showed that outcome expectations about both the benefits of TV and Internet use and the cons of not limiting TV and Internet use correlate with self-reported TV and Internet use in a sample of adults from Belgium. They also showed that self-efficacy to limit these sedentary behaviors was a large correlate (negative relationship) with behavior. This finding has also been shown with adolescents in the United States (Zabinski, Norman, Sallis, Calfas, & Patrick, 2007). Perhaps most interesting is the potential link between screen viewing and families. A recent study by Jago, Sebire, Edwards, and Thompson (2013) showed that children were five times more likely to engage in excessive screen time behavior if their parents also reported high screen time themselves. Furthermore, the researchers found that parental self-efficacy to limit screen time had a large link to child-reported screen time. The findings illustrate how social cognitive theory may interact with reciprocal determination (parental behavior to child behavior) in a family setting.

There have also been promising results in intervention trials to reduce sedentary behavior using approaches that target outcome expectations and self-efficacy. Studies from older adults (Gardiner, Eakin, Healy, & Owen, 2011) to adolescents (Bergh et al., 2012; Dewar et al., 2014) to preschool children (Zimmerman, Ortiz, Christakis, & Elkun, 2012) have all shown that social cognitive theory–based interventions can reduce sedentary behavior. The exact mechanism, however, for the behavior change is less understood. For example, while Zimmerman and colleagues work with preschool children and their parents showed that screen time was limited via a change in the negative outcome expectation from letting children watch TV, the studies with adolescents were unable to show why sedentary behavior decreased. None of these studies have yet linked these changes to self-efficacy, which is considered the most important variable in social cognitive theory.

CRITICAL THINKING ACTIVITY 3-4

© ecco/Shutterstock, Inc.

The strength and level aspects of self-efficacy suggest that it is relevant to skilled behaviors such as physical activities, but does it correspond within the context of sedentary behavior? For example, does it make sense that TV viewing behavior is dictated by the confidence to carry out pressing the power button on the remote, or does it seem more likely that sedentary behavior is influenced by outcome expectations, such as the expected pleasure versus guilt from sitting and watching TV for long periods of time? What sedentary behaviors might contain enough skill to involve self-efficacy, and what sedentary behaviors seem less efficacy-driven?

■ Summary

Bandura (1997) has defined self-efficacy as the belief that one is capable of organizing and executing the courses of action required to produce an outcome. It is thought to be influenced by a variety of factors, including mastery experiences, vicarious experiences (i.e., observational learning), imagery experiences, verbal persuasion, physiological states, and mood. In the context of exercise and physical activity, self-efficacy has been assessed with a variety of operational definitions, including barrier efficacy (capability of overcoming obstacles to physical activity), scheduling efficacy (capability of scheduling physical activity into routine), disease-specific/health behavior efficacy (capability of successfully engaging in incremental bouts of physical activity for a specific disease), and task efficacy (degree of personal control over completing the physical task).

Efficacy plays an important role in exercise and physical activity and may play a role in limiting sedentary behavior. For example, it has been shown to be positively associated with physical activity generally, as well as with the initiation of a program of physical activity, maintenance of involvement, and expenditure of effort during participation. Also, more efficacious individuals also are likely to report more positive and less negative affect following acute bouts of activity and more enjoyment. Finally, efficacy is positively related to the personal qualities of optimism and self-esteem. Despite these findings, there are still some areas of self-efficacy research with mixed findings. Some researchers have demonstrated that self-efficacy may measure motivation and willingness more than capability. The experimental evidence on self-efficacy and physical activity is also mixed, showing that correlations are not necessarily causation. Changing self-efficacy has proven difficult in our current interventions, and changes in self-efficacy do not always link to subsequent changes in behavior. Furthermore, contemporary evidence suggests that vicarious experience and positive feedback may be even stronger sources of self-efficacy than graded mastery experiences.

KEY TERMS

barrier efficacy
mastery experiences
mood states
outcome expectations
physiological state
reciprocal determinism

scheduling efficacy
self-efficacy
task efficacy
verbal persuasion
vicarious experiences

REVIEW QUESTIONS

1. According to Bandura's social cognitive theory, what are the most important reasons for performing or not performing physical activity?

2. What are the main causes of self-efficacy beliefs? Which causes are most important?

3. Explain the three dimensions of self-efficacy measurement.

4. What types of self-efficacy are important to physical activity?

APPLYING THE CONCEPTS

1. How did Jennifer's heart attack change her efficacy and outcome expectations toward exercise?

2. What types of experiences might Jennifer need to have in order to join her friends in spin class and make exercise a more regular part of her life?

REFERENCES

Armstrong, C. A., Sallis, J. F., Hovell, M. F., & Hofstetter, C. R. (1993). Stages of change, self-efficacy, and the adoption of vigorous exercise: A prospective analysis. *Journal of Sport and Exercise Psychology, 15*, 390–402.

Ashford, S., Edmunds, J., & French, D. P. (2010). What is the best way to change self-efficacy to promote lifestyle and recreational physical activity? A systematic review with meta-analysis. *British Journal of Health Psychology, 15*, 265–288.

Bandura, A. (1977). Self-efficacy: Toward a unifying theory of behavioral change. *Psychological Review, 84*, 191–215.

Bandura, A. (1986). *Social foundations of thought and action: A social-cognitive theory.* Englewood Cliffs, NJ: Prentice-Hall.

Bandura, A. (1995). On rectifying conceptual ecumenism. In J. E. Maddux (Ed.), *Self-efficacy, adaptation, and adjustment: Theory, research, and application.* New York, NY: Plenum.

Bandura, A. (1997). *Self-efficacy, the exercise of control.* New York, NY: Freeman.

Bandura, A. (1998). Health promotion from the perspective of social cognitive theory. *Psychology and Health, 13*, 623–649.

Bandura, A. (2004). Health promotion by social cognitive means. *Health Education and Behavior, 31*, 143–164.

Baranowski, T., Anderson, C., & Carmack, C. (1998). Mediating variable framework in physical activity interventions: How are we doing? How might we do better? *American Journal of Preventive Medicine, 15*, 266–297.

Bergh, I. H., Bjelland, M., Grydeland, M., Lien, N., Andersen, L. F., Klepp, K. I., … Ommundsen, Y. (2012). Mid-way and post-intervention effects on potential determinants of physical activity and sedentary behavior, results of the HEIA study—a multi-component school-based randomized trial. *International Journal of Behavioral Nutrition and Physical Activity, 9*, 63.

Blanchard, C. M., Fortier, M. S., Sweet, S. N., O'Sullivan, T. L., Hogg, W., Reid, R. D., & Sigal, R. J. (2007). Explaining physical activity levels from a self-efficacy perspective: The physical activity counseling trial. *Annals of Behavioral Medicine, 34*, 323–328.

Blanchard, C. M., Rodgers, W., Courneya, K. S., Daub, B., & Knapik, G. (2002). Does barrier efficacy mediate the gender/exercise adherence relationship during phase II cardiac rehabilitation? *Rehabilitation Psychology, 47*, 106–120.

Cahill, S. P., Gallo, L. A., Lisman, S. A., & Weinstein, A. (2006). Willing or able? The meanings of self-efficacy. *Journal of Social and Clinical Psychology, 25*, 196–209.

Conn, V. S., Hafdahl, A. R., & Mehr, D. R. (2011). Interventions to increase physical activity among healthy adults: Meta-analysis of outcomes. *American Journal of Public Health, 101,* 751–758.

Dewar, D. L., Morgan, P. J., Plotnikoff, R. C., Okely, A. D., Batterhamd, M., & Lubans, D. R. (2014). Exploring changes in physical activity, sedentary behaviors and hypothesized mediators in the NEAT girls group randomized controlled trial. *Journal of Science and Medicine in Sport, 17,* 39–46.

French, D. P., Olander, E. K., Chisholm, A., & Mc Sharry, J. (2014). Which behaviour change techniques are most effective at increasing older adults' self-efficacy and physical activity behaviour? A systematic review. *Annals of Behavioral Medicine, 48*(2), 225–234.

Gardiner, P. A., Eakin, E. G., Healy, G. N., & Owen, N. (2011). Feasibility of reducing older adult's sedentary time. *American Journal of Preventive Medicine, 41,* 174–177.

Higgins, T. J., Middleton, K. R., Winner, L., & Janelle, C. M. (2014). Physical activity interventions differentially affect exercise task and barrier self-efficacy: A meta-analysis. *Health Psychology, 33,* 891–903.

Jago, R., Sebire, S. J., Edwards, M. J., & Thompson, J. L. (2013). Parental TV viewing, parental self-efficacy, media equipment, and TV viewing among preschool children. *European Journal of Pediatrics, 172,* 1543–1545.

Kavussanu, M., & McAuley, E. (1995). Exercise and optimism: Are highly active individuals more optimistic? *Journal of Sport and Exercise Psychology, 17,* 246–258.

Kirsch, I. (1982). Efficacy expectations or response predictions: The meaning of efficacy ratings as a function of task characteristics. *Journal of Personality and Social Psychology, 42,* 132–136.

Kirsch, I. (1995). Self-efficacy and outcome expectancy: A concluding commentary. In J. E. Maddux (Ed.), *Self-efficacy, adaptation, and adjustment: Theory, research, and application* (pp. 341–345). New York, NY: Plenum.

Lubans, D. R., Foster, C., & Biddle, S. J. H. (2008). A review of mediators of behavior in interventions to promote physical activity among children and adolescents. *Preventive Medicine, 47,* 463–470.

Maddux, J. E. (1995). Looking for common ground: A comment on Kirsch and Bandura. In J. E. Maddux (Ed.), *Self-efficacy, adaptation, and adjustment: Theory, research, and application* (pp. 377–386). New York, NY: Plenum.

McAuley, E. (1994). Enhancing psychological health through physical activity. In H. A. Quinney, L. Gauvin, & A. E. T. Wall (Eds.), *Toward active living: Proceedings of the International Conference on Physical Activity, Fitness, and Health* (pp. 83–90). Champaign, IL: Human Kinetics.

McAuley, E., & Blissmer, B. (2000). Self-efficacy determinants and consequences of physical activity. *Exercise and Sport Sciences Reviews, 28,* 85–88.

McAuley, E., Katula, J. A., Mihalko, S. L., Blissmer, B., Duncan, T. E., Pena, M., & Dunn, E. (1999). Mode of physical activity and self-efficacy in older adults: A latent growth curve analysis. *Journal of Gerontology: Psychological Sciences, 54B,* 283–292.

McAuley, E., & Mihalko, S. (1998). Measuring exercise-related self-efficacy. In J. Duda (Ed.), *Advances in sport and exercise psychology* (pp. 371–390). Morgantown, WV: Fitness Information Technology.

McAuley, E., Shaffer, S. M., & Rudolph, D. (1995). Affective responses to acute exercise in elderly impaired males: The moderating effects of self-efficacy and age. *International Journal of Aging and Human Development, 41,* 13–27.

McAuley, E., Wraith, S., & Duncan, T. E. (1991). Self-efficacy, perceptions of success, and intrinsic motivation for exercise. *Journal of Applied Social Psychology, 21,* 139–155.

Oman, R. F., & King, A. C. (1998). Predicting the adoption and maintenance of exercise participation using self-efficacy and previous exercise participation rates. *American Journal of Health Promotion, 12,* 154–161.

Prestwich, A., Sniehotta, F. F., Whittington, C., Dombrowski, S. U., Rogers, L., & Michie, S. (2014). Does theory influence the effectiveness of health behavior interventions? Meta-analysis. *Health Psychology, 33*(5), 465–474.

Rhodes, R. E., & Blanchard, C. M. (2007). What do confidence items measure in the physical activity domain? *Journal of Applied Social Psychology, 37,* 753–768.

Rhodes, R. E., & Courneya, K. S. (2003). Self-efficacy, controllability, and intention in the theory of planned behavior: Measurement redundancy or causal independence? *Psychology and Health, 18,* 79–91.

Rhodes, R. E., & Courneya, K. S. (2004). Differentiating motivation and control in the theory of planned behavior. *Psychology, Health, and Medicine, 9,* 205–215.

Rhodes, R. E., & Nasuti, G. (2011). Trends and changes in research on the psychology of physical activity across 20 years: A quantitative analysis of 10 journals. *Preventive Medicine, 53*(1–2), 17–23.

Rhodes, R. E., & Pfaeffli, L. A. (2010). Mediators of physical activity behaviour change among adult nonclinical populations: A review update. *International Journal of Behavioral Nutrition and Physical Activity, 7,* 37.

Rhodes, R. E., Temmel, C., & Mark, R. (2012). Correlates of adult sedentary behaviour: A systematic review. *American Journal of Preventive Medicine, 42,* e3–e28.

Sonstroem, R. J., Harlow, L. L., & Josephs, L. (1994). Exercise and self-esteem: Validity of model expansion and exercise associations. *Journal of Sport and Exercise Psychology, 16,* 29–42.

Spence, J. C., Burgess, J. A., Cutumisu, N., Lee, J. G., Moylan, B., Taylor, L., & Witcher, C. S. (2006). Self-efficacy and physical activity: A quantitative review. *Journal of Sport and Exercise Psychology, 28,* S172.

Terlecki, M., Brown, J., Harner-Steciw, L., Irvin-Hannum, J., Marchetto-Ryan, N., Ruhl, L., & Wiggins, J. (2011). Sex differences and similarities in video game experience, preferences, and self-efficacy: Implications for the gaming industry. *Current Psychology, 30,* 22–33.

Van Dyck, D., Cardon, G., Deforche, B., Owen, N., De Cocker, K., Wijndaele, K., & De Bourdeaudhuij, I. (2011). Socio-demographic, psychosocial, and home environmental attributes associated with adults' domestic screen time. *BMC Public Health, 11,* 668.

Williams, D. M., Anderson, E. S., & Winett, R. A. (2005). A review of the outcome expectancy construct in physical activity research. *Annals of Behavioral Medicine, 29,* 70–79.

Williams, D. M., & Rhodes, R. E. (2014). The confounded self-efficacy construct: Review, conceptual analysis, and recommendations for future research. *Health Psychology Review,* 1–16.

Zabinski, M. F., Norman, G. J., Sallis, J. F., Calfas, K. J., & Patrick, K. (2007). Patterns of sedentary behaviour among adolescents. *Health Psychology, 26,* 113–120.

Zimmerman, F. J., Ortiz, S. E., Christakis, D. A., & Elkun, D. (2012). The value of social-cognitive theory to reducing preschool TV viewing: A pilot randomized trial. *Preventive Medicine, 54,* 212–218.

Motivational Theories

Runner © Izf/Shutterstock

Vignette: Bryan

I was sitting on my couch with a half-eaten Carvel cake and an overflowing ashtray on my coffee table when I got the call. My mother never contacted anyone after 10:00 p.m., so I assumed something was very wrong. She didn't even say hello when I answered. When I picked up all I heard was, "Dad's in the emergency room. Again."

My father was a lifelong smoker, having begun around age 12. I picked up his bad habit during my first year of high school, during which time I'd also learned to mimic his pure aversion to all things physical. In his opinion, time spent playing sports was time wasted. (Better to rally your friends for a trip to the library or look for an after-school job than whittle away hours getting sweaty.)

To call dad a workaholic would have been an understatement. He got up early in the morning to drive from our suburban home to his city law office, often came home late (unless he booked a hotel for the night to be closer to work), and made it clear to me that if I didn't get into an Ivy League college he wouldn't pay for my education. (Thanks to the fortitude of my SAT scores and high school resume, I ended up making the mark. But I nearly had a nervous breakdown midway through freshman year due to all the pressure.)

LEARNING OBJECTIVES

After completing this chapter, you will be able to

- Describe the constructs of the health belief model, protection motivation theory, and self-determination theory.
- Describe research that has applied these theories to physical activity.
- Discuss the advantages and limitations of the health belief model, protection motivation theory, and self-determination theory.

In a typical day, dad would go through a pack and a half of menthols. Cheeseburgers, pizza, and steak topped his list of favorite meal choices. And, as I'd come to find out only after graduating from college, he frequently polished off a bottle of gin every week.

It wasn't surprising to anyone that he had his first heart attack at age 47. Because he only followed his cardiologist's orders to take up a thrice-weekly walking regimen for a month—and moderated his diet only by asking for an extra tomato with his usual burger orders—he was back in the hospital for a second heart attack about a year later. He got a stent put in during that visit and left the cardiac rehabilitation center with a new prescription for blood thinners atop an even stronger admonishment from his doctor to alter a lifestyle that was bound to keep his health mired in disaster.

Still, my dad didn't heed the doctors' advice. "They don't understand how I operate," he would say to mom and I, referring to his unstoppable work ethic—without which, he claimed, he'd never have founded his own successful law firm. Maybe he could see the link between his lack of adequate exercise and poor eating habits—not to mention the steady stream of alcohol and cigarettes into his bloodstream. But he didn't believe that starting a regular physical activity regimen or swapping French fries for salad would make a worthwhile impact on his well-being.

My grandfather—also a lawyer—led a lifestyle similar to my dad's. (Go figure that his behaviors got handed down one generation.) Grandpa suffered comparable medical issues but remained professionally successful well into his late 60s, when he finally succumbed to cardiac arrest. My father admired him more than anyone and endorsed the same attitude toward not making lifestyle changes that my grandfather did when he was ill: "I'd rather leave on a high note, without slacking," my father would often say, reiterating his belief that because exercise got in the way of work it was a futile endeavor.

I had a feeling that the fourth time he landed in the ER—this time from complications due to the colon cancer he'd been diagnosed with shortly after his 58th birthday—it might be a red flag indicating his precipitous end. He was 63 at the time. On that fateful phone call mom told me the cancer had metastasized to his lungs. Though heartbroken, I wasn't surprised.

After a night of little to no sleep due to worrying, I arranged to meet my parents at the hospital the following morning. (This required me to call in sick to work, a decision I knew dad would decry.) On my way there in the car I could no longer avoid a horrifying reality. I was living an inactive lifestyle riddled with poor nutrition and tobacco. Though I wasn't as inflexible as my father in the belief that work should be the be-all-end-all of a man's existence, nor was I as much of a boozer as he was, in terms of lifestyle we were strikingly similar. I was on track to end up cycling through hospital doors in about a decade, just like him. And at 32 years of age, if I didn't do anything to change my habits I might already be halfway done with my life.

Dad finally succumbed to lung cancer before I turned 33. It was a devastating loss, but one neither my mother nor I could say we didn't expect. Up until his final days he remained irate—despite the morphine and other drugs he was on to numb his chronic pain and keep him alive—that the nurses wouldn't let him work from his hospital room.

I visited him each day in that hospital. And though it took a chunk out of my stamina at work, those months I spent with him toward the end of his life were the most meaningful time I think we ever had together. What's more, that was a period where I started walking each morning for 15 to 30 minutes, bought a couple weights, and hired a personal trainer to show me some basic weight training exercises I could do in my own home, after work.

Once I shed enough pounds to feel comfortable entering a gym without the stigma of being the largest one in there, I committed to spending at least 30 minutes on machines there every other day. I was bound and determined not to end up like my dad. Watching the decline of his health throughout my early adult life and seeing him die before he was even old enough to retire was more incentive than I could have ever asked for. (Not that it made pushing myself to be active after decades of laziness any easier. But I was convinced that I could actually take charge of my own health and thereby live longer, perhaps much longer, than dad.)

I've been exercising regularly for the past decade. (I'm turning 44 next month.) I can comfortably say it hasn't, as dad feared, negatively interfered with my work. I'm currently a partner at an impressive law firm. And, if anything, exercise has made me sharper, more energized, and less burnt out on the job.

I'd say smoking has been the hardest habit to give up. But I periodically attend a smoking-cessation support group and I've cut back to a few cigarettes a week. Of course, what helps keep me on track with my diet and fitness goals isn't just the knowledge that I might, in so doing, have a different life outcome than my dad. I can't deny that the influence of my wife—a part-time yoga teacher and special education instructor who I (can you believe it?) met at the gym!—has also been immensely helpful.

That we anticipate the arrival of our baby daughter in about 4 months is probably the most enormous motivator of all. I plan on being an available father for her. And that means doing whatever it takes for my health so as to be alive when she herself has children.

■ Introduction

Fred Kerlinger (1973), in a discussion on the scientific process, noted that, "the basic aim of science is theory … perhaps less cryptic, the basic aim of science is to explain natural phenomena" (p. 8). A similar observation was made by Leonardo da Vinci hundreds of years ago. Science generally, and the theories of science specifically, provide the rudder or compass to guide practice. In this chapter, we highlight one of the first theories applied to understand physical activity and finish the chapter with a theory that has begun to receive much contemporary research.

A natural phenomena that scientists and public health practitioners are trying to explain is why more people are not physically active. Physically inactive people are at risk for several chronic disorders, such as heart disease, stroke, obesity, and diabetes (Warburton, Nicol, & Bredin, 2006). Moreover, even though these individuals are at risk, they may not experience any symptoms associated with these diseases. Thus, they may not consider it necessary to discuss their inactive lifestyle with a physician or increase their physical activity level. Two scientific theories—the health belief model (Rosenstock, 1974) and protection motivation theory (Rogers, 1983)—have been used to explain physical (in)activity.

■ Health Belief Model

The health belief model is generally acknowledged as the first model that adapted theory from the behavioral sciences to health problems, and it remains one of the most widely recognized conceptual frameworks for health behavior. It was introduced in the 1950s by social psychologists Godfrey Hochbaum, Stephen Kegels, and Irwin Rosenstock, who all worked for the United States Public Health Service. During the early 1950s, the Public Health Service was oriented toward prevention of disease rather than treatment of disease. Thus, the originators of the health belief model were concerned with the widespread failure of individuals to engage in preventive health measures, such as getting a flu vaccine. They postulated that individuals will comply with preventive regimens if they possess minimal levels of relevant health motivation and knowledge, perceive themselves as potentially vulnerable, view the disease as severe, are convinced that the preventive regimen is effective, and see few difficulties or barriers in undertaking the regimen. In addition, internal or external cues that individuals associate with taking health-related actions are considered to be an essential catalyst.

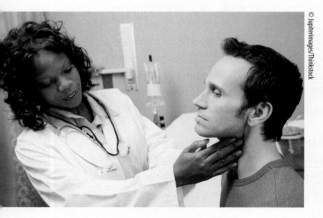

© Jupiterimages/Thinkstock

The first research based on the health belief model was initiated by Godrey Hochbaum (1952). He attempted to identify factors underlying the decision to obtain the then available preventive service of a chest x-ray for the early detection of tuberculosis. Subsequently, the model has been applied to screening utilization rates for high blood pressure, cervical cancer, dental disease, polio, and influenza. It has now been applied to predict patient responses to symptoms (Kirscht, 1974) and to compliance with prescribed medical and health regimens (Becker, 1974), such as hypertension medication, diet, and physical activity (Aho, 1979; Frewen,

Schomer, & Dunne, 1994; Hayslick, Weigand, Weinberg, Richardson, & Jackson, 1996; Tirrell & Hart, 1980). In short, the health belief model has become a major framework for explaining and predicting the reasons people engage in a variety of preventive health behaviors.

Health Belief Model Constructs

The basic components of the health belief model suggest that behavior depends mainly upon two variables: (1) the value placed by an individual on a particular behavioral goal, and (2) the individual's estimate of the likelihood that a given action will achieve that goal (Janz & Becker, 1984). When these two variables were conceptualized in the context of health-related behavior, the focus was on either (1) the desire to avoid illness, or if ill, to get well, or (2) the belief that a specific health action will prevent or improve illness.

The model was originally composed of the following four constructs: perceived susceptibility, perceived severity, perceived benefits, and perceived barriers. These concepts were proposed as accounting for people's "readiness to act." An added concept, cues to action, would activate that readiness and stimulate the actual behavior. A recent addition to the model is self-efficacy, or one's confidence in the ability to successfully perform a behavior. Self-efficacy was included in the model by Irwin Rosenstock and his colleagues (Rosenstock, Stretcher, & Becker, 1988) to accommodate the challenges of changing unhealthy behaviors, such as being sedentary, smoking, or overeating, to healthy behaviors. In addition to these constructs, the following three other variables are considered important for predicting health behavior: (1) demographic factors, such as age, sex, and race; (2) psychosocial factors, such as personality and peer pressure; and (3) structural factors, such as knowledge (Rosenstock et al., 1988). **FIGURE 4-1** provides a schematic of the health belief model. Each of the model's constructs is described in detail in the following discussion. (Also see **TABLE 4-1** for definitions and applications of the health belief model constructs.)

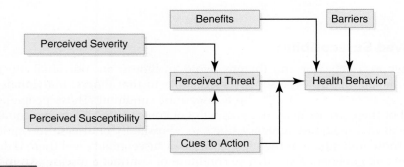

FIGURE 4-1   Health Belief Model

Data from Janz, N., & Becker, M. (1984). The health belief model: A decade later. *Health Education Quarterly, 11*, 1–47.

TABLE 4-1   Definitions, Applications, and Examples of the Health Belief Model Constructs

Construct	Definition	Application	Example
Perceived susceptibility	Person's opinion of the chances of getting a disease.	Define populations at risk. Personalize risk based on a person's features or behavior. Heighten perceived susceptibility if too low.	My chances of getting cardiovascular disease are high because I am sedentary and overweight.
Perceived severity	Person's opinion of the seriousness of a condition and its consequences.	Specify consequences of the risk and condition.	Cardiovascular disease is a serious illness that may cost me my life.
Perceived benefits	Person's opinion of the efficacy of the advised action to reduce risk or seriousness of impact.	Define when, where, and how to take action. Clarify the positive effects to be expected.	I will walk for a half-hour 6 days a week. Becoming physically active will make me healthier and reduce my chances of a heart attack.
Perceived barriers	Person's opinion of the physical and psychological costs of the advised action.	Identify and reduce barriers through reassurance, incentives, and assistance.	Becoming physically active will take time away from others things I enjoy doing.
Cues to action	Strategies to activate "readiness."	Provide how-to information, promote awareness, give reminders.	I will buy physical activity videos and magazines and post reminder notes on the fridge.
Self-efficacy	Confidence in one's ability to take action.	Provide training and guidance in performing action.	I will start slow and gradually increase my frequency, intensity, and duration of walking.

Perceived Susceptibility

To engage in a behavior and thereby avoid an illness, an individual must first believe that he or she is personally susceptible to that illness. Individuals vary in their **perceived susceptibility** to a disease or condition. Those people at the low end of the extreme deny the possibility of contracting an adverse condition. Individuals in a moderate category admit to a possibility of disease susceptibility. Finally, those individuals at the high extreme of susceptibility feel there is danger that they will experience an adverse condition or contract a disease. An individual's perception of personal susceptibility is related to a variety of health behaviors, including immunization (Cummings, Jette, Brock, & Haefner, 1979), dental visits (Becker, Kaback, Rosenstock, & Ruth, 1975), and screening for tuberculosis (Haefner & Kirscht, 1970). In regard to physical activity, if a person believes she is at-risk for cardiovascular disease, she may begin an exercise regimen to reduce her perceived susceptibility to the disease.

Perceived Seriousness or Severity

Perceived severity refers to an individual's feelings concerning the seriousness of a health condition if it is contracted or treatment is not obtained, or both. Feelings concerning the seriousness of contracting an illness (or leaving it untreated) also vary from person to person. These feelings can be considered from the point of view of the difficulties that an illness (or potential illness) would create. For example, an individual may evaluate the severity of cancer in terms of the following: (1) medical consequences, such as pain, discomfort, death, and disability; (2) social consequences, such as difficulties with family, friends, and significant others; and (3) occupational consequences, such as loss of work time and financial burdens (Rosenstock, 1990).

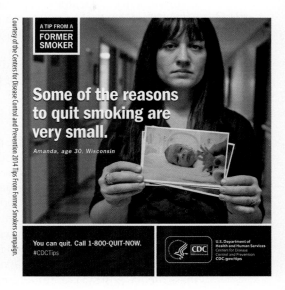

Courtesy of the Centers for Disease Control and Prevention 2014 Tips From Former Smokers campaign.

Perceived Benefits of Taking Action

Perceived benefits is the efficacy of the advised action to reduce risk or seriousness of impact. The direction of action that a person chooses will be influenced by his or her beliefs regarding the action. For example, a sedentary individual at high risk for cardiovascular disease would not be expected to increase his or her physical activity level unless it was perceived as feasible and efficacious. Perceived benefits are conceptually identical to the concept of outcome expectation construct of Bandura's social cognitive theory (Bandura, 2004).

Self-Efficacy

Self-efficacy is a judgment regarding one's ability to perform a behavior required to achieve a certain outcome, and it is an important component of behavior change (Bandura, 1997). Due to its recent inclusion in the health belief model, self-efficacy has not been evaluated as extensively as the other constructs. Researchers, however, who have examined self-efficacy with the model have found overwhelming support for it. For example, Chen, Neufeld, Feely, and Skinner (1998) found that self-efficacy was the only health belief model construct to predict exercise compliance among patients with upper-extremity impairment.

Perceived Barriers to Take Action

It is important to note that action may not take place even though the individual believes that the benefits to taking action are effective, and he or she possesses self-efficacy about performing that behavior. This inactivity may be due to **perceived barriers**. Common barriers to undertaking physical activity include low motivation, inconvenience of facilities, expense, lack of time, and discomfort (e.g., muscle soreness). These barriers may cause a person to not engage in the health behavior. For example, an individual may acknowledge the severity of type 2 diabetes, and know that she is at risk for the disease. She may also believe that physical activity will reduce her chance of developing diabetes. However, she may not become active due to the perceived barrier of lack of time to engage in physical activity.

Cues to Action

An individual's perception of the degree of both susceptibility and severity provide his or her desire to take action, and the perceptions of benefits provide the preferred path of action. However, an event or cue is necessary to trigger the decision-making process and motivate an individual's readiness to take action. These **cues to action** might be internal, external, or both. Internal cues could include perceptions of bodily states such as dizziness, elevated heart rate, and shortness of breath. External cues could include mass media communications (e.g., watching a physical activity video or television commercial) or receiving a postcard from a physician that outlines the health benefits of exercise (Rosenstock, 1974). Such factors as use of mass media, postcard reminders, and the presence of symptoms have been found to influence people to take a recommended health action (Rosenstock, 1974).

The following example illustrates how the components of the health belief model are hypothesized to predict behavior. An inactive person believes that he or she could have a heart attack (*is susceptible*), that inactivity can lead to heart attack (*the severity is great*), and that becoming physically active will reduce the risk (*benefits*) without negative side effects or excessive difficulty (*barriers*). Print materials and letters of reminder sent to the person might promote physical activity adherence (*cues to action*). And, if the individual has had a hard time being active in the past, a strategy involving the use of behavioral contracts could be used to establish achievable short-term goals so that the person's confidence (*self-efficacy*) to engage in physical activity increases.

CRITICAL THINKING ACTIVITY 4-1

© ecco/Shutterstock, Inc.

The cues to action construct is relatively unique to the health belief model. It suggests that there are defining events in our lives that push us into action to change our behavior. Consider your own life and any big changes you have made over the last 2 years. Were there any cues to action?

Application of the Health Belief Model to Physical Activity

Harrison, Mullen, and Green (1992) conducted a meta-analysis of studies using the health belief model with adults. The conclusions of this review were that there is a lack of standardized definitions of the six constructs of the health belief model, and, as a result, the strength of the theory as a psychological framework is decreased. The review found small and varied effect sizes for the constructs of the health belief model. It was also found that retrospective studies had significantly larger effect sizes than prospective studies.

Researchers have also found that health beliefs differ across health behaviors. This was illustrated in a study by Janelle O'Connell and his colleagues (1985). They tested 69 obese and 100 nonobese adolescents to determine if both dieting and exercise behavior could be predicted using the health belief model constructs. The health beliefs examined included knowledge of the (1) etiology, pathology, and demographic variables associated with obesity; (2) proper means of losing weight by dieting and exercising; (3) perceived severity of obesity; (4) perceived susceptibility to the causes of obesity; (5) cues to losing weight by dieting and exercising; (6) benefits of losing weight by dieting and exercising; (7) barriers to losing weight by dieting and exercising; and (8) social support for dieting and exercise. To determine salient beliefs within the health belief model, an elicitation study was undertaken with 58 obese and nonobese adolescents. The most prevalent responses elicited were then used to construct a health belief model questionnaire.

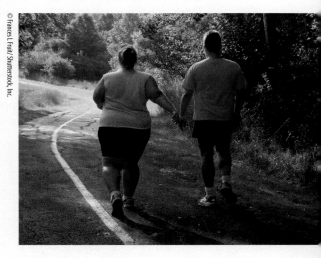

© Frances L Fruit/ Shutterstock, Inc.

It was found that knowledge of the benefits of dieting was the most powerful predictor of dieting for the obese adolescents, whereas knowledge of the susceptibility to the causes of obesity best explained the current dieting practices of the nonobese adolescents. Exercising behavior of obese teenagers was best explained by cues to exercising. The salient cues for exercising included the external cue of peer pressure and the internal cues of poor health and poor muscle tone. None of the health belief model constructs were significant predictors of exercise behavior of nonobese adolescents. The authors concluded that weight-control programs for obese children should attempt to emphasize cues to exercising to encourage participation in aerobic exercise. The cues should be provided in the form of both internal and external stimuli for maximal results. The authors also concluded, however, that the utility of the health belief model was limited for explaining exercise behavior.

In another prospective study, Neil Oldridge and David Streiner (1990) examined the ability of the health belief model to predict exercise compliance and dropout in a cardiac rehabilitation population. They also examined whether the model added predictive utility to routinely assessed patient demographics and health behaviors such as age, weight, occupation type, and smoking status. The health beliefs of 120 male patients with coronary artery disease assessed were the severity of the disease, perceptions of susceptibility to the disease, perceptions of effectiveness of exercise, barriers to exercise, and cues to action. A 6-month exercise program was introduced consisting of twice-weekly supervised exercise sessions lasting approximately 90 minutes. Home-based exercise also was recommended for at least 3 days a week. At the end of the program, the patients were divided into either compliers or dropouts. Dropouts were defined as those participants who either missed more than 50% of all the sessions or more than eight consecutive sessions. Dropouts were then further classified as either unavoidable or avoidable. Reasons for unavoidable dropout included cardiac complications, death, and moving away. Reasons for avoidable dropouts included loss of motivation/interest, inconvenience, and fatigue.

They found that 62 patients (52%) dropped out of the program. Of those who dropped out, 34 were categorized as avoidable and 28 were classified as unavoidable. Compliers were more likely to be nonsmokers, have a white-collar occupation, have active leisure habits, and be younger than the dropouts. In regard to the health belief model constructs, the only significant difference between the compliers and dropouts was in perceptions of the severity of the

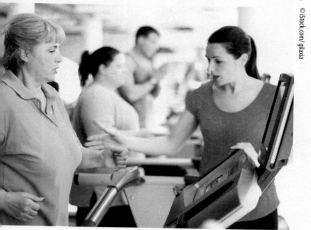

© iStock.com/gilaxia

disease, but this was in the opposite direction of what was hypothesized; that is, the compliers perceived less susceptibility than the dropouts. The predictive ability of the health belief model was found to be very small. Thus, the authors concluded that the results of the study provided limited evidence for the usefulness of the health belief model in accounting for compliance behavior. Not surprisingly, there are few contemporary tests of the health belief model and limited use of the model in physical activity interventions. Given the disease-based focus of the model, there has also been limited application of the model to understand sedentary behavior.

Protection Motivation Theory

Television advertisements often attempt to instill fear in observers in order to change their attitudes and behavior. For example, a dramatic car crash is followed by the observation that drinking and driving do not mix. But appeals based on fear do not consistently result in attitude and behavior changes. The protection motivation theory was originally developed to explain inconsistencies in research on fear appeals and attitude change (Rogers, 1983), but since this time it has been employed primarily as a model to explain health decision making and action. Protection motivation theory is concerned with the decision to protect oneself from harmful or stressful life events, although it can also be viewed as a theory of coping with such events. In the protection motivation theory, decisions to engage (or not engage) in health-related behaviors are thought to be influenced by two primary cognitive processes: (1) **threat appraisal**, which is an evaluation of the factors that influence the likelihood of engaging in an unhealthy behavior (e.g., smoking, sedentary lifestyle), and (2) **coping appraisal**, which is an evaluation of the factors that influence the likelihood of engaging in a recommended preventive response (e.g., physical activity). The most common index of protection motivation is a measure of *intentions* to perform the recommended preventive behavior, with behavior as the ultimate outcome. **FIGURE 4-2** provides an illustration of the constructs of protection motivation theory.

The threat appraisal component depends on (1) **perceived vulnerability**, which is a person's estimate of the degree of personal risk for a specific health hazard if a current unhealthy behavior is continued (e.g., risk for developing lung cancer if one continues smoking), and (2) *perceived severity*, which is a person's estimate of the threat of the disease (e.g., perceived severity of lung cancer). It is assumed that as perceptions of vulnerability and severity increase, the likelihood of engaging in the unhealthy behavior decreases.

Coping appraisal consists of (1) *response efficacy*, the person's expectancy that complying with recommendations will remove the threat (e.g., quitting smoking

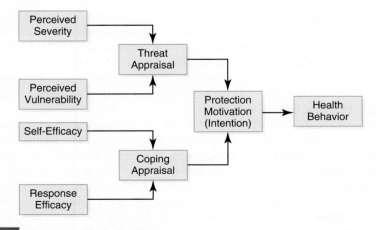

FIGURE 4-2 Protection Motivation Theory

Data from Rogers, R. W. (1983). Cognitive and physiological processes in fear appeals and attitude change: A revised theory of protection motivation. In J. T. Cacioppo & R. E. Petty (Eds.), *Social psychophysiology* (pp. 153–176). New York, NY: Guilford Press.

will reduce one's risk for lung cancer), and (2) *self-efficacy*, the person's belief in his or her ability to implement the recommended coping behavior or strategy (e.g., belief that one can quit smoking). As response efficacy and self-efficacy increase, so does the likelihood of engaging in the recommended preventive behavior.

Protection motivation theory assumes that the motivation to protect oneself from danger is a positive linear function of four cognitive beliefs. That is, when the individual perceives that (1) the threat is severe, (2) he or she is personally vulnerable to the threat, (3) the coping response is effective to avert the threat, and (4) he or she has the ability to perform the coping response, then motivation to implement the coping response is at its maximum. Thus, the emotional state of fear is thought to influence threat and change behavior indirectly through the appraisal of the severity.

Application of the Protection Motivation Theory to Physical Activity

Two meta-analytic reviews on protection motivation theory representing over 20 health issues, including exercise and physical activity, have found some support for the utility of the theory (Floyd, Prentice-Dunn, & Rogers, 2000; Milne, Sheeran, & Orbell, 2000). A relatively recent review of 14 studies on protection motivation theory and physical activity (Plotnikoff & Trinh, 2010) also identified some support for the theory. The meta-analysis carried out by Donna Floyd and her colleagues (2000) on 65 studies (with 29,650 participants) found that, in accordance with the theory, increases in threat severity, threat vulnerability, response efficacy, and self-efficacy facilitated adaptive intentions and behaviors. The magnitude of the effect sizes obtained was in the moderate range.

In the meta-analysis undertaken by Sarah Milne and her colleagues (2000), more stringent criteria for including studies were used. As a result, only 29 studies with approximately 7,700 participants were analyzed. Nonetheless, Milne et al. obtained results that were similar to those of Floyd et al. (2000) of effect sizes in the small to moderate range. Specifically, Milne et al. (2000) found that the threat and coping appraisal components of the protection motivation theory were useful in predicting ongoing behavior.

The review by Plotnikoff and Trinh (2010) concluded similar findings for protection motivation theory and physical activity as other health behaviors. Overall, the authors found little support for the threat component of the model but did find support for the coping constructs as predictors of both physical activity intention and behavior. For example, Plotnikoff and Higginbotham (1998) examined the relative contributions of the protection motivation theory to predict intentions to engage in both a low-fat diet and exercise for the prevention of further cardiovascular heart disease in 151 patients who had recently suffered a heart attack. The participants completed baseline measures of threat appraisal (i.e., vulnerability and susceptibility) during their hospital stay following a heart attack. Six months later the participants completed measures of threat appraisal and coping appraisal (i.e., self-efficacy and response efficacy) via mail. It was found that self-efficacy was the strongest predictor of exercise and diet intentions and behaviors. The authors concluded that health education for this population should promote self-efficacy enhancing activities for such behaviors.

© iStock.com/ Dean Mitchell

Protection Motivation Theory and Physical Activity Intervention

The application of protection motivation theory to intervening upon actual physical activity behavior has had limited attention and mixed results. Typically, researchers use persuasive communications to manipulate the threat of a disease, and the subsequent effectiveness of physical activity can aid in coping. For example, Sandy Wurtele and James Maddux (1987) examined the relative effectiveness of threat (i.e., severity and vulnerability) and coping (i.e., self-efficacy and response efficacy) appraisals for increasing exercise behavior in 160 nonexercising undergraduate females. Nonexercisers were defined as engaging in fewer than two bouts of exercise per week. Each participant received a written persuasive message containing none, one, two, three, or four of the protection motivation theory components (see **TABLE 4-2** for examples of the persuasive messages). After reading the message, all participants completed a postexperiment questionnaire. Participants were then given a list of suggested means of achieving aerobic fitness. Two weeks later the participants reported on any changes in their exercise behavior since the initiation of the study.

It was found that perceptions of both vulnerability and self-efficacy enhanced exercise intentions and behaviors. Furthermore, intentions predicted changes in exercise behavior. It was also found that the participants adopted a "precaution strategy"; that is, they intended to adopt exercise even though they held weak beliefs about its effectiveness and were not convinced of their at-risk status.

This result was not replicated, however, by Milne and colleagues (2002). Their intervention using threat and coping messages in a persuasive communication among 248 undergraduates resulted in higher intentions to exercise but not actual exercise when compared to a control group. More recently, however, Anca Gaston and Harry Prapavessis (2009) also examined protection motivation threat and coping messaging among 208 pregnant women and found intention and exercise 1 week later were significantly higher than the control group or a group that received nutritional information. The results suggest that protection motivation information was at least successful in producing very short-term changes in behavior. Still, this limited and mixed research on the usefulness of

TABLE 4-2 Persuasive Messages Read by the Participants of Wurtele and Maddux's Experiment on Protective Motivation Theory		
Appraisal Construct	**Message Focus**	**Example**
Severity	The seriousness of remaining sedentary by describing the immediate and long-term effects of having a heart attack or stroke.	"Suddenly, the victim is overwhelmed with a crushing pain in the chest as if the ribs were being squeezed in a vise.... Nauseated, the victim vomits; pink foam comes out of the mouth. The face turns an ashen gray, sweat rolls down the face, and the victim, very weak, staggers to the floor."
Vulnerability	The susceptibility to developing heart disease and circulatory problems.	"Because you do not exercise regularly, your cardiovascular system has already begun deteriorating, which puts the health of your body in jeopardy."
Response efficacy	The importance and efficacy of exercising in preventing health problems by presenting evidence that the physiological changes in the body resulting from a regular exercise program serve vital protection functions.	"Since exercise leads to higher levels of high-density lipoprotein, which in turn lowers the level of cholesterol, exercising thus prevents heart attacks."
Self-efficacy	Reasons why women would be able to begin and continue with a regular exercise program.	"We all have a built-in urge for physical activity, and this basic human physical need will serve as an energizer.... At your age you now have the cognitive abilities to commit yourself to a long-term exercise program."

Modified from Wurtele, S. K., & Maddux, J. E. (1987). Relative contributions of protection motivation theory components in predicting exercise intentions and behavior. *Health Psychology, 6*, 453–466.

protection motivation theory suggests that very little is known about whether it has usefulness in the maintenance of physical activity.

Limitations of the Health Belief Model and Protection Motivation Theory

An important construct in both the health belief model (Rosenstock, 1974) and protection motivation theory (Rogers, 1983) is perceived severity; that is, an individual's feelings about the seriousness of a health condition if it is contracted or not treated. However, researchers have been unable to consistently find that perceived severity is an important construct for motivation to engage in physical activity. People may agree that being physically inactive can contribute to severe coronary problems, but there is a limited link between perceptions of the severity of the problem and the tendency to adopt a physically active lifestyle.

One of the problems that has plagued both the health belief model and protection motivation theory is the fundamental assumption that people engage in health behaviors such as regular physical activity for its protective health benefits. To be fair, it should be noted that the models were originally designed for risk-avoiding, not health-promoting, behaviors. A behavior such as physical activity has several other reasons for its performance beyond health, such as social aspects, physical appearance enhancement, and pure enjoyment (Symons Downs & Hausenblas, 2005). Indeed, the affective reasons for physical activity, such as enjoyment, have been shown to be a much larger and more reliable correlate of physical activity performance than health (Rhodes, Fiala, & Conner, 2009). The disease focus, rather than enjoyment focus, also explains why the models have not been applied to understand sedentary behavior. It is enjoyment for performing physical activity compared to outside interests that forms the basis for the theory that concludes this chapter.

CRITICAL THINKING THEORY 4-2

© ecco/Shutterstock, Inc.

Although not all health behaviors seem likely to be performed just for health protective reasons, some may fit the theory better than others. Write a list of 10 health behaviors. Which ones do you think work well for the health belief model and protection motivation theory? Which ones might not due to motives other than health?

Self-Determination Theory

Self-determination theory (Deci & Ryan, 1985) has its origins in the search for understanding the relative influence of intrinsic interest and extrinsic rewards on human behavior. As a consequence, attention was directed toward understanding the function of rewards. A generalization that resulted from the earliest work was that extrinsic rewards can be perceived by a recipient in one of two ways. One way pertains to receiving information about *competence*. Thus, for example, a young child who receives a special treat for playing well in a competition likely would perceive that reward as an affirmation that he or she is competent. Another pertains to receiving information about *control*. If that same young child is given the special treat as an inducement to participate in the competition, that reward could be perceived to be a bribe to have him or her compete. Rewards that convey information to the individual that he or she is highly competent enhance intrinsic motivation. Conversely, however, rewards that convey information that the recipient is no longer fully in control of the reasons for behavior reduce intrinsic motivation.

Sources of Motivation

Early research emphasized the independence of intrinsic and extrinsic motivation; if one was present, it was assumed that the other could not be. However, when research showed that this approach did not adequately explain human behavior, Edward Deci and Richard Ryan (1985, 2000) developed self-determination theory. In the theory, extrinsic and intrinsic motivation are assumed to fall along a continuum (see **FIGURE 4-3**). At one end of the continuum is **amotivation**—the absence of motivation toward an activity.

In the middle of the continuum lies **extrinsic motivation**. According to self-determination theorists, extrinsic motivation is best viewed as multidimensional in nature. One dimension is called **external regulation**, the "purest" form of extrinsic motivation. The individual engages in a behavior solely to receive a reward or to avoid punishment. Consider the case of a person who has been told by his or her physician that an immediate consequence of continued inactivity could be hospitalization. So, grudgingly, a program of physical activity is initiated. That person could be considered to be motivated through external regulation.

A dimension that is slightly further along the continuum is called **introjected regulation**. It represents the incomplete internalization of a regulation that was previously solely external. Returning to our example, the individual might eventually progress to where he or she was no longer at high risk. However, if the physical activity program was maintained because of a sense of "should" or "must," the source of motivation would be introjected regulation. The distinction

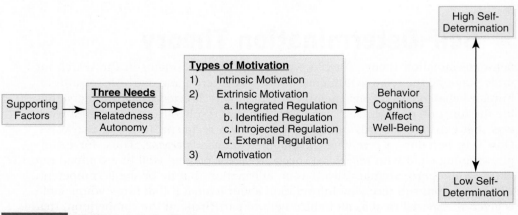

FIGURE 4-3 Self-Determination Theory

Deci, E. L., & Ryan, R. M. (1985). *Intrinsic motivation and self-determination in human behavior.* New York, NY: Plenum Press.

between external and introjected regulation lies in the fact that in the latter case the individual has begun to internalize the motivation for the behavior.

A third extrinsic motivation dimension that is slightly further along the continuum is called **identified regulation**. Here, the individual freely chooses to carry out an activity that is not considered to be enjoyable per se, but which is thought to be important to achieve a personal goal. The individual internalizes the sentiment "I want to." Identified regulation would be illustrated by an individual who is regularly physically active, does not enjoy the activity in the least, but views it as essential for weight control.

The final extrinsic regulation construct is called **integrated regulation**. When identified regulations are well coordinated with other values, it is said to be integrated regulation, which can be a powerful form of regulation because it represents a choice to carry out the activity congruent with other behaviors and choices in one's life.

At another extreme on the continuum is **intrinsic motivation**, which is the motivation to do an activity for its own sake or the pleasure it provides. Robert Vallerand and his colleagues (Vallerand, 1997; Vallerand, Deci, & Ryan, 1987; Vallerand et al., 1993) have proposed that intrinsic motivation is also multidimensional in nature. One form is reflected in intrinsic motivation toward *knowledge*—the pleasure of engaging in an activity to learn something new or about the activity. An individual who chooses to run a marathon to learn how his or her body will respond under that stress would be an example of this form of intrinsic motivation. A second type is intrinsic motivation toward *accomplishment*. The same would-be marathoner used in our earlier example might also want to have the satisfaction of completing such a long distance. Finally, the third type is reflected in intrinsic motivation toward *stimulation*. It represents motivation to experience the pleasant sensations derived from the activity itself. An individual who is physically active because of the bodily sensations accompanying physical activity—sweating, elevated heart rate, muscles responding to the increased load—would be an example of intrinsic motivation toward stimulation.

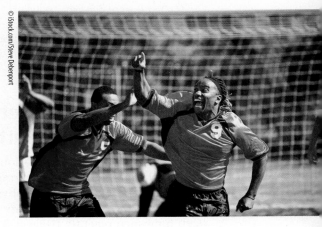
© iStock.com/Steve Debenport

The Antecedents of Intrinsic and Extrinsic Motivation

Figure 4-3 provides an overview of self-determination theory. According to Deci and Ryan (1985), the various motives that individuals have for an activity are driven by psychological needs that have as their basis a striving toward growth and the actualization of personal potential.

The need for *autonomy* refers to the desire to be self-initiating in the regulation of personal behavior. If a sense of autonomy is present, intrinsic motivation is facilitated. The need for *competence* reflects the fact that individuals want to interact effectively within their environment. As is the case with autonomy, if an activity provides the individual with a sense of competence, intrinsic motivation is facilitated. Thus, for example, if exercisers begin to attend a step class and discover that they are never able to coordinate their actions with the rest of their classmates, they are likely to seek out another form of physical activity. Finally, the need for *relatedness* reflects the fact that individuals want to feel connected to others. When relatedness is perceived to be present, intrinsic motivation is facilitated.

According to Deci and Ryan (1985), the various types of motivation are intimately related to perceptions of self-determination (refer back to Figure 4-3). When self-determination is absent, amotivation (i.e., an absence of motivation) exists. Also, when an activity is undertaken for extrinsic motives, minimal perceptions of self-determination are present. Finally, at the extreme end of the continuum, complete self-determination is associated with the various manifestations of intrinsic motivation.

CRITICAL THINKING ACTIVITY 4-3

© ecco/Shutterstock, Inc.

The three needs outlined in self-determination theory are based on sound research and validation. Still, think about the behaviors you will perform this week, from watching TV to taking a nap. Are there other needs that these behaviors may meet? What other needs can you think of that might also drive behavior?

Research on Self–Determination Theory in Physical Activity Settings

Research using self-determination theory to understand sedentary behavior is scant at this point, but self-determination theory is now one of the most popular models applied to understand physical activity. Several mini-reviews and narratives on self-determination theory applied to the setting of physical activity have been published recently (Hagger & Chatzisarantis, 2007; Ryan, Williams, Patrick, & Deci, 2009; Wilson, Mack, & Grattan, 2008), as well as a systematic review (Teixeira, Carraça, Markland, Silva, & Ryan, 2012). Much of the earliest research into intrinsic and extrinsic motivation was carried out in laboratory, school, and sport settings. However, researchers have begun to assess the applicability of the theory in physical activity and exercise settings. Teixeira and colleagues (2012) reviewed 66 studies that have applied the model to understand physical activity. The findings showed clear support for more autonomous forms of motivation (intrinsic, integrated, identified) and a correlation with physical activity performance over more controlled forms of motivation (introjected, external). This is in clear support of the tenets of self-determination theory. Interestingly, however, not all of the three psychological needs have been associated with physical activity. Indeed, the need for relatedness is almost always null in its relationship with physical activity, and autonomy has been inconsistent. Only the need for competence has been a consistent correlate of physical activity (Teixeira et al., 2012).

The measurement of self-determination theory constructs has generally been obtained through use of the Behavioral Regulation in Exercise Questionnaire (Markland & Tobin, 2004) or the exercise motivation scale. For example, Fuzhong Li (1999) used the exercise motivation scale to examine 371 male and female college students who varied in their frequency of exercise. Interestingly, Li found differences between males and females in underlying motivations for exercise. Females reported higher levels of intrinsic motivation and the self-determined forms of motivation illustrated in Figure 4-3. Frequent exercisers (i.e., individuals who were active two or more times per week) also showed higher levels of intrinsic motivation and self-determined forms of motivation than infrequent exercisers (i.e., individuals who were active either one or no times per week).

Li also tested self-determination theory to determine how perceptions of competence, autonomy, and relatedness about physical activity were related to the various forms of motivation illustrated in Figure 4-3. He found that consistent with what would be predicted from self-determination theory, perceptions of competence, autonomy, and relatedness were positively related to the three types of intrinsic motivation (i.e., to learn, to accomplish tasks, and to experience sensations) and negatively related to amotivation.

Similarly, Phil Wilson and colleagues (Wilson, Rodgers, Blanchard, & Gessell, 2003) used the Behavioral Regulation in Exercise Questionnaire to assess 53 community-dwelling adults in Western Canada. The results suggested that identified and intrinsic regulation were large correlates of exercise behavior, while identified regulation correlated with autonomy and competence and intrinsic regulation correlated with competence. The results lend some support to the importance of self-determined motivation and the potential impact of autonomy and competence.

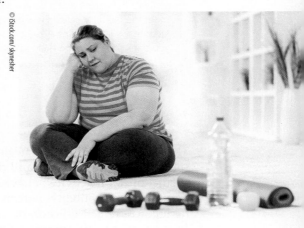

© iStock.com/ skynesher

Self-Determination Theory in Physical Activity Intervention

At present, interventions using self-determination theory have been small-sample pilot studies, although the scope and number are increasing. Teixeira and colleagues (2012) identified seven interventions in their comprehensive review. All have centered primarily on the autonomy support construct (manipulations of choice in physical activity) in the sociocontextual environment of physical activity (Fortier, Duda, Guerin, & Teixeira, 2012; Wilson et al., 2008). For example, Fortier, Sweet, O'Sullivan, and Williams (2007) used a primary care intervention setting and found that the intervention that focused on supporting participant autonomy had an effect on exercise behavior and self-determined motivation. Research that has attempted to change self-determination with persuasive messages has shown less success. For example, Levy and Cardinal (2004) employed a print-mail intervention and did not see changes in self-determined motivations or exercise behavior. Still, the bulk of interventions have been successful at demonstrating changes in physical activity when compared to control groups. The longest experiment to date was implemented in 239 overweight women through 30 weekly group sessions for 1 year, with a 3-year follow up (Silva et al., 2011). Results showed that the intervention was perceived as need supportive; it increased perceptions of competence and autonomy for exercise, intrinsic and identified motivation, and subsequent exercise behavior.

CRITICAL THINKING ACTIVITY 4-4

© ecco/Shutterstock, Inc.

Self-determination theory intervenes on three needs (autonomy, competence, relatedness) in order to affect the quality of motivation toward a behavior. As these needs are met, the behavior is likely to become more self-determined. One challenge with this approach may be limits to the extent that a behavior can meet certain needs. For example, running may not meet the need for relatedness as well as team sports or going to the local pub. Think of your favorite leisure activities. Are there some that meet your three needs more than others? Do you think this would be likely to change with modifications to that behavior?

■ Summary

This chapter examined the health belief model, protection motivation theory, and self-determination theory and the research utilizing these models to explain and predict physical activity behavior. The components of the health belief model are perceived susceptibility, perceived seriousness or severity, perceived benefits of taking action, self-efficacy, perceived barriers to take action, and cues to action. In comparison, the premise for protection motivation theory is that decisions to engage in exercise are influenced by threat appraisals and coping appraisals. Despite limitations of both theories, they provide unique insights into physical activity behaviors, in particular perceived severity (i.e., an individual's feelings about the seriousness of a health condition if it is contracted or not treated). In short, the health belief model and protection motivation theory have provided a compass to guide research to explain exercise behavior.

Self-determination theory is based on the premise that activities are more likely to be selected and maintained if they satisfy three psychological needs: competence, self-determination, and relatedness. Behavior occurs as a result of extrinsic motivation (external regulation, introjected regulation, identified regulation, or integrated regulation) or intrinsic motivation. The various types of motivation are associated with perceptions of self-determination, and perceptions of self-determination are associated with satisfaction and behavior. Initial research has shown support for the theory as a means of understanding and intervening upon behavior in the context of exercise and physical activity.

KEY TERMS

amotivation
coping appraisal
cues to action
external regulation
extrinsic motivation
identified regulation
integrated regulation
intrinsic motivation

introjected regulation
perceived barriers
perceived benefits
perceived severity
perceived susceptibility (perceived vulnerability)
self-efficacy
threat appraisal

REVIEW QUESTIONS

1. According to the health belief model, what are the two main reasons one would engage in health behaviors?

2. People may perceive severe consequences from a health condition, consider they are susceptible, and see clear benefits to engaging in a health behavior, but not take action. According to the health belief model, what additional construct is needed to take action?

3. Protection motivation theory outlines two key appraisals needed to initiate health behavior intentions. What are these appraisals?

4. Self-determination theory suggests that a behavior is performed based on whether it satisfies three basic needs. What are these needs?

APPLYING THE CONCEPTS

1. What constructs of the health motivation model did Bryan's decision to change his diet and exercise behaviors illustrate?

2. How does the protection motivation theory help explain Bryan's motivational shift toward physical activity?

REFERENCES

Aho, W. R. (1979). Smoking, dieting, and exercise: Age differences in attitudes and behavior to selected health belief model variables. *Rhode Island Medical Journal, 62*, 85–92.

Bandura, A. (1997). *Self-efficacy, the exercise of control.* New York, NY: Freeman.

Bandura, A. (2004). Health promotion by social cognitive means. *Health Education and Behavior, 31*, 143–164.

Becker, M. H., Kaback, M., Rosenstock, I. M., & Ruth, M. (1975). Some influences on public participation in a genetic screening program. *Journal of Community Health, 1*, 3–14.

Chen, C., Strecker Neufeld, P., Feely, C. A., & Sugg Skinner, C. (1998). Factors influencing compliance with home exercise programs among patients with upper-extremity impairment. *American Journal of Occupational Therapy, 153*, 171–180.

Cummings, K. M., Jette, A. M., Brock, B. M., & Haefner, D. P. (1979). Psychological determinants of immunization behavior in a swine influenza campaign. *Medical Care, 17*, 639–649.

Deci, E. L., & Ryan, R. M. (1985). *Intrinsic motivation and self-determination in human behavior.* New York, NY: Plenum Press.

Deci, E. L., & Ryan, R. M. (2000). The "what" and "why" of goal pursuits: Human needs and the self-determination of behaviour. *Psychological Inquiry, 11*, 227–268.

Floyd, D. L., Prentice-Dunn, S., & Rogers, R. W. (2000). A meta-analysis of research on protection motivation theory. *Journal of Applied Social Psychology, 30*, 407–429.

Fortier, M. S., Duda, J., Guerin, E., & Teixeira, P. J. (2012). Promoting physical activity: development and testing of self-determination theory-based interventions. *International Journal of Behavioral Nutrition and Physical Activity, 9*, 20.

Fortier, M. S., Sweet, S. N., O'Sullivan, T. L., & Williams, G. C. (2007). A self-determination process model of physical activity adoption in the context of a randomized controlled trial. *Psychology of Sport and Exercise, 8*, 741–757.

Frewen, S., Schomer, H., & Dunne, T. (1994). Health belief model interpretation of compliance factors in a weight loss and cardiac rehabilitation programme. *South African Journal of Psychology, 24*, 39–43.

Haefner, P., & Kirscht, J. P. (1970). Motivational and behavioral effects of modifying health beliefs. *Public Health Reports, 85*, 478–484.

Hagger, M., & Chatzisarantis, N. L. D. (Eds.). (2007). *Intrinsic motivation and self-determination in exercise and sport.* Champaign, IL: Human Kinetics.

Harrison, J. A., Mullen, P. D., & Green, L. W. (1992). A meta-analysis of studies of the health belief model with adults. *Health Education Research, 7*, 107–116.

Hayslick, B., Weigand, D., Weinberg, R., Richardson, P., & Jackson, A. (1996). The development of new scales for assessing health belief model constructs in adulthood. *Journal of Aging and Physical Activity, 4*, 307–323.

Hochbaum, G., Rosenstock, I., and Kegels, S. (1952). "Health Belief Model," United States Public Health Service, 1952.

Janz, N., & Becker, M. (1984). The health belief model: A decade later. *Health Education Quarterly, 11*, 1–47.

Kerlinger, F. N. (1973). *Foundations of behavioral research.* (2nd ed.). New York, NY: Holt, Rinehart & Winston.

Kirscht, J. P. (1974). The health belief model and illness behavior. *Health Education Monograph, 2*, 387–408.

Levy, S. S., & Cardinal, B. J. (2004). Effects of a self-determination theory-based mail-mediated intervention on adults' exercise behavior. *American Journal of Health Promotion, 18*, 345–349.

Li, F. (1999). The Exercise Motivation Scale: Its multifaceted structure and construct validity. *Journal of Applied Sport Psychology, 11*, 97–115.

Markland, D., & Tobin, V. (2004). A modification to the Behavioural Regulation in Exercise Questionnaire to include an assessment of amotivation. *Journal of Sport and Exercise Psychology, 26*, 191–196.

Milne, S., Sheeran, P., & Orbell, S. (2000). Prediction and intervention in health-related behavior: A meta-analytic review of protection motivation theory. *Journal of Applied Social Psychology, 30*, 106–143.

O'Connell, J. K., Price, J. H., Roberts, S. M., Jurs, S. G., & McKinely, R. (1985). Utilizing the health belief model to predict dieting and exercising behavior of obese and nonobese adolescents. *Health Education Quarterly, 12*, 343–351.

Oldridge, N. B., & Streiner, D. L. (1990). The health belief model: Predicting compliance and dropout in cardiac rehabilitation. *Medicine and Science in Sports and Exercise, 22*, 678–683.

Plotnikoff, R. C., & Higginbotham, N. (1998). Protection motivation theory and the prediction of exercise and low-fat diet behaviors among Australian cardiac patients. *Psychology and Health, 13*, 411–429.

Plotnikoff, R. C., & Trinh, L. (2010). Protection motivation theory: Is this a worthwhile theory for physical activity promotion? *Exercise and Sport Sciences Reviews, 38*, 91–98.

Rhodes, R. E., Fiala, B., & Conner, M. (2009). Affective judgments and physical activity: A review and meta-analysis. *Annals of Behavioral Medicine, 38*, 180–204.

Rogers, R. W. (1983). Cognitive and physiological processes in fear appeals and attitude change: A revised theory of protection motivation. In J. T. Cacioppo & R. E. Petty (Eds.), *Social psychophysiology* (pp. 153–176). New York, NY: Guilford Press.

Rosenstock, I. M. (1974). Historical origins of the health belief model. *Health Education Monographs, 2*, 1–9.

Rosenstock, I. M. (1990). The health belief model: Explaining health behavior through expectancies. In K. Glanz, F. Lewis, & B. Rimer (Eds.), *Health behavior and health education* (pp. 39–62). San Francisco, CA: Jossey-Bass.

Rosenstock, I. M., Stretcher, V. J., & Becker, M. (1988). Social learning theory and the health belief model. *Health Education Quarterly, 15*, 175–183.

Ryan, R. M., Williams, G. C., Patrick, H., & Deci, E. L. (2009). Self-determination theory and physical activity: The dynamics of motivation in development and wellness. *Hellenic Journal of Psychology, 6*, 107–124.

Symons Downs, D., & Hausenblas, H. A. (2005). Elicitation studies and the theory of planned behavior: A systematic review of exercise beliefs. *Psychology of Sport and Exercise, 6*, 1–31.

Teixeira, P. J., Carraça, E. V., Markland, D., Silva, M. N., & Ryan, R. M. (2012). Exercise, physical activity, and self-determination theory: A systematic review. *International Journal of Behavioral Nutrition and Physical Activity, 9*, 78.

Tirrell, B. E., & Hart, L. K. (1980). The relationship of health beliefs and knowledge to exercise compliance in patients after coronary bypass. *Heart Lung, 9*, 487–493.

Vallerand, R. J. (1997). Toward a hierarchical model of intrinsic and extrinsic motivation. In M. J. Zanna (Ed.), *Advances in experimental and social psychology* (pp. 271–360). New York, NY: Plenum.

Vallerand, R. J., Deci, E., & Ryan, R. (1987). Intrinsic motivation in sport. In K. B. Pandolf (Ed.), *Exercise and sport science reviews* (pp. 389–425). New York, NY: Macmillan.

Vallerand, R. J., Pelletier, L. G., Blais, M. R., Brière, N. M., Senécal, C. B., & Vallières, E. F. (1993). On the assessment of intrinsic, extrinsic, and amotivation in education: Evidence on the concurrent and construct validity of the Academic Motivation Scale. *Educational and Psychological Measurement, 53,* 159–172.

Warburton, D. E. R., Nicol, C., & Bredin, S. S. (2006). Health benefits of physical activity: The evidence. *Canadian Medical Association Journal, 174*(6), 801–809.

Wilson, P. M., Mack, D. E., & Grattan, K. P. (2008). Understanding motivation for exercise: A self-determination theory perspective. *Canadian Psychology, 49,* 250–256.

Wilson, P. M., Rodgers, W. M., Blanchard, C. M., & Gessell, J. G. (2003). The relationships between psychological needs, self-determined motivation, exercise attitudes, and physical fitness. *Journal of Applied Social Psychology, 33,* 2373–2392.

Wurtele, S. K., & Maddux, J. E. (1987). Relative contributions of protection motivation theory components in predicting exercise intentions and behavior. *Health Psychology, 6,* 453–466.

Theory of Planned Behavior

Runner: © lzf/Shutterstock

Vignette: Rachel

One of the first things my mother said to me after I told her I'd finally gotten pregnant was, "Well, then you should probably stop running."

About 6 months before my husband and I verified our forthcoming baby's heartbeat, I completed my first marathon. I was thrilled when I finally crossed the finish line! Learning how to stay properly fueled and come into race day fully prepared was an incredible learning process—terrifying at times (not to mention arduous), but ultimately one of the most rewarding periods of my life.

My mother did not approve of my marathon training. She was concerned it would reignite the eating disorder I briefly grappled with during college—even though this episode of my life had taken place over a decade ago.

I'd always been the chubby girl in middle and high school. So once I moved across country for undergrad, I was hell bent on proving to my new friends that I, too, could squeeze into a pair of size 2 jeans. I went overboard on restricting what I ate, in part, because I wasn't exactly sure what a healthy diet should entail. And I was unaware there were severe health consequences associated with massively reducing your caloric intake like I did.

LEARNING OBJECTIVES

After completing this chapter, you will be able to

- Describe the theory of planned behavior variables.
- Discuss the research that has applied the theory of planned behavior to physical activity and sedentary behavior.
- Identify the advantages and limitations of the theory of planned behavior.
- Incorporate how the theory of planned behavior can be used to develop physical activity and sedentary behavior interventions.

I had tried out for the track team shortly after beginning my first semester of classes because I thought this would help keep my weight down. But once my weight fell so low that I stopped getting my period, I had to quit. I didn't have the stamina, and my body simply couldn't take the daily meets.

After working with a nutritionist and psychologist at my college's health center, I was able to figure out a more moderate daily meal plan. I never had to leave school or take any drastic measures to get better, like enrolling in an inpatient clinic. I got my weight back up to a normal level and resumed running. This time with the cross-country team.

I've managed to keep a steady training regimen ever since graduating, paying particular attention to my nutritional needs so as not to mess up my system again. If nothing else, I feel that my running schedule has helped improve my body image concerns, because the mileage I cover each week makes me feel more empowered in my skin.

But doubt began wending its way into my devotion to running when my husband and I initially tried to conceive. Because it didn't happen immediately, I started to worry that my daily runs might be interfering with the process of getting pregnant. It was hard not to think that my exercise habits were to blame, even though I was regularly menstruating and maintaining a healthy BMI.

But my OB/GYN, an exercise physiologist I worked with, and a nutritionist all told me it was okay to keep exercising as I had been while attempting to get pregnant. I wanted to trust them, but weekly insinuations from mom that running was rendering me unable to foster new life inside of me really messed with my head.

I guess habit won out, though. No, I didn't jump into gearing up for marathon number two once I switched into baby mode, but until my pregnancy tests turned up positive I was logging between 5 and 8 miles on most days of the week. I dialed down my mileage after getting the good news. I'll admit: I was nervous that hitting the trail near my home might induce a miscarriage, even though my OB/GYN reiterated that the chances of this were so low as to be negligible. But throughout my first trimester I was still able to complete a 5K.

What truly changed my behavior wasn't the social stigma of being told I was insane for not staunching my runs (and not just by my mother, but also by other family members and some colleagues at work), it was the morning sickness and fatigue that got in the way. And once the second trimester rolled around, the discomfort in my lower back—coupled with an elevated need of trips to the ladies' room during my workouts—eventually took me back to walking and taking advantage of the elliptical machine at my gym.

Despite the fear and the negative attitudes from my family and some coworkers, I really did believe in my ability to make it through my pregnancy without giving up physical activity altogether. Though during the final few weeks of it I was really only able to do prenatal Pilates and yoga in between a few light spurts on the elliptical, I started each morning with the intention to do whatever I could.

I gave birth to a healthy baby girl on schedule and with no complications. (I had worried that, like my mother had to do when I was born, I would have to deliver via a C-section. But this wasn't necessary.)

That baby girl is now turning 5 and I've gotten back to running 10Ks ever since she was a year old. And the only reason I'm not training for another marathon is that her brother is now on his way into the world.

The best part? Over the holidays the discussion of running came up over a family dinner with my mother. I watched her open her mouth as she looked from her new granddaughter to my husband, then to me. "You know how I feel about you still doing those races," she said to me. Then added, "but I guess you proved me wrong."

■ Introduction

This chapter examines the theory of planned behavior, a social cognitive theory that has guided a large majority of the theory-based research on physical activity (Ajzen, 1985, 1988, 1991). The **theory of planned behavior** is an extension of the **theory of reasoned action** developed by Martin Fishbein and Icek Ajzen (Ajzen & Fishbein, 1980; Fishbein & Ajzen, 1975). Since its introduction about 30 years ago, the theory of planned behavior has become one of the most frequently cited and influential models for predicting human behavior. This theory has been applied to many health behaviors, including breastfeeding, alcohol use, smoking, illegal drug use, safe sex, eating a healthy diet, wearing a seat belt, and oral hygiene, to name just a few. Of course, the focus of this chapter is the application of the theory of planned behavior for physical activity and sedentary behavior.

The theory of planned behavior is concerned with the link between our attitudes and our behaviors. The following quote by William James (1842–1910), a pioneering American psychologist, highlights the effects that our attitudes have on our behaviors: "It is our attitude at the beginning of a difficult task, which, more than anything else, will affect its successful outcome (n.d.)." The theory of planned behavior also assumes that individuals are capable of forethought and making rational decisions about their behavior and its consequences when they have perceived control over their intentions and behaviors.

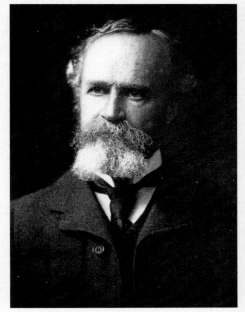

William James (1842–1910), an American philosopher and psychologist, is often called the Father of American Psychology.

Courtesy of U.S. National Library of Medicine.

The theory of planned behavior specifies that the following four psychological variables may influence our behavior: intention, attitude, subjective norm, and perceived behavioral control. The combination of an individual's expectations about performing a particular behavior and the value attached to that behavior form the conceptual basis of this theory. This expectation-by-value approach provides a framework for understanding the relationship between people's attitudes and their underlying beliefs.

■ Theory of Planned Behavior Variables

FIGURE 5-1 presents the main variables of the theory of planned behavior. Let's take a look at each of these main variables in more detail.

Intention

A person's **intention** to perform a behavior is the central determinant of whether he or she engages in that behavior. Intention is reflected in a person's willingness and how much effort he or she is planning to exert to perform the behavior. The stronger a person's intention to perform a behavior, the more likely he or she will be to engage in that behavior. Thus, if someone has a strong intent to go for a walk this afternoon, he or she is likely to go for that walk. In comparison, if a person has a strong intent to watch television after work today, he or she will most likely be sitting on the couch and enjoying his or her favorite television show.

As might be expected, a person's intention can weaken over time. The longer the time between intention and behavior, the greater the likelihood that unforeseen events will produce changes in people's intention. For example, a young adult may intend to be a regular lifetime runner. However, after running for a few years, this person may become bored with the activity and start to swim

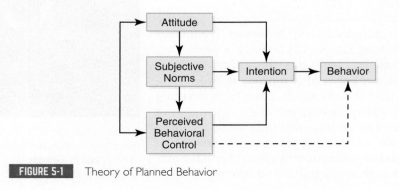

FIGURE 5-1   Theory of Planned Behavior

instead. She did not expect boredom to affect her intention to run. A person's behavioral intentions are influenced by his or her attitudes about the behavior, the perceived social pressures to perform the behavior (i.e., subjective norm), and the amount of perceived control over performing the behavior (i.e., perceived behavioral control).

Attitude

Attitude represents an individual's positive or negative evaluation of performing a behavior. Do you find regular exercise useless or useful, harmful or beneficial, boring or interesting? An older adult may have a negative attitude toward engaging in a vigorous physical activity such as running, but have a positive attitude toward walking in the neighborhood. Our attitude toward a specific behavior is a function of our **behavioral beliefs**, which are the perceived consequences of carrying out a specific action and our evaluation of each of these consequences. A college student's beliefs about playing doubles tennis could be represented by both positive expectations (e.g., it will improve my social life because I will meet lots of people) and negative expectations (e.g., it will reduce my time to study). In shaping a physical activity behavior, the person evaluates the consequences attached to each of these beliefs. Common behavioral beliefs for physical activity include that it improves fitness/health, enhances physical appearance, provides enjoyment, increases social interactions, and improves psychological health (Symons Downs & Hausenblas, 2005a).

Subjective Norm

Subjective norm reflects the perceived social pressure that individuals feel to perform or not perform a particular behavior. Subjective norm is believed to be a function of **normative beliefs**, which are determined by the perceived expectations of important significant others (e.g., family, friends, physician, priest) or groups (e.g., classmates, teammates, church members) and by the individual's motivation to comply with the expectations of these important significant others. For example, an individual may feel that his wife thinks he should exercise three times a week. The husband, however, may not be inclined to act according to these perceived beliefs. Common normative beliefs for physical activity include family members, friends, and healthcare professionals (Symons Downs & Hausenblas, 2005a).

Perceived Behavioral Control

Perceived behavioral control represents the perceived ease or difficulty of performing a behavior. Perceived behavioral control influences behavior either directly or indirectly through intention. People may hold positive attitudes toward a behavior and believe that important others would approve of their behavior. However, they are not likely to form a strong intention to perform that behavior if they believe they do not have the resources or opportunities to do so (Ajzen, 1991). You may have a positive attitude and enjoy swimming; however, if you do not have access to a pool you will not be able to perform this behavior.

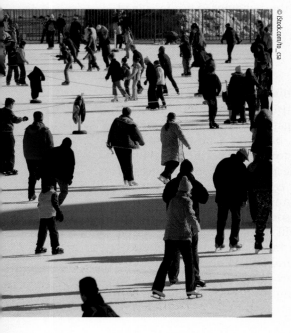

Perceived behavioral control is a function of control beliefs. **Control beliefs** represent the perceived presence or absence of required resources and opportunities (e.g., there is a road race this weekend), the anticipated obstacles or impediments to behavior (e.g., the probability of rain on the weekend is 90%), and the perceived power of a particular control factor to facilitate or inhibit performance of the behavior (e.g., even if it rains this weekend, I can still participate in the road race; Ajzen & Driver, 1991). The most common control beliefs for physical activity include lack of time, lack of energy, and lack of motivation (Symons Downs & Hausenblas, 2005a). **TABLE 5-1** contains sample items for measuring the theory of planned behavior constructs in relation to regularly exercising

TABLE 5-1 Theory of Planned Behavior Sample Items for Exercise

Construct	Item	Scaling						
Attitude	For me to exercise regularly during the winter will be:	Useless				Useful		
		1	2	3	4	5	6	7
Intention	I intend to exercise regularly during winter.	Strongly disagree				Strongly agree		
		1	2	3	4	5	6	7
Subjective norm	Most people who are important to me would like me to exercise regularly during the winter.	Strongly disagree				Strongly agree		
		1	2	3	4	5	6	7
Perceived behavioral control	How much control do I have over exercising during the winter?	Very little control				Complete control		
		1	2	3	4	5	6	7

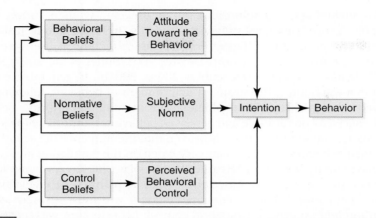

FIGURE 5-2 Relationship of the Theory of Planned Behavior Constructs (including beliefs) with Behavior

Reproduced from Ajzen, I. (1985). From intentions to actions: A theory of planned behavior. In J. Kuhl & J. Beckman (Eds.), *Action-control: From cognition to behavior* (pp. 11–39). With permission of Springer Science+Business Media.

during the winter. **FIGURE 5-2** highlights the relationships among the beliefs and the other theory of planned behavior constructs.

CRITICAL THINKING ACTIVITY 5-1

© ecco/Shutterstock, Inc.

Read the vignette about Rachel at the beginning of this chapter. Describe in detail her attitude, perceived behavioral control, subjective norm, and intention. How did these constructs change over time to influence her exercise behavior?

■ Theory of Planned Behavior Research

Researchers have used the theory of planned behavior in attempts to examine physical activity as well as sedentary activity. Some of this research is described in more detail in the following sections.

Physical Activity Research

Several meta-analytic and narrative reviews have supported the theory of planned behavior for explaining and predicting a variety of physical activities in a variety of populations, including ethnic minorities, youth, pregnant women, cancer patients, diabetic adults, cancer survivors, university students, and older adults, just to name a few (Blanchard et al., 2008; Hagger & Chatzisarantis, 2009; Hausenblas, Carron, & Mack, 1997; Hausenblas & Symons Downs, 2004; Jones et al., 2007; Karvinen et al., 2007; Symons Downs & Hausenblas, 2005a, 2005b). In general, the research has found that intention is the strongest determinant of behavior, followed closely by perceived behavioral control. In addition, our intention to perform a behavior is largely influenced by our attitude and perceived behavioral control, followed by subjective norm. It is important to note, however, that the influence of each of the theory of planned behavior constructs can vary based on the population and context.

Danielle Symons Downs and Heather Hausenblas (2005b) reviewed 111 studies in a meta-analysis that examined the theory of planned behavior and physical activity. They found that (1) exercise behavior was most strongly associated with intention and perceived behavioral control; (2) intention was most strongly associated with attitude; and (3) intention predicted exercise behavior and attitude and perceived behavioral control predicted intention (see **TABLE 5-2** for the effect sizes). These results support the tenets of the theory of planned behavior and reveal that people's intention is the strongest determinant of their exercise behavior, with attitude most strongly influencing their exercise intention. This information is important for designing exercise interventions because it illustrates that how people feel about exercise (i.e., their attitude) has the greatest impact on whether they will plan to exercise (i.e., their intention).

Robert Chaney and his colleagues (Chaney, Bernard, & Wilson, 2014) examined active travel among college students using the theory of planned behavior. Students ($N = 1,280$) from a large Midwestern university were recruited through the university registrar's office and emailed an electronic survey assessing the theory of planned behavior constructs for active travel. Active travel is traveling

TABLE 5-2   Effect Size for Symons Downs and Hausenblas's Meta-Analysis on the Theory of Planned Behavior for Exercise

Variables		Mean Effect Size
Behavior and		
	Intention	1.01
	Perceived behavioral control	0.51
Intention and		
	Perceived behavioral control	0.90
	Attitude	1.07
	Subjective norm	0.59

Data from Symons Downs, D., & Hausenblas, H. A. (2005b). Exercise behavior and the theories of reasoned action and planned behavior: A meta-analytic update. *Journal of Physical Activity and Health, 2,* 76–97.

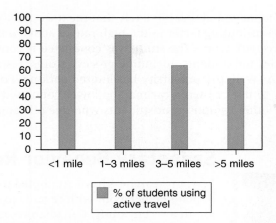

FIGURE 5-3   Differences in Proportion of Active Travel Users by Distance from Campus

Note: The proportion of students using AT decreases the further they live from campus. Statistical differences in the proportion of AT users as distance increased were seen up to three miles. After that point, differences between proportions of AT users were insignificant.

Data from Chaney, R. A., Bernard, A. L., & Wilson, B. R. A. (2014). Characterizing active transportation (e.g., bicycling) behavior among college students using the theory of planned behavior. *International Quarterly of Community Health Education, 34*, 283–294.

that focuses on physical activity (such as walking, bicycling, and skateboarding) as opposed to motorized means (such as cars, buses, and trains).

The researchers found that the students used active travel an average of 4.38 times a week. Not surprisingly, as students lived further from the campus, the less likely they were to be active travel users. In fact, as seen in **FIGURE 5-3** the proportion of students using active travel decreased the further the students lived from campus. The statistical differences in the proportion of students using active travel as distance increased were seen up to three miles. After that point, differences between the proportions of students using active travel were insignificant.

The researchers also found significant differences between the active travel users versus the nonactive-travel users for most of the theory of planned behavior constructs. More specifically, all the theory of planned behavior constructs except perceived behavior control had statistically higher scores for active travel users. In other words, the active travel users had higher attitude, subjective norms, and intention scores than the nonactive-travel users.

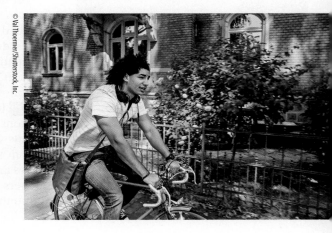

© Val Thoermer/Shutterstock, Inc.

The researchers suggested that it is likely that the university's dense urban setting was a major contributing factor to the high rate of active travel use among its students. The university where the study was conducted is conveniently located to several amenities for students, including grocery stores, restaurants, and recreation facilities. As well, the university has limited parking. For this reason, the need for students to use or own a car may be lower compared to other populations, students on other campuses, or students who live off campus.

Sedentary Behavior Research

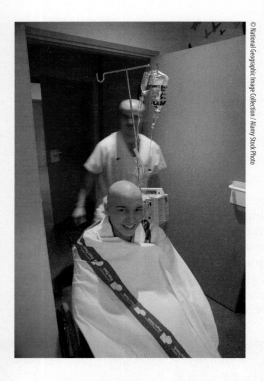
© National Geographic Image Collection / Alamy Stock Photo

Fewer researchers have attempted to study the theory of planned behavior with regards to sedentary behavior. In a recent study, Canadian researchers examined the theory of planned behavior correlates of sedentary behavior in 31 advanced cancer patients with brain metastases (Lowe et al., 2015). The patients completed a survey interview that assessed the theory of planned behavior variables as well as medical and demographic information. The cancer patients also wore an accelerometer that objectively recorded their time spent lying down (i.e., supine), sitting, standing, and stepping during 7 days of active treatment.

The researchers found that the time spent lying down or sitting was correlated with attitude toward physical activity. More specifically, patients who sat or were supine for greater than 20.7 hour per day reported significantly lower attitudes than patients who sat less. As well, patients who were older than 60 years of age spent more time sitting or being supine.

In another study, Harry Prapavessis and his colleagues (2015) examined the utility of the theory of planned behavior for predicting sedentary intention and sedentary time with 372 adults. Using a Web-based survey design, the participants completed a modified version of the Sedentary Behavior Questionnaire. In addition, the participants self-reported their attitude, subjective norm, intention, and perceived behavioral control toward sedentary behavior (see **TABLE 5-3** for sample questionnaire items). The researchers found more positive cognitions and greater intentions to engage in leisure and recreation sedentary pursuits on weekends versus weekdays. The authors suggested that this may stem from the fact that Western society values academic and career success, and weekdays are typically reserved for work, school, or family responsibilities. The researchers also found that the strongest and most consistent predictor of sedentary intention and behavior were subjective norm and intentions.

TABLE 5-3	Sample Theory of Planned Behavior Items for Sedentary Behavior
Construct	**Sample Item**
Intention	How much time do you intend to spend sitting for work, school, or leisure or recreational pursuits (e.g., watching TV; using the computer; doing office or school work; reading; talking on the phone; sitting in lectures or meetings; sitting in a car, train, or bus; eating; socializing; sitting for religious or spiritual pursuits) per day in the coming week?
Attitude	For you to sit for work, school, or leisure or recreational pursuits (e.g., watching TV; using the computer; doing office or school work; reading; talking on the phone; sitting in lectures or meetings; sitting in a car, train, or bus; eating; socializing; sitting for religious or spiritual pursuits) FOR 0-4 HOURS PER DAY (none to one-quarter of your waking hours) would be… Pleasant Unpleasant 1 2 3 4 5 6 7
Subjective norm	The people in my life whose opinions I value would approve of my sitting for work, school, or leisure or recreational pursuits (e.g., watching TV; using the computer; doing office or school work; reading; talking on the phone; sitting in lectures or meetings; sitting in a car, train, or bus; eating; socializing; sitting for religious or spiritual pursuits) for _____ per day.
Perceived behavioral control	How much control do you have over the amount of time you spend sitting for work, school, or leisure or recreational pursuits (e.g., watching TV; using the computer; doing office or school work; reading; talking on the phone; sitting in lectures or meetings; sitting in a car, train, or bus; eating; socializing; sitting for religious or spiritual pursuits) per day? No control Complete control 1 2 3 4 5 6 7

Data from Prapavessis, H., Gaston, A., & DeJesus, S. (2015). The theory of planned behavior as a model for understanding sedentary behavior. *Psychology of Sport and Exercise, 19*, 23–32.

CRITICAL THINKING ACTIVITY 5-2

© ecco/Shutterstock, Inc.

Which of the theory of planned behavior constructs are most effective in predicting exercise behavior?

▇ Elicitation Studies

A main strength of the theory of planned behavior is that an elicitation study forms the basis for developing questions to assess the theory's variables in a specific population. The elicitation study enables a practitioner to determine the specific beliefs for a specific population. This is important because we know that beliefs vary by population and even by activity. For example, the main behavioral beliefs for breast cancer survivors are that exercise gets their mind off cancer and treatment, makes them feel better, improves their well-being, and helps them maintain a normal lifestyle (Courneya, Jones, Mackey, & Fairey, 2006). In comparison, the main behavioral beliefs for pregnant women are related to pregnancy-specific issues, such as having a healthier pregnancy and an easier labor and delivery (Hausenblas, Giacobbi, Cook, Rhodes, & Cruz, 2011).

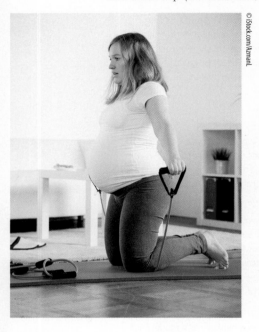

© iStock.com/Azmanl

Because beliefs vary by population, researchers and practitioners are encouraged to refer to research that has already determined the physical activity beliefs of their specific intervention population (e.g., postpartum women, cancer survivors, high school students). If physical activity beliefs for a specific population of interest have not been determined, then it is recommended that the practitioner or researcher conduct an elicitation study to determine the main beliefs for the population of interest. **TABLE 5-4** provides an example of open-ended items used to assess the beliefs of pregnant women during their first trimester. Women during their first trimester would be asked to list about three to five responses for each of the items. Then a content analysis (i.e., a simple frequency count) is undertaken to determine which beliefs are most salient. Finally, a structured belief questionnaire is developed based on the salient beliefs that were identified.

Structured items that arise from the elicitation study should be specific to the target at which the

TABLE 5-4 **Assessing the Theory of Planned Behavior Beliefs in Pregnant Women During Their First Trimester**

Belief	Item
Behavioral beliefs	List the main advantages of exercising during your first trimester.
	List the main disadvantages of exercising during your first trimester.
Control beliefs	List the main factors that prevented you from exercising during your first trimester.
	List the main factors that helped you to exercise during your first trimester.
Normative beliefs	List the individuals or groups who were/are most important to you when you thought/think about exercising during your first trimester.

behavior is directed, the action or specificity of the behavior under study, and the context and time in which the behavior is being performed (Ajzen & Fishbein, 1980). This means, for example, that when trying to develop a walking intervention for older adults, you should ask a sample of older adults to "List the advantages of walking briskly three times a week for 30 minutes outside during the summer." This information will help researchers to develop an intervention based on the salient behavioral beliefs of these older adults that is specific to the behavior. According to the theory of planned behavior, once beliefs are modified, intention will be altered, and the desired behavior change will occur (Symons Downs & Hausenblas, 2005a, 2005b). The relative contribution of the theory of planned behavior constructs may fluctuate from context to context. Thus, before interventions using this framework are implemented, the predictive ability of these constructs with the specific population and specific context should first be tested. **TABLE 5-5** contains belief items that assess the main variables of the theory of planned behavior for pregnant women (Hausenblas et al., 2011).

CRITICAL THINKING ACTIVITY 5-3

© ecco/Shutterstock, Inc.

Describe how the theory of planned behavior beliefs may vary from pregnant women to older adults. What implications does this have for developing exercise interventions with these two populations?

■ Using Theory for Practice

The theory of planned behavior (Ajzen, 1991) is one of the most validated theories for explaining and predicting physical activity behavior (Symons Downs & Hausenblas, 2005a, 2005b), as evidenced by meta-analyses that reveal the strong descriptive and predictive ability of the theory of planned behavior for explaining physical activity intention and behavior and variables that moderate this relationship (Hagger, Chatzisarantis, & Biddle, 2002; Hausenblas, Carron, & Mack, 1997; Plotnikoff, Costigan, Karunamuni, & Lubans, 2013; Symons Downs & Hausenblas, 2005a, 2005b). This large volume of research testing the predictive ability of the theory of planned behavior (more than 300 published studies) has resulted in strong implementation of theory of planned behavior–based intervention research with clinical and nonclinical populations.

The theory of planned behavior is useful in identifying psychosocial determinants of physical activity. Therefore, it has been useful for developing community and individual exercise programs. For example, people intend to exercise when they hold a positive attitude toward exercise. Exercise programs that offer a positive experience would likely increase people's intention to exercise, which would likely positively influence their exercise behavior. Positive behavioral beliefs and their evaluation may be enhanced if people are given experiences with enjoyable

TABLE 5-5 Example of Theory of Planned Behavior Belief Items for Pregnant Women

Part D Instructions. The following questions pertain to your **first trimester** exercise behavior. Using the scales below, please indicate your answer by placing it in the space provided after each statement.

1	2	3	4	5	6	7
Extremely Unlikely					Extremely Likely	

Exercising regularly in my first trimester will:

Help control my weight _____
Improve my physical health _____
Make me feel better _____
Increase my energy _____
Improve my appearance/body image _____
Improve my fitness _____
Make my labor and delivery easier _____
Get me outside (fresh air) _____
Relieve my stress _____
Reduce my nausea _____
Improve my baby's health _____
Improve my circulation/blood flow _____
Take too much time _____
Increase my risk of injury _____

1	2	3	4	5	6	7
Strongly Disagree					Strongly Agree	

Would the following people approve of me exercising regularly in my first trimester:

Spouse/Significant Other _____
Friends _____
Children _____
Co-workers _____
Parents _____
Doctors _____
Siblings _____

1	2	3	4	5	6	7
Strongly Disagree					Strongly Agree	

I will be able to exercise regularly during my first trimester despite:

Health issues (injury/pain) _____
No time to exercise _____
Being tired (having no energy) _____
Bad weather _____
Limited knowledge about exercising during my pregnancy _____
Other children to care for _____
Limited social support _____
Pregnancy-specific discomforts (e.g., breast soreness) _____
Fear of miscarriage/harming baby _____
Headaches _____
Morning sickness/nausea _____

types of physical activities and then gradually encouraged to increase the intensity,
duration, and frequency of those activities.
Perceived behavioral control is an important
factor in intention to be physically active
(Plotnikoff, Lippke, Courneya, Birkett, &
Sigal, 2010). When people perceive physical activity as difficult to do, their intention
is low. Assisting people to overcome barriers
such as time involvement, other obligations,
or feelings of inability should enhance perceptions of control about exercising. We will
now take a closer look at a physical activity
intervention called "Wheeling Walks" that
was guided by the theory of planned behavior.

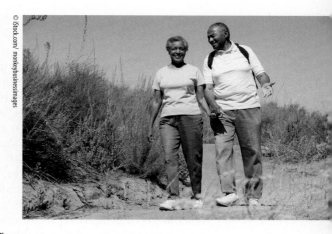

Wheeling Walks was an 8-week mass media walking campaign developed
by Bill Reger and his colleagues (2002). The main goal of the intervention was
to promote walking among sedentary adults aged 50 to 65 years in the city of
Wheeling, West Virginia (Reger-Nash et al., 2005). This communication intervention used the theory of planned behavior constructs to try to change sedentary
adults' behavior by promoting 30 minutes of daily walking through paid media,
public relations, and public health activities. A main goal of the interventions was
to effect a 10% increase in the proportion of adults meeting the physical activity
guidelines of moderate-intensity walking. The impact of the campaign was determined by pre- and postintervention telephone surveys with 719 adults in the
intervention community and 753 adults in the comparison community, as well as
the observations of walkers at 10 community sites.

The city of Wheeling, West Virginia, a community of 31,420 people, was chosen because of its adequate and affordable media (i.e., 2 local network television
stations, 2 daily newspapers, 12 radio stations) and the cooperation of local health
agencies. Parkersburg, West Virginia, population 33,099, served as the comparison community. Parkersburg is located 92 miles from Wheeling. It has a separate
media market, and the residents are not exposed to media from the Wheeling
media market. The researchers used a **quasi-experimental design** because they
could not randomly assign people to either the treatment or control group. Quasi-
experimental studies take on many forms, but may best be defined as lacking key
components of a true experiment, such as randomization.

To develop the messages to be used in the intervention, the theory of planned
behavior was used to determine the salient beliefs that should be targeted during
the walking intervention. The researchers found that sedentary and irregularly
active people shared similar behavioral beliefs (i.e., attitude) and normative beliefs
(i.e., subjective norm) with regular exercisers, but showed very strong differences
on control beliefs (i.e., perceived behavioral control). For the control beliefs, sedentary adults believed that they had less control over their time and scheduling of
exercise compared to regular exercisers. Thus, the campaign messages focused on

changing sedentary adults' control beliefs by emphasizing that they do have the time to walk for 30 minutes a day.

The Wheeling Walks campaign activities included paid advertising, special public relations events designed to generate additional media coverage, and public health educational activities at worksites, churches, and local organizations. The paid advertisements consisted of two newspaper ads, two 30-second television ads, and two 60-second radio ads. Wheeling Walks promoted 30 minutes or more of moderate intensity walking on almost every day for better health and feeling more energetic. To address the "I don't have time" belief, which was identified as a primary barrier to physical activity, the ads suggested "start walking 10 minutes a day at first, then 20 minutes ..." and compared the 30-minute time period to that of "one TV program." Each ad ended with the tagline, "Isn't it time you started walking?" Transcripts of the ads are available on their website at http://www .wheelingwalks.org/WW_TrainingManual/appendix/appendix-2.asp.

Behavioral observation showed a 23% increase in the number of walkers in the intervention community versus no change in the comparison community. The researchers also found that 32% of the baseline sedentary population in the intervention community reported meeting the physical activity guidelines by walking at least 30 minutes at least five times per week versus 18% in the comparison community (see **FIGURE 5-4**).

In a follow-up study at 3 months postintervention, Gebel, Baumen, Regen-Nash, and Leydon (2011) found that the changes in walking after the mass media campaign were influenced by the perceived environment; that is, people living in neighborhoods with nice aesthetics, benches or other places to rest, high connectivity, and lots of other walkers increased their walking levels significantly more

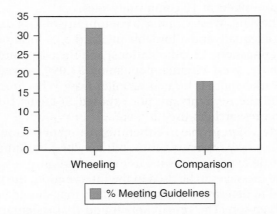

FIGURE 5-4   Percentage of Older Adults Meeting the Physical Activity Guidelines

Note: Pre to post changes in self-reported physical activity among sedentary older adults.

Adapted from Reger, B., Cooper, L., Booth-Butterfield, S., Smith, H., Bauman, A., Wootan, M., Middlestadt, S., Marcus, B., & Greer, F. (2001). Wheeling Walks: A community campaign using paid media to encourage walking among sedentary older adults. *Preventive Medicine, 35,* 285–292.

than those whose environments were less walkable. For the factor of aesthetics and facilities, people in the more walkable environment increased walking by 87 minutes more than those in less walkable environments (Gebel et al., 2011).

Important research questions are: Did the increased walking last by the adults in Wheeling? And can these results be replicated in other communities? The answer to both of these questions is yes. A follow-up study revealed that the campaign succeeded in sustaining the increase in walking 12 months after the intervention. As well, the campaign has been successfully replicated in other communities, including rural and larger communities (> 200,000 people; Reger-Nash et al., 2006, 2008).

CRITICAL THINKING ACTIVITY 5-4

© ecco/Shutterstock, Inc.

How would you modify the Wheeling Walks intervention to include sedentary behavior? Using the theory of planned behavior as a guide, how would you assess the constructs for sedentary behavior and then apply the findings to conduct a sedentary behavior intervention?

Limitations of the Theory of Planned Behavior

Although the theory of planned behavior has been successful in explaining and predicting physical activity behavior, limitations of research examining the theory exist (Sniehotta, Presseau, & Araujo-Sores, 2014). As Icek Ajzen (2011) stated: "Yet, for all its popularity, or perhaps because of it, the theory of planned behavior [TPB] has also been the target of much criticism and debate" (p. 1113). Some researchers reject the theory of planned behavior outright as an adequate explanation of behavior (Wegner, 2002). Most critics, however, accept the theory's basic assumptions but either question its sufficiency or inquire into its limiting conditions (Ajzen, 2011). We will briefly discuss some of the theory's potential limitations.

Other Variables

First, factors such as personality, affect, mood, demographic variables (e.g., age, gender, socioeconomic status), past exercise behavior, and habit are not directly taken into consideration within the theory of planned behavior (Ajzen, 2011; McEachan, Conner, Taylor, & Lawton, 2011). This is a limitation because researchers examining the determinants of physical activity have consistently found, for example, that the percentage of the population reporting no physical activity is higher among female than male populations, among older adults than younger adults, among extroverts than neurotics, and among the less affluent than the more affluent (U.S. Department of Health and Human Services, 2000).

Researchers have examined the relationship of some of the aforementioned variables with the theory of planned behavior for exercise (Blanchard et al., 2008; Rhodes, Blanchard, & Blacklock, 2008; Rhodes & Courneya, 2003; Courneya, Friedenreich, Sela, Quinney, & Rhodes, 2002). Study findings are revealing that these variables tend to improve the explanatory value of the theory of planned behavior (Whitford & Jones, 2011). For example, a recent study by Kwan and Bryan (2011) found that positive affective response to acute bouts of exercise can improve exercise motivation. These researchers tested whether affective response to exercise leads to greater motivation in terms of attitudes, subjective norms, self-efficacy, and intentions to exercise. They had 127 participants complete self-reported information on the theory of planned behavior constructs and their exercise behavior at baseline and 3 months later. The participants also provided reports of their exercise-related affect during a 30-minute bout of moderate-intensity treadmill exercise at baseline.

The researchers found that participants who experienced greater improvements in positive affect, negative affect, and fatigue during exercise tended to report more positive attitudes, exercise self-efficacy, and intentions to exercise 3 months later. They also found that affective response was not predictive of subjective norms.

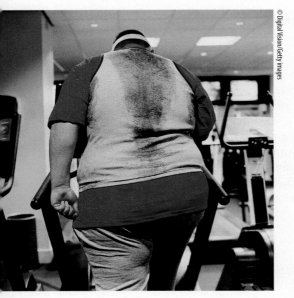

© Digital Vision/Getty images

With regard to past behavior, Ron Plotnikoff and his colleagues (2010) examined the utility of the theory of planned behavior constructs and past behavior in understanding physical activity in adults with type 1 and type 2 diabetes. They had 2,311 adults complete the theory of planned behavior constructs of attitude, subjective norm, perceived behavioral control, intention, and physical activity at baseline. At the 6-month follow up they had 1,717 adults complete a physical activity behavior measure. After adjusting for past physical activity behavior (i.e., adults' physical activity behavior at baseline), they found that the impact of perceived behavior control and intention for predicting exercise behavior was reduced. In other words, our past exercise behavior is a strong predictor of whether we will be exercising in the future.

Perceived Behavioral Control Issues

Second, there is ambiguity regarding how to define perceived behavioral control, and this creates measurement problems (see Ajzen, 2002a). In fact, Paul Estabrooks and Albert Carron (1998) noted that Icek Ajzen (1985, 1987, 1991) has been inconsistent in the manner in which he has defined perceived behavioral control, representing it as both self-efficacy and as the perceived ease or difficulty of performing the specific behavior. Because there is no agreed-upon protocol for the assessment of perceived behavioral control, Estabrooks and Carron (1998) compared the relative merits of three different measures in a study using the theory of planned behavior to examine the physical activity of older adults (average age 68 years).

In one approach, the participants indicated their confidence in their ability to schedule exercise into their daily routine. This was referred to as *scheduling self-efficacy*. In another approach, the participants indicated their confidence in their ability to overcome barriers that might arise to inhibit attendance. This was called *barrier self-efficacy*. For the third approach, the participants rated the ease or difficulty of attending exercise classes. The third approach was labeled as *perceived behavioral control*. Estabrooks and Carron found that scheduling self-efficacy was the best predictor of exercise behavior.

Ajzen (2002a) stated that the term *perceived behavioral control* may be misleading and to avoid misunderstanding he suggested that perceived behavioral control should be read as "perceived control over performance of a behavior." Ajzen further noted that perceived behavioral control is composed of the following two components: (1) self-efficacy (i.e., ease or difficulty of performing the behavior) and (2) controllability (i.e., beliefs about the extent to which performing the behavior is up to the person). Thus, measures of perceived behavioral control should contain items that assess both self-efficacy and controllability.

Terry and O'Leary (1995), in a prospective study examining the theory of planned behavior constructs' ability to predict regular exercise over a 2-week period, found support for the two components of perceived behavioral control. They also reported that self-efficacy predicted intention but not behavior, whereas perceived controllability predicted behavior but not intention.

Intention–Behavior Gap

Third, the longer the time interval between intention and behavior, the less likely the behavior will occur (Ajzen & Fishbein, 1980; McEachan et al., 2011; Symons Downs & Hausenblas 2005b). Fishbein and Ajzen (1975) argued that the predictive power of intention will vary inversely with the time between the measurement of intention and performance of the behavior. They also suggested that the longer the time interval between intention and behavior, the more likely intention is to change with newly available information. As time passes, an increasing number of intervening events can change people's behavioral, normative, or control beliefs and modify attitudes, subjective norms, or perceptions of control, thus generating revised intentions. Changes of this kind will tend to reduce the predictive validity of intentions that were assessed before the changes took place. This new information would result in a diminished relationship between intention and behavior. Consistent with this argument, shorter intervals between assessment of intentions and behavior are associated with stronger correlations than longer time intervals.

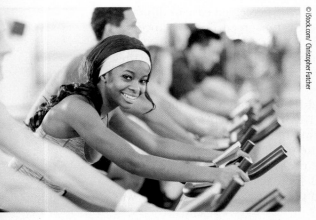

Kerry Courneya and Edward McAuley (1993) found support for this contention. They examined 42 undergraduate students' short-term (i.e., 2 days) and long-term (i.e., 4 weeks) intention to engage in physical activity. Short-range intention was assessed by asking the students to respond to the question: "Do you intend to be physically active between this class and next class?" Two days later the students reported their physical activity behavior. Long-range intention was assessed by having the students respond to the statement: "During the next 4 weeks I intend to be physically active _____ times."

Four weeks later the students listed their physical activity for the past month. The correlations between short- and long-range intention and physical activity were .59 and .39, respectively, confirming the expectation that short-range intention is a better predictor of physical activity than is long-range intention.

Habit and Planning

While measurement aspects such as the time range between intention and behavior assessments may account for some of the reason for the intention behavior gap, some theorists have suggested that other key variables are missing from the theory of planned behavior. Two of the most researched variables include habit and planning. **Habit** refers to the automatic performance of a behavior from consistent cues and practice (Gardner, 2014). The simplest way to think about habit may be with a behavior like driving, where people often get into their car and navigate to work or some routine destination without much thought. The act is so routine that it almost performs itself, below awareness. Habits are often easy to understand when one tries to break them. Have you ever intended to change your driving route, say to pick something up from the store, and find yourself forgetting to make that change? This is likely the power of habit. In physical activity, habit is a more controversial construct than something like driving. It seems difficult to imagine performing vigorous exercise, for example, completely below awareness! Still, some of the routine aspects of physical activity, from preparing workout clothes, to driving to a facility, or even the repetitive act of some physical activities (such as running or walking routes) may have some automatic function brought upon by cues and not always motivation.

Ben Gardner and his colleagues (Gardner, de Bruijn, & Lally, 2011) showed some evidence for this possibility in a meta-analysis of habit and physical activity. In 10 studies, they showed that habit positively correlated with leisure-time physical activity ($r = 0.44$) and active transport ($r = 0.70$). The strength of these correlations rivaled or exceeded behavioral intentions. This means that habit is a strong (or even stronger in some instances) correlate of our physical activity behavior than intention. Rhodes, de Bruijn, and Matheson (2010) also showed that habit is an independent predictor of physical activity when accounting for intention, suggesting that we may have both motivated and habit factors that contribute to our activity behaviors.

Another well-researched factor that may account for the intention–behavior gap is planning behavior and/or strategies employed to keep intentions on track. It has been recognized for a long time (Ach, 1905) that forming intentions and translating intentions into action may be two distinct factors. Researchers have argued that the motivation to perform a behavior is still dependent of the volitional act of creating a good plan to enact the behavior (e.g., Gollwitzer & Brandstatter, 1997; Heckhausen & Gollwitzer, 1987). These have typically included action plans (i.e., planning how, when, where, and what to do), implementation intentions (i.e., if-then plans linking the behavior to environment and cues), and coping plans (i.e., plans to overcome barriers) (Hagger & Luszczynska, 2014; Schwarzer, 2008). However, self-monitoring of behavior, enlisting support, making cues to act, and formulating plans to prepare for a behavior are also potentially important to bridge the intention–behavior gap (Rhodes & de Bruijn, 2013a, 2013b). Research in the physical activity domain has supported this theorizing.

For example, Carraro and Gaudreau (2013) conducted a meta-analysis of 23 studies and showed that both action planning and coping planning had effects on physical activity behavior that partially mediated the intention relationship. A review on the physical activity intention–behavior gap also showed that the use of strategies employed to help maintain intentions, such as plans and monitoring of behavior, was one of the most reliable factors that closed the gap (Rhodes & de Bruijn, 2013a). These findings suggest that strategy variables, such as plans, may be needed beyond good intentions.

Sparked by the intention–behavior gap, several recent models that attempt to explain this relationship with habit, planning, or other factors have begun to gain attention by physical activity researchers, such as the health action process approach (Schwarzer, 2008), the multiprocess action control model (Rhodes & de Bruijn, 2013a, 2013b), the integrated behavior change model (Hagger & Chatzisarantis, 2014), the I-change model (de Vries, Mesters, van de Steeg, & Honing, 2005), the motivational/volitional process model (Fuchs, 1996), and temporal self-regulation theory (Hall & Fong, 2007). Only time and testing will tell whether these approaches replace the theory of planned behavior for understanding physical activity.

Subjective Norm Issues

Another potential limitation pertains to the construct of subjective norm. Consistent throughout the physical activity literature, the theory of planned behavior variables of attitude and perceived behavioral control have been significant predictors of intention. Subjective norm, however, is generally a weaker predictor of intention (Symons Downs & Hausenblas, 2005a, 2005b). One reason that has been offered by Nicole Culos-Reed and her colleagues (Culos-Reed, Gyurcsik, & Brawley, 2001) for the inconsistent usefulness of subjective norm is that the role of significant others may not be important in encouraging participation of physically active individuals. Support for this view comes from the fact that subjective norm is a stronger predictor of intention for other health behaviors, such as contraceptive use, where the role of significant others is deemed to be more important for the decisions made, and thus cannot be ignored (Culos-Reed et al., 2001).

A second reason for the weak contribution of subjective norm to the prediction of physical activity might lie in its operationalization (Manning, 2009). Some authors have suggested that a better operational definition for subjective norm might be one that more closely approximates the concept of **social support** (e.g., Courneya, Plotnikoff, Hotz, & Birkett, 2000): Is your motivation (or intention) to be involved in physical activity more the result of your belief that important others wish you to do so (i.e., subjective norm), or is it more the result of the support and praise you receive from others who are significant in your life (i.e., social support)? That is, the conceptual distinction between these two social influence constructs is that subjective norm refers to the perceived pressure to perform a behavior that comes from observing what important others say and/or do, whereas social support implies the perception of assistance in performing the behavior (Courneya et al., 2000). Physical activity scientists increasingly favor the latter alternative.

CRITICAL THINKING ACTIVITY 5-5

© ecco/Shutterstock, Inc.

What are the main differences between subjective norm and social support? What are the implications of using social support in place of subjective norm in the theory of planned behavior?

The theoretical argument for why social support should be superior to subjective norm in the exercise domain is due to exercise behavior not being under complete volitional control (i.e., not capable of being done at will or free of practical constraints). Thus, subjective norm may be the most relevant social influence construct for behaviors that are under complete volitional control because for such behaviors a person only needs to know whether important others approve of the behavior. By definition, they do not need any help. For behaviors that are incompletely volitional, however (such as exercise), it is likely that assistance from others for performing the behavior (i.e., social support) would be helpful beyond knowing that they approve of the behavior.

Research by Ryan Rhodes and his colleagues (Rhodes, Jones, & Courneya, 2002) supports the importance of social support for predicting exercise intentions and behaviors. Using a prospective design, they had 192 undergraduate students complete self-report measures of the theory of planned behavior variables and social support. And then 2 weeks later the students completed a follow-up measure of their exercise behavior. The researchers found that social support had a significant effect on intention, along with perceived behavioral control and attitude. This suggests that individuals are influenced by perceived support for exercise when forming exercise intentions independent of attitudes, subjective norms, and perceptions of behavioral control. They also found that social support exerted a significant direct effect upon strenuous exercise behavior when controlling for the significant effects of intention and perceived behavioral control. This finding supports the research and theorizing by Courneya et al. (2000) suggesting that exercise behavior, not being under complete volitional control, is influenced by assistance from others (i.e., social support).

■ Summary

Changing people's behaviors is very difficult to do, especially when dealing with a complex health behavior such as physical activity. To increase the success of predicting, understanding, explaining, and changing physical activity behavior, researchers and practitioners should use a theoretical framework such as the theory of planned behavior as a guide (Vallance, Courneya, Plotnikoff, Mackey, 2008). Researchers have found support for the utility of attitudes, perceived behavioral control, and, to a lesser extent, subjective norms in explaining people's intention to becoming physically active. Emerging research is revealing that the theory of planned behavior may be effective in explaining and predicting sedentary behavior.

Research has also found a strong relationship between someone's intention to be active and his or her engaging in the behavior. Furthermore, a person's perception of the control they have over engaging in physical activity can also directly predict behavior. In general, there is strong evidence that the theory of planned behavior can explain and predict people's physical activity intentions and behaviors. In summary, because of the success of the theory of planned behavior to explain and predict exercise behavior, intervention research reveals that it is also a useful framework to guide physical activity interventions.

KEY TERMS

attitude
behavioral beliefs
control beliefs
habit
intention
normative beliefs

perceived behavioral control
quasi-experimental design
social support
subjective norm
theory of planned behavior
theory of reasoned action

REVIEW QUESTIONS

1. Define the theory of planned behavior variables that explain exercise intention.

2. Define the theory of planned behavior variables that explain exercise behavior.

3. Describe three limitations of the theory of planned behavior.

4. Outline the methods used in an elicitation study.

5. Describe the theory of planned behavior beliefs.

6. Jerry is a 65-year-old adult who is a cancer survivor. Based on his physician's recommendation, he has started to walk daily for 30 minutes. He has been walking daily now for 4 months. He is very motivated to walk every day, and his wife also walks with him for support. He really enjoys walking, and he likes how it makes him feel. He is worried that with the winter months approaching it will be more difficult to walk when it is cold out. Using the theory of planned behavior, describe Jerry's intention, perceived behavioral control, attitude, and subjective norm toward his behavior of daily walking for 30 minutes.

APPLYING THE CONCEPTS

1. Which variable(s) of the theory of planned behavior best explain Rachel's ability to stick to her running regimen throughout her pregnancy?

2. Apart from the variables in the theory of planned behavior, what else might account for Rachel's ability to maintain her commitment to running?

REFERENCES

Ach, N. (1905). *Uber die Willenstatigkeit und das Denken*. Gottingen: Vandenhoeck & Ruprecht.

Ajzen, I. (1985). From intentions to actions: A theory of planned behavior. In J. Kuhl & J. Beckman (Eds.), *Action-control: From cognition to behavior* (pp. 11–39). Heidelberg: Springer.

Ajzen, I. (1988). *Attitudes, personality, and behavior*. Milton Keynes: Open University Press.

Ajzen, I. (1991). The theory of planned behavior. *Organizational Behavior and Human Decision Processes*, *50*, 179–211.

Ajzen, I. (2002a). Perceived behavioral control, self-efficacy, locus of control, and the theory of planned behavior. *Journal of Applied Social Psychology, 32*, 665–683.

Ajzen, I. (2002b). Construction of a standard questionnaire for the theory of planned behavior. Retrieved August 2002 from http://www-unix.oit.umass.edu/~aizen

Ajzen, I. (2011). The theory of planned behavior: Reactions and reflections. *Psychology and Health, 26*, 1113–1127.

Ajzen, I., & Driver, B. L. (1991). Prediction of leisure participation from behavioral, normative, and control beliefs: An application of the theory of planned behavior. *Leisure Sciences, 13*, 185–204.

Ajzen, I., & Fishbein, M. (1980). *Understanding attitudes and predicting social behavior.* Englewood-Cliffs, NJ: Prentice-Hall.

Blanchard, C., Fisher, J., Sparling, P., Nehl, E., Rhodes, R., Courneay, K., & Baker, F. (2008). Understanding physical activity behavior in African American and Caucasian college students: An application of the theory of planned behavior. *Journal of American College Health, 56*, 341–346.

Carraro, N. & Gaudreau, P. (2013). Spontaneous and experimentally induced action planning and coping planning for physical activity: A meta-analysis. *Psychology of Sport and Exercise, 14*, 228–248.

Chaney, R. A., Bernard, A. L., & Wilson, B. R. A. (2014). Characterizing active transportation (e.g., bicycling) behavior among college students using the theory of planned behavior. *International Quarterly of Community Health Education, 34*, 283–294.

Courneya, K. S., Friedenteich, C. M., Sela, R. A., Quinney, H. A., & Rhodes, R. E. (2002). Correlates of adherence and contamination in a randomized controlled trial of exercise in cancer survivors: An application of the theory of planned behavior and the five factor model of personality. *Annals of Behavioral Medicine, 24*, 257–268.

Courneya, K. S., Jones, L. W., Mackey, J. R., & Fairey, A. S. (2006). Exercise beliefs of breast cancer survivors before and after participation in a randomized controlled trial. *International Journal of Behavioral Medicine, 13*, 259–264.

Courneya, K. S., & McAuley, E. (1993). Can short-range intentions predict physical activity participation? *Perceptual and Motor Skills, 77*, 115–122.

Courneya, K. S., Plotnikoff, R. C., Hotz, S. B., & Birkett, N. J. (2000). Social support and the theory of planned behavior in the exercise domain. *American Journal of Health Promotion, 24*, 300–308.

Culos-Reed, S. N., Gyurcsik, N. C., & Brawley, L. R. (2001). Using theories of motivated behavior to understand physical activity: Perspectives on their influence. In R. N. Singer, H. A. Hausenblas, & C. M. Janelle (Eds.), *Handbook of research on sport psychology* (2nd ed.) (pp. 695-717). New York, NY: John Wiley.

de Vries, H., Mesters, I., van de Steeg, H., & Honing, C. (2005). The general public's information needs and perceptions regarding hereditary cancer: An application of the integrated change model. *Patient Education and Counseling, 56*, 154–165.

Estabrooks, P. A. & Carron, A. V. (1998). The conceptualization and effect of control beliefs on exercise attendance in the elderly. *Journal of Aging and Health, 10*, 441–457.

Fishbein, M. & Ajzen, I. (1975). *Belief, attitude, intention, and behavior.* Don Mills, NY: Addison-Wesley.

Fuchs, R. (1996). Causal models of physical exercise participation: Testing the predictive power of the construct "pressure to change." *Journal Applied Social Psychology, 26*, 1931–1960.

Gardner, B. (2014). A review and analysis of the use of 'habit' in understanding, predicting, and influencing health-related behaviour. *Health Psychology Review*. doi:10.1080/17437199.2013.876238

Gardner, B., de Bruijn, G. J., & Lally, P. (2011). A systematic review and meta-analysis of applications of the Self-Report Habit Index to nutrition and physical activity behaviors. *Annals of Behavioral Medicine, 42*, 174–187.

Gebel, K., Bauman, A. E., Reger-Nash, B., & Leydon, K. M. (2011). Does the environment moderate the impact of a mass media campaign to promote walking? *American Journal of Health Promotion, 26*, 45–48.

Gollwitzer, P. M., & Brandstatter, V. (1997). Implementation intentions and effective goal pursuit. *Journal of Personality and Social Psychology, 73*, 186–199.

Hagger, M. S., Chatzisarantis, N. L., & Biddle, S. J. (2002). The influence of autonomous and controlling motives on physical activity intentions with the theory of planned behavior. *British Journal of Health Psychology, 7*, 283 – 297.

Hagger, M. S., & Chatzisarantis, N. L. (2009). Integrating the theory of planned behaviour and self-determination theory in health behaviour: A meta-analysis. *British Journal of Health Psychology, 14*, 275–302.

Hagger, M., & Chatzisarantis, N. L. D. (2014). An integrated behavior-change model for physical activity. *Exercise and Sport Sciences Reviews, 42*, 62–69.

Hagger, M., & Luszczynska, A. (2014). Implementation intention and action planning interventions in health contexts: State of the research and proposals for the way forward. *Applied Psychology: Health and Well-Being, 6*, 1–47.

Hall, P. A., & Fong, G. T. (2007). Temporal self-regulation theory: A model for individual health behavior. *Health Psychology Review, 1*, 6–52.

Hausenblas, H. A., Carron, A. V., & Mack, D. (1997). Application of theories of reasoned action and planned behavior to exercise behavior: A meta-analysis. *Journal of Sport & Exercise Psychology, 19*, 36 – 51.

Hausenblas, H. A., Giacobbi, P., Cook, B., Rhodes, R., & Cruz, A. (2011). Prospective examination of pregnant and nonpregnant women's physical activity beliefs and behaviors. *Journal of Infant and Reproductive Psychology, 29*, 308–319.

Hausenblas, H. A., & Symons Downs, D. (2004). Prospective examination of the theory of planned behavior applied to exercise behavior during women's first trimester of pregnancy. *Journal of Reproductive and Infant Psychology, 22*, 199–210.

Heckhausen, H., & Gollwitzer, P. M. (1987). Thought contents and cognitive functioning in motivational and volitional states of mind. *Motivation and Emotion, 11*, 101–120. doi:10.1007/BF00992338

James, W. (n. d.). *BrainyQuote.com*. Retrieved August 19, 2015, from BrainyQuote.com website: http://www.brainyquote.com/quotes/quotes/w/williamjam157168.html. Read more at http://www.brainyquote.com/citation/quotes/quotes/w/williamjam157168.html#x8DpS5ooSp37bJjR.99

Jones, L. W., Guill, B., Keir, S. T., Carter, K., Friedman, H. S., Bigner, D. D., & Reardon, D. A. (2007). Using the theory of planned behavior to understand the determinants of exercise intention in patients diagnosed with primary brain cancer. *Psycho-Oncology, 16*, 232–240.

Karvinen, K. H., Courneya, K. S., Campbell, K. L., Pearcey, R. G., Dundas, G., Capstick, V., & Tonkin, K. (2007). Correlates of exercise motivation and behavior in a population-based sample of endometrial cancer survivors: An application of the theory of planned behavior. *International Journal of Behavioral Nutrition and Physical Activity, 4*, 20–30.

Kwan, B. M., & Bryan, A. D. (2010). Affective response to exercise as a component of exercise motivation: Attitudes, norms, self-efficacy, and temporal stability on intentions. *Psychology of Sport and Exercise, 11*, 71–79.

Lowe, S. S., Danielson, B., Beaumont, C., Watanabe, S. M., Baracos, V. W., & Courneya, K. S. (2015). Correlates of objectively measured sedentary behavior in cancer patients with brain metastases: An application of the theory of planned behavior. *Psycho-Oncology*. doi:10.1002/pon.3641

Manning, M. (2009). The effects of subjective norms on behaviour in the theory of planned behaviour: A meta-analysis. *British Journal of Social Psychology, 48*, 649–705.

McEachan, R. R. C., Conner, M., Taylor, N., & Lawton, R.J. (2011). Prospective prediction of health-related behaviors with the theory of planned behavior: A meta-analysis. *Health Psychology Review, 5*, 97–144.

Plotnikoff, R. C., Costigan, S. A., Karunamuni, N., & Lubans, D. R. (2013). Social cognitive theories used to explain physical activity behavior in adolescents: A systematic review and meta-analysis. *Preventive Medicine, 56*, 245–253.

Plotnikoff, R. C., Lippke, S., Courneya, K., Birkett, N., & Sigal, R. (2010). Physical activity and diabetes: An application of the theory of planned behavior to explain physical activity for type 1 and type 2 diabetes in an adult population sample. *Psychology and Health, 25*, 7–23.

Prapavessis, H., Gaston, A., & DeJesus, S. (2015). The theory of planned behavior as a model for understanding sedentary behavior. *Psychology of Sport and Exercise, 19*, 23–32.

Reger, B., Cooper, L., Booth-Butterfield, S., Smith, H., Bauman, A., Wootan, M., … Greer, F. (2002). Wheeling Walks: A community campaign using paid media to encourage walking among sedentary older adults. *Preventive Medicine, 35*, 285–292.

Reger-Nash, B., Bauman, A., Booth-Butterfield, S., Cooper, L., & Smith, H. (2005). Wheeling Walks. Evaluation of a media-based community intervention. *Family & Community Health, 28*, 64–78.

Reger-Nash, B., Bauman, A., Cooper, L., Chey, T., Simon, K. J., Brann, M., & Leyden, K. M. (2008). WV Walks: Replication with expanded reach. *Journal of Physical Activity and Health, 5*, 19–27.

Reger-Nash, B., Fell, P., Spicer, D., Fisher, B. D., Cooper, L., Chey, T., & Bauman, A. (2006). BC Walks: Replication of a communitywide physical activity campaign. *Preventing Chronic Disease, 3*, 1–12.

Rhodes, R. E., Blanchard, C. M., & Blacklock, R. E. (2008). Do physical activity beliefs differ by age and gender? *Journal of Sport and Exercise Psychology, 30*, 412–423.

Rhodes, R. E., & Courneya, K. S. (2002). Relationships between personality, an extended theory of planned behaviour model, and exercise behaviour. *British Journal of Health Psychology, 8*, 19–36.

Rhodes, R. E., & de Bruijn, G. J. (2013a). What predicts intention-behavior discordance? A review of the action control framework. *Exercise and Sports Sciences Reviews, 41*, 201–207.

Rhodes, R. E., & de Bruijn, G. J. (2013b). How big is the physical activity intention-behaviour gap? A meta-analysis using the action control framework. *British Journal of Health Psychology, 18*, 296–309.

Rhodes, R. E., Jones, L. W., & Courneya, K. S. (2002). Extending the theory of planned behavior in the exercise domain: A comparison of social support and subjective norm. *Research Quarterly in Exercise and Sport, 73*, 193–199.

Schwarzer, R. (2008). Modeling health behavior change: How to predict and modify the adoption and maintenance of health behaviors. *Applied Psychology, 57*, 1–29.

Symons Downs, D., & Hausenblas, H. A. (2005a). Elicitation studies and the theory of planned behavior: A systematic review of exercise beliefs. *Psychology of Sport and Exercise, 6*, 1–31.

Symons Downs, D., & Hausenblas, H. A. (2005b). Exercise behavior and the theories of reasoned action and planned behavior: A meta-analytic update. *Journal of Physical Activity and Health, 2*, 76–97.

Sniehotta, F. F., Presseau, J., & Araujo-Soares, V. (2014). Time to retire the theory of planned behavior. *Health Psychology Review, 8*, 1–7.

Sweet, S. N., Martin Ginis, K. A., & Latimer-Cheung, A. E. (2012). Examining physical activity trajectories for people with spinal cord injury. *Health Psychology, 31*, 728–732.

Terry, D. J., & O'Leary, J. E. (1995). The theory of planned behaviour: The effects of perceived behavioural control and self-efficacy. *British Journal of Social Psychology, 34*, 199–220.

Vallance, J. K., Courneya, K. S., Plotnikoff, R. C., & Mackey, J. R. (2008). Analyzing theoretical mechanisms of physical activity behavior change in breast cancer survivors: Results from the activity promotion (ACTION) trial. *Annals of Behavioral Medicine, 35*, 150–158.

Wegner, D. M. (2002). *The illusion of conscious will*. Cambridge, MA: MIT Press.

Whitford, H. M., & Jones, M. (2011). An exploration of the motivation of pregnant women to perform pelvic floor exercises using the revised theory of planned behaviour. *British Journal of Health Psychology, 16*, 761–778.

Transtheoretical Model

Runner: © lzf/Shutterstock

Vignette: Gina

The way I saw it, the sole purpose of going to the gym or forcing yourself to run, walk, or bike outdoors was just to be skinny. Because I was never a fan of the outdoors the idea that one could engage in sustained physical activity for pleasure struck me as absurd. And since I could always shimmy into a size 4 dress I didn't see why I'd have to start an exercise program—especially since I'd made it to my 30s maintaining a healthy weight.

But then my doctor discovered I had high blood pressure, high blood sugar, and high cholesterol during an annual physical. I was floored. "Doesn't this only happen to people who are overweight?" I asked her. Apparently not.

During that visit—and after a fair bit of Googling "normal weight obesity"—I learned that even if a person (such as myself) has a normal BMI and thin frame, she could still be at risk for cardiovascular disease, hypertension, and metabolic syndrome. It comes down to how much body fat she has on her—not just her weight.

Apparently, my body fat levels were higher than I wanted to admit. And because a few of my maternal aunts and uncles suffered from heart disease, my doctor urged me to try walking or biking to and from work, possibly joining a gym, or investing in some kind of cardio trainer for my home.

My initial reaction was "yeah, right." I thought *maybe* I could cut back on the penne al forno and other cheesy pasta

LEARNING OBJECTIVES

After completing this chapter, you will be able to

- Describe the constructs of the transtheoretical model.
- Discuss the physical activity research that has applied the transtheoretical model.
- Discuss the advantages and limitations of the transtheoretical model.

dishes that had been staples of my diet since my Italian grandmother taught me how to make them when I was a kid. But join a gym? I barely owned a functional pair of sneakers.

The doctor thought maybe yoga or a stationary bike would be better alternatives. I decided to give the former a shot but after three agonizing classes where I could barely hold a "downward-facing dog" for 15 seconds, I called it quits. Exercise simply wasn't for me.

But then the recession hit, and I was laid off from my full-time high school teaching position. For many months, I was only able to secure part-time work, and I ended up facing long stretches of free time that I truly didn't know what on earth I'd do with.

A girlfriend of mine implored me to come take some dance class with her called *Zumba* that she'd grown increasingly obsessed with. I refused countless times until she promised to take me for gelato afterwards if I came with her on a Saturday. I acquiesced and ended up humiliating myself in a roomful of women far more adept at moving to a beat than I was.

When that same friend suggested we go for a hike the following week, my initial reaction was a resounding "no." But she offered to make it more about photography and brought along her fancy XLR digital camera. Because there was something artistic involved I thought, *fine.*

I enjoyed the hike. Mostly because it was with my friend and there weren't any intimidating fitness instructors barking orders at us to keep moving. (Nor was there a gaggle of women far fitter than myself that might judge me for being out of sync with any music.)

Over the next few months, we'd regularly meet on weekend mornings to lightly trek the trails and state parks within a reasonable driving distance from our homes in Cincinnati. It got to the point where I even had to buy a new pair of sneakers in order to sustain the growing habit. And eventually, I was really coming to look forward to these hikes—sometimes even doing them on my own on days where I didn't have work or my friend wasn't available.

My doctor was pretty pleased with my progress as well. When I returned to her for the my next annual physical, my cholesterol and blood sugar levels had come down a bit and my body fat percentage had gone down.

And then I was offered a full-time teaching job at a charter school in Indiana, requiring me to relocate away from my friend and away from our stomping grounds.

I took the job. I had to. I desperately needed the money, and the position was one I'd been hoping to land for months. I planned on staying active after I'd settled into my new (thankfully, larger) home, an apartment within walking distance of the new school. But once classes began and the stresses of adapting to a new environment piled up, my interest in finding a new hiking trail and recommitting to regular walks vastly diminished. By the end of my first year at the new job, I'd gone back to spending weekends cooking high-fat, high-carb recipes; avoiding physical activity; and feeling my body succumb to fatigue.

I've been working in Indiana for over a year now. And periodically I get back in the habit of exercising. (Usually, during the summers, when I don't have to teach full time.) I have a gym membership to a fitness center, and every so often I'll go there to watch television while I cycle on a stationary bike or elliptical machine. But I'm sorry to say that it's harder to maintain my interest in fitness when I don't have a friend motivating me nor an innate love of physical activity.

To help keep myself moving (not because I love to but because I feel like I should for my health—and my new doctor agrees), I did, however, take a measure that's proven to be quite effective. A few months ago I adopted a rambunctious Boston terrier from my local humane society.

Having to take this adorable pup out in the morning, afternoon, and evening forces me to be on my feet. And as soon as he gets accustomed to his new abode, like I had to, I plan on taking him with me on some of the nearby hiking trails I've been researching. (I will, of course, be sending my former friend back in Ohio any and all pictures I end up snapping on the refurbished XLR she sent me for my birthday several weeks ago.)

■ Introduction

For most people, changing unhealthy behaviors to healthy behaviors is often challenging. Change usually does not occur all at once; it may be a lengthy process that involves progressing through several stages. The concept of stages—or a "one size does not fit all" philosophy (Marcus, King, Clark, Pinto, & Bock, 1996)—forms the basis for the transtheoretical model of behavior change (also sometimes referred to as the *stages of change model*) developed by James Prochaska and his colleagues at the University of Rhode Island. This model emerged from a comparative analysis of leading theories of psychotherapy and behavior change. In developing the model, the goal was to provide a systematic integration of a field that had fragmented into more than 300 theories of psychotherapy (Marcus et al., 1996). The transtheoretical model includes five constructs—stages of change, decisional balance, processes of change, self-efficacy, and temptation—that are considered important in understanding the process of volitional change. After its initial application with smoking cessation, the model was extended in an attempt to better understand a broad range of health and mental health behaviors such as nutrition, weight control, alcohol abuse, eating disorders, unplanned pregnancy protection, mammography screening, sun exposure, substance abuse, and physical activity (Prochaska & Velicer, 1997). The latter, of course, represents the focus in this chapter.

■ Constructs of the Transtheoretical Model

The transtheoretical model has five main constructs: stages of change, decisional balance, processes of change, self-efficacy, and temptation. Each of these constructs is outlined in greater detail in this section.

Stages of Change

One of the major contributions of the transtheoretical model to the health field is the suggestion that behavior change unfolds slowly over time through a series of stages. Benjamin Franklin recognized this fact over 300 years ago when he noted:

> To get the bad customs of a country changed and new ones, thought better, introduced, it is necessary first to remove the prejudices of the people, enlighten their ignorance, and convince them that their interests will be promoted by the proposed changes; and this is not the work of a day.
> (cited in U.S. Department of Health and Human Services, 1999, p. 73)

The **stages of change** construct has three aspects. First, stages fall somewhere between traits and states. Traits are stable and are not open to immediate change. States, in contrast, are readily changeable and typically lack stability. Thus, for example, an individual who is chronically anxious would be characterized as having have high trait anxiety. Conversely, an individual who has severe butterflies before a race would be known to possess high state anxiety.

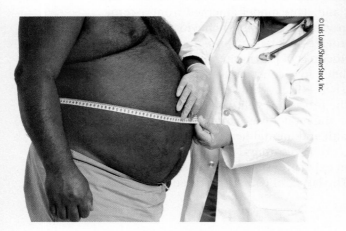

© iStock.com/Terry J Alcorn

© Luis Louro/ShutterStock, Inc.

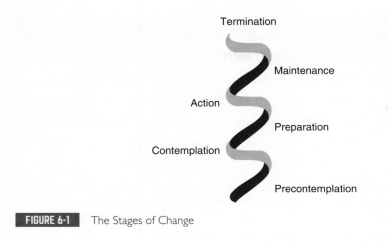

FIGURE 6-1   The Stages of Change

Second, stages are both stable and dynamic; that is, although stages may last for a considerable period, they are susceptible to change. Prochaska and DiClemente (1982, 1986) have hypothesized that as individuals change from an unhealthy to a healthy behavior they move through a number of stages at varying rates and in a cyclical fashion, with periods of progression and relapse. For example, a sedentary person may begin to think about the benefits (e.g., have more energy) and costs (e.g., time away from watching television) of physical activity. Then, a few months later, he or she may buy a pair of walking shoes. Six months later he or she may go walking three times a week. After a year of walking regularly, however, this individual may become overwhelmed with the stress of work and stop walking. The cessation of physical activity would represent a regression to an earlier stage. In short, individuals going through the process of behavioral change are thought to cycle (or progress and relapse) through a series of stages as they recognize the need to change, contemplate making a change, make the change, and, finally, sustain the new behavior. **FIGURE 6-1** provides a graphic illustration of the stages of change.

Third, people pass through six stages in attempting any health behavior change: (1) precontemplation (not intending to make changes); (2) contemplation (intending to make changes within the foreseeable future, which is defined as the next 6 months); (3) preparation (intending to change in the immediate future, which is defined as within 1 month); (4) action (actively engaging in the new behavior); (5) maintenance (sustaining change over time); and (6) termination (the probability of relapse is eliminated) (Reed, Velicer, Prochaska, Rossi, & Marcus, 1997). Operational definitions for the various stages are outlined in **TABLE 6-1**. A more comprehensive description of each stage is provided in the following discussion.

TABLE 6-1	Operational Definitions of the Stages of Exercise Change
Stage	**Operational Definition**
Precontemplation	I do not intend to begin exercising in the next 6 months.
Contemplation	I intend to begin exercising in the next 6 months.
Preparation	I intend to begin exercising regularly in the next 30 days.
Action	I have been exercising, but for less than 6 months.
Maintenance	I have been exercising for more than 6 months.

Adapted from Reed, G. R., Velicer, W. F., Prochaska, J. O., Rossi, J. S., & Marcus, B. H. (1997). What makes a good staging algorithm: Examples from regular exercise. *American Journal of Health Promotion, 12*, 57–66.

Precontemplation ("I won't" or "I can't")

People in the precontemplation stage are not considering change or do not want to change their behavior. The so-called "couch potato" is an example of someone who may fall into the precontemplation stage. Precontemplators typically deny having a problem and have no intention of making a behavior change in the fore-seeable future. As Table 6-1 states, "the foreseeable future" is typically defined as within the next 6 months—the period of time most people might use if they are considering a behavior change (Prochaska & Velicer, 1997).

The hallmark of precontemplation is a lack of intention to take action, regardless of the reason or excuse (Reed et al., 1997). Thus, insofar as adopting physical activity is concerned, an individual may be in precontemplation because he or she does not think it is valuable or thinks it is valuable but may be overwhelmed by barriers such as lack of time. Precontemplators are considered the most difficult people to stimulate into behavioral change.

Gabriella Reed (1999) reported the existence of two types of precontempla-tors, each of whom have different reasons for not planning to engage in physical activity. Precontemplation *nonbelievers* either do not believe in regular physical activity or do not see the value of engaging in it. Precontemplation *believers* do believe that physical activity is a worthwhile behavior; however, they cannot seem to start intending to participate in it. The precontemplation nonbelievers would conceivably need to become aware of and learn to appreciate the "pros," or benefits, of physical activity, such as improving mood states and energy levels. By contrast, precontemplation believers need help overcoming the "cons," or costs, of exercising, such as taking time away from other activities (Reed, 1999).

Contemplation ("I might")

Individuals in the contemplation stage are thinking about changing their behavior sometime within the next 6 months. They see a need for change because they are aware of the costs and benefits of changing their behavior. For example, they may realize that physical activity reduces their risk of developing heart disease (this represents a benefit of exercise). However, they also acknowledge that physical activity will take time away from doing other things, such as working and spending time with family and friends (this represents a cost of exercise). Contemplators are conceived as being open to new information and interested in knowing more about the benefits of change. At this stage, however, people are not committed to the change; they are only contemplating or thinking about it. Therefore, they may become "chronic contemplators," never moving beyond the information-gathering phase (Prochaska & Velicer, 1997; Reed, 1999).

Preparation ("I will")

In the preparation stage, people are seriously considering or planning to change their activity level in near the future, usually within the next month. The preparation stage has both a behavioral and an intentional component. For example, preparers may have bought a pair of running shoes, joined a running club, and even gone for a half hour walk once a week. They may also intend to increase the frequency of their walk from once a week to three times a week within the next month. These individuals often have strong incentives to change based upon optimistic views about the beneficial outcomes. Preparation is a relatively unstable stage because people in this stage are more likely than precontemplators or contemplators to progress over the next 6 months. Not surprisingly, this stage is the most controversial in terms of measurement because it can represent both behavioral (e.g., some physical activity, but not regular activity) and/or intentional properties (e.g., intend to act within the month but not doing physical activity) (Reed et al., 1997).

Action ("I am")

Individuals who have recently changed their behavior (i.e., within the last 6 months) are considered to be in the action stage. This is the stage that requires the greatest commitment of time and energy. To be classified within the action stage insofar as physical activity is concerned, the individual must meet the minimal physical activity recommendations developed by public health agencies (Canadian Society for Exercise Physiology, 2011; USDHHS, 2010). For example, in Canada and the United States, recommendations state that adults should accumulate 150 minutes or more of at least moderate-intensity (e.g., brisk walking) physical activity each week. Because the person in the action stage has only recently established the new activity pattern, attentiveness is necessary because relapse is probable (Reed, 1999).

Maintenance ("I have")

Once the individual has been regularly active for 6 consecutive months, he or she is deemed to have progressed into the maintenance stage. Although the new behavior has become better established, boredom and a loss of focus could become a danger to relapse. The constant vigilance initially required to establish a new activity pattern is exhausting and difficult to sustain. It is at this time that a person works to reinforce the gains made through the various stages of change and strives to prevent lapses and relapses (Nigg et al., 2011; Reed, 1999).

Termination

Once a behavior has been maintained for over 5 years, the individual is considered to have exited from the cycle of change, and a fear of relapse is eliminated. This stage is the ultimate goal for all people searching for a healthier lifestyle. Termination is the stage in which the person has no temptation to engage in the old behavior and shows 100% self-efficacy in all previously tempting situations.

CRITICAL THINKING ACTIVITY 6-1

© ecco/Shutterstock, Inc.

The termination stage seems relevant for cessation behaviors where a person is just trying to stop a behavior, such as smoking, but does it make sense for acquisition behaviors, where the goal is to keep on going? Can you ever really be "invulnerable" to missing physical activity?

Decisional Balance

Decision making was first conceptualized by Janis and Mann (1977) as a decisional "balance sheet" that assesses the importance that an individual places on the potential advantages, or pros, and disadvantages, or cons, of a behavior. The balance between the pros and cons varies depending on which stage of change the individual is in. When the cons of exercise (e.g., takes time away from other activities) are of greater importance than the pros of exercise (e.g., improves psycho-

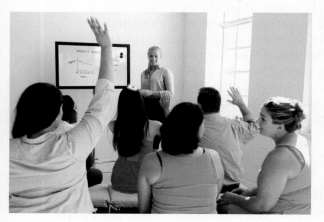

logical well-being), motivation to change behavior (i.e., to move from being inactive to engaging in physical activity) is thought to be low. Thus, for example, in the precontemplation and contemplation stages, the cons are assumed to outweigh the pros. In the preparation stage, the pros and cons are believed to be relatively equal. Finally, in the action, maintenance, and termination stages, the pros are thought to outweigh the cons. Carlos DiClemente and his colleagues (1991) proposed that assessing the pros and cons is relevant for understanding and predicting transitions among the first three stages of change (i.e., precontemplation, contemplation, and preparation). During the action and maintenance stages, however, these **decisional balance** measures are thought to be much less important predictors of progress.

Processes of Change

According to the transtheoretical model, the 10 **processes of change** represent the behaviors, cognitions, and emotions that people engage in during the course of changing a behavior. These have been proposed to collapse into five experiential processes and five behavioral processes (Prochaska & Velicer, 1997). The experiential processes include: (1) consciousness raising (gathering information and determining the pros and cons of the positive behavior); (2) counterconditioning (substituting a positive behavior for a negative one); (3) dramatic relief (experiencing and expressing feelings about the consequences of the positive behavior); (4) environmental reevaluation (being a role model and considering how the negative behavior impacts significant others); and (5) self-reevaluation (instilling the positive behaviors as an integral component of self-image). The behavioral processes include: (1) helping relationships (getting social support and using significant others to effect change); (2) reinforcement management (being rewarded by the self or others for engaging in the positive behavior); (3) social liberation (taking advantage of social situations that encourage the positive behavior); (4) stimulus control (using cues as a catalyst for the positive behavior); and (5) self-liberation (becoming committed to the positive behavior). It is postulated that the experiential processes are more important to the earlier three stages, whereas the later stages rely on the behavioral process of change to move to the next stage. **TABLE 6-2** outlines the various processes of change and provides a description for each. The processes of change provide information on *how* shifts in behavior occur.

CRITICAL THINKING ACTIVITY 6-2

© ecco/Shutterstock, Inc.

The processes of change represent behavioral and mental strategies that people use to change their behavior. Think of some behaviors you have changed in the past. What strategies did you employ to make the change, if any? Do they resemble the processes of change outlined in the transtheoretical model, or were they different?

Self-Efficacy

Self-efficacy is a judgment regarding one's ability to perform a behavior required to achieve a certain outcome. Not surprisingly, it is believed to be critical to behavior change (Bandura, 1997). Self-efficacy is proposed to change with each stage, presumably increasing as the individual gains confidence (Prochaska & DiClemente, 1982). Conversely, self-efficacy may decrease if an individual falters and spirals back to an earlier stage.

TABLE 6-2	**The Processes of Change**
Classic Term	**Description**
Consciousness raising	Gathering information about regular physical activity (learning the pros and cons of exercising)
Counterconditioning	Substituting sedentary behavior with activity
Dramatic relief	Experiencing and expressing feelings about the consequences of the positive behavior
Environmental reevaluation	Consideration and assessment of how inactivity affects friends, family, and citizens
Helping relationships	Getting support for your intention to exercise
Self-reevaluation	Appraising one's self-image as a healthy regular exerciser
Social liberation	Taking advantage of social policy, customs, and mores that enhance physical activity (e.g., New Year's resolutions)
Reinforcement management	Rewarding oneself or being rewarded by others for making changes
Stimulus control	Using cues to remember to engage in physical activity
Self-liberation	Committing oneself to becoming or staying a regular exerciser

Adapted from Reed, G. R. (1999). Adherence to exercise and the transtheoretical model of behavior change. In S. Bull (Ed.), *Adherence issues in sport and exercise* (pp. 19–46). New York, NY: John Wiley & Sons.

Temptation

Temptation represents the intensity of the urges to engage in a specific behavior when in the midst of difficult situations (Grimley, Prochaska, Velicer, Blais, & DiClemente, 1994). Temptation and self-efficacy function inversely across the stages of change, with temptation proposed as a predictor of relapses and self-efficacy as a predictor of progression.

◼ Advantages and Limitations of the Transtheoretical Model

Advantages

The advantages of the transtheoretical model to understanding physical activity behavior change have been detailed in various commentaries across the years

(Armitage, 2009; Nigg et al., 2011; Reed, 1999). Claudio Nigg and colleagues (2011) have commented on the intuitive appeal of the model for allied health professions when understanding readiness for change, and this was also noted by Gabrielle Reed (1999) in earlier work. The staging construct provides for the opportunity to match interventions to the different needs of individuals. As a consequence, researchers and healthcare professionals are able to target specific interventions for the total population (i.e., those who have not yet made a behavior change and are at risk, as well as those who have changed but may be at risk of relapse). For example, limited success has been observed for traditional interventions in terms of promoting the adoption and maintenance of a physically active lifestyle. According to the transtheoretical model, this lack of success may be attributed, in part, to the fact that an educational focus has been utilized rather than a behavioral and motivational focus. Many inactive individuals are not ready to adopt regular exercise because they are unmotivated. Thus, providing them with advice and a physical activity prescription is unlikely to lead to behavior change. Therefore, the traditional physical activity intervention may fail to recruit the vast majority of inactive individuals because they have no intention of becoming active. This reflects an incongruity between what is typically offered (action-oriented programs) and population motivational readiness to change (inactive and not intending to become active). Consequently, it is important to customize interventions to meet the specific motivational needs of the majority of individuals who are either inactive or underactive.

A second advantage is that adopting a stages of change approach provides for the opportunity to subdivide the at-risk population into precontemplation, contemplation, and preparation stages. This identification of the three types of people at risk allows healthcare professionals to proactively try to recruit individuals who are most in need but the least likely to react to a physical activity program (i.e., precontemplators and contemplators).

A third advantage is associated with recruitment and retention. An individual's readiness to change can predict the likelihood that that person will successfully adopt and maintain a healthy lifestyle. Recruitment of people at earlier stages can be successful if (1) health professionals proactively target them and (2) an intervention is used that is matched to the specific stage of change. Proactive recruitment by either telephone or a personal letter coupled with stage-matched interventions has resulted in good participation rates (Reed, 1999). As Bess Marcus and her colleagues (2000) stated, "'One-size-fits-all' programs are rarely as effective as programs that tailor treatment to at least some aspects of the individual or group" (p. 39).

Chris Armitage (2009) has also noted the innovation present in the processes of change constructs. Almost all other models applied to understanding physical activity behavior use constructs that attempt to explain "why" people will perform the behavior. The transtheoretical model employs constructs that attempt to explain "why" people change or are resistant to change with constructs such as self-efficacy, decisional balance, and temptation, but it also includes constructs that attempt to understand "how" people change with the processes of change.

These are relatively unique to the model (Armitage, 2009). Interestingly, reviews of the factors linked to physical activity behavior change have supported the utility of the behavioral processes of change over all other constructs at present (Lewis, Marcus, Pate, & Dunn, 2002; Lubans, Foster, & Biddle, 2008; Rhodes & Pfaeffli, 2010). This supports the innovation of the processes of change within the model.

Limitations

Despite some of the strengths of the model, the validity of the transtheoretical model has been a frequent source of debate over the last 15 years (Adams & White, 2003; Bandura, 1998; Brug et al., 2005; Weinstein, Rothman, & Sutton, 1998). Interested readers are encouraged to seek out these original papers, but the main points of critique are focused on whether a stage of change actually has validity and whether the constructs of the model actually represent a meaningful theoretical framework.

Most of the tests conducted with the stages of change model are descriptive, as opposed to explanatory, and involve cross-sectional designs (Nigg et al., 2011). These descriptive designs have been successful at showing that constructs such as self-efficacy are significantly different across people who report they are at different stages of change. There is far less evidence to demonstrate that people actually go through these stages of change in longitudinal designs. It may be that these stages just describe the population more than they explain the change process. For example, Bandura (1998) stated that stages should reflect qualitative change and provide an invariant and nonreversible sequence. People's progression, however, through the stages of change of the transtheoretical model is reversible (i.e., people can relapse), and advancing from one stage to the next does not reflect a qualitative change (Weinstein, Rothman, & Sutton, 1998). Another related critique of the model is from the sequential differences of the same constructs across the stages rather than different constructs showing importance at single stages but not others. For example, mean values for self-efficacy increase across the stages, but more compelling evidence would be where self-efficacy is only important for one stage transition. Finally, the stages of change construct has been criticized for the time frames attached to each stage (e.g., the action stage is the first 6 months). Certainly, some people could move from action to maintenance much faster than 6 months or move from contemplation to preparation to action in time frames different from that of the current staging. Nigg and colleagues (2011), recognizing the arbitrariness of the time frames, have called for the abandonment of them in favor of other criteria.

The stages of change construct has received the most criticism in the model, but the other constructs and their interrelationships have also received critique. Support for the relationship between the processes of change and decisional balance and the stages of change is equivocal. There is not a consistent pattern for how these constructs change across the stages and whether they have differential predictive utility (Spencer, Adams, Malone, Roy, & Yost, 2006). The transtheoretical model also fails to include the influence of moderator variables (e.g., gender, age, ethnicity) within its frame. Finally, the integration of various theories (e.g., self-efficacy, decisional balance) to develop the transtheoretical model places these theories at odds with each other within the model. An understanding of the ordering for how these constructs interact is not defined, and too often these constructs are treated as single (univariate) variables rather than as a complex (multivariate) theory.

CRITICAL THINKING ACTIVITY 6-3

© ecco/Shutterstock, Inc.

The stages of change construct suggests a deliberative and ongoing progression to change behavior, with 6 months to contemplate, additional time to prepare, and then 6 months to move from action to maintenance. This raises the question about people who change cold turkey. The transtheoretical model does not explain this type of rapid change. Have you ever just changed a behavior very quickly?

■ Physical Activity Research Examining the Transtheoretical Model

Research that uses the transtheoretical model to understand sedentary behavior or sedentary-limiting behaviors (e.g., resisting screen time) is not available at this time, but the model has considerable application in understanding physical activity. The transtheoretical model was first applied to physical activity in the late 1980s by Robert Sonstroem (1987), and since then its popularity in examining physical activity has grown. Bess Marcus and her colleagues were the first to develop self-report instruments to measure the constructs of the transtheoretical model. Through a series of studies, they developed measures for stages of change, self-efficacy, process of change, and decisional balance (Marcus, Selby, Niaura, & Rossi, 1992). Over the last decade, the model has been used to examine physical activity in cross-sectional studies, and to a lesser extent in longitudinal and quasi-experimental intervention studies. The application of the transtheoretical model to physical activity was reviewed in the form of a meta-analysis several years ago (Marshall & Biddle, 2001). More recently, there have been two systematic reviews of the literature (Hutchison, Breckon, & Johnston, 2009; Spencer et al., 2006) and a recent review of future research practices (Nigg et al., 2011).

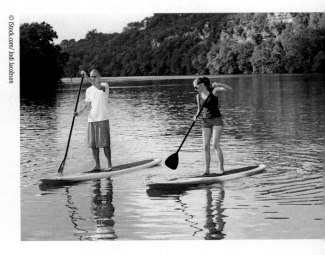

© iStock.com/Jodi Jacobson

Observational Studies

Most of the existing research on the transtheoretical model has been conducted with cross-sectional or short longitudinal designs (Marshall & Biddle, 2001; Spencer et al., 2006). In general, these studies have shown that mean differences occur across stage membership for the constructs of self-efficacy, decisional balance, and processes of change (Marshall & Biddle, 2001; Spencer et al., 2006). Probably the most consistent construct to show differences by stages of change is self-efficacy. For example, Gorely and Godon (1995) in a study of Australian adults 50 to 65 years of age found that self-efficacy to overcome barriers to exercise increased systematically from precontemplation to contemplation to preparation to action to maintenance.

Some research has demonstrated possible deviations of the transtheoretical model from smoking research when compared to physical activity. For example, research on the termination stage for physical activity is limited and generally suggests that it may not be applicable to many people. Courneya and Bobick (2000) found no evidence for this stage. Cardinal (1999) also examined if a termination stage exists for physical activity, surveying 551 adults, and found that only 16.6% were classified within the termination stage.

Similar findings have been identified with the temptation construct. For example, Nigg and colleagues recently showed that the temptation construct was not predictive of stage of change after considering self-efficacy in the prediction equation (Nigg, McCurdy, et al., 2009). It may be that temptation is more relevant to smoking cessation.

Perhaps the biggest deviation from smoking has been with the processes of change construct. Reviews and specific analyses show that the currently conceived processes of change do not work well with physical activity in their proposed structure (i.e., five behavioral and five experiential) or potentially their content (Marshall & Biddle, 2001; Nigg, Norman, Rossi, & Benisovich, 1999; Nigg, Lippke, & Maddock, 2009; Rhodes, Berry, Naylor, & Wharf Higgins, 2004). This would make sense, as different strategies for changing physical activity compared to smoking seem possible. Continued work on creating relevant constructs for the processes of change has been recommended (Nigg et al., 2011).

CRITICAL THINKING ACTIVITY 6-4

© ecco/Shutterstock, Inc.

The transtheoretical model suggests that different people need different types of intervention depending on their readiness for physical activity. This model suggests that these differences are based on decisional balance, self-efficacy, and the processes of change; however, there may be other aspects of an intervention: Consider culture, health status, age, gender, and physical activity background aspects. What might you change for people who differ on these variables? Would those changes be limited to just the constructs of the transtheoretical model?

Intervention Research

Two systematic reviews have identified experimental evidence for the transtheoretical model to evaluate whether interventions can move people to later stages of change. Spencer and colleagues (2006) outlined 38 studies from which to draw conclusions about the model, while Hutchinson and colleagues (2009) used 34 studies. Bess Marcus and her colleagues (1992) conducted the first intervention study based on the transtheoretical model. The intervention was designed to increase the adoption of physical activity among 610 community volunteers. At baseline, 39% of the participants were in the contemplation stage, 37% were in the preparation stage, and 24% were in the action stage. A 6-week stage-matched intervention consisting of three different sets of self-help materials, a resource manual describing activity options, and weekly fun walks and activity nights were delivered. A subsample of 236 participants were telephoned following the study to determine the efficacy of the intervention. The results showed that 17% of subjects were in contemplation, 24% were in preparation, and 59% were in action, thus demonstrating that subjects had become significantly more active during the intervention.

Hutchinson and colleagues (2009) point out that many of the interventions have not focused on trying to change all of the constructs in the model, which could limit its ability to change physical activity. They note that all interventions have used the stages of change in intervention development, but more interventions have used the processes of change (71%) and pros/cons (63%) than self-efficacy (33%) in interventions. They further note that 86% of the interventions that used all of the transtheoretical model constructs in the intervention were successful at showing physical activity change, whereas only 71% of the studies that applied a few of the constructs were successful.

The most compelling validation for the transtheoretical model comes from experimental tests to attempt to "match" or "mismatch" people on their interventions, corresponding to their stage of change. For example, people who are in the contemplation stage receive either an intervention package targeting the contemplation stage (match) or a package targeting the maintenance stage (mismatch), and the success of the intervention in moving people to preparation is evaluated. To this end, Spencer and colleagues (2006) identified 15 studies in their systematic review that had examined this procedure. Nine of these studies showed some evidence for the superiority of the stage-matched intervention, indicating some support for the internal validity of the transtheoretical model. These effects were within the small effect size range, but they spanned all stages (Nigg et al., 2011). Thus, there is enough evidence to continue research on the stages of change construct, but more of these tests are recommended before any definitive conclusions can be drawn as to whether the stages of change construct is valid (Nigg et al., 2011).

For example, in a worksite intervention study, Bess Marcus and her colleagues (1998) used the transtheoretical model constructs to design an intervention to increase the initiation, adoption, and maintenance of physical activity among 1,559 employees. The employees were randomized into either a stage-matched

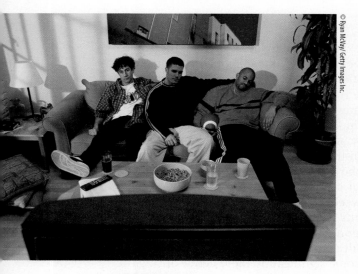

© Ryan McVay/ Getty Images Inc.

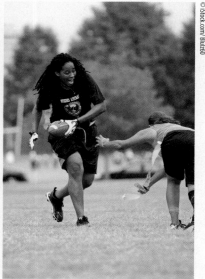

© iStock.com/ Blulz60

self-help intervention or a standard self-help intervention. Printed physical activity promotion materials were given to subjects at baseline and again 1 month later. The stage-matched group received a motivationally tailored intervention that consisted of five manuals. Each manual focused on one of the stages of change. In comparison, the standard self-help intervention consisted of five manuals on physical activity developed by the American Heart Association. These manuals were used because they represent typical action-oriented material available to the public. Assessments of motivational readiness for physical activity and time spent in physical activity participation were conducted at the beginning of the program and 3 months later. At the 3-month follow-up, more individuals in the stage-matched group demonstrated positive changes than individuals in the standard self-help group. Conversely, more individuals in the standard self-help group failed to progress to another stage or even showed regression to an earlier stage compared to the stage-matched group.

■ Summary

This chapter examined the transtheoretical model and its application to physical activity behavior. Over the last decade, the transtheoretical model has been increasingly applied to examine physical activity behavior in cross-sectional studies and to a lesser extent in longitudinal and quasi-experimental intervention studies. The core constructs of the model are the stages of change, processes of change, decisional balance, self-efficacy, and temptation. The most frequently examined construct of the transtheoretical model in the exercise domain has been the stages of change construct. The stages of change construct assesses people's progression and regression through five main stages as they attempt to become physically active: precontemplation (not intending to make changes), contemplation (intending to make changes in the foreseeable future), preparation (immediate intention to change), action (actively engaging in the new behavior), and maintenance (sustaining change over time).

The processes of change are the overt and covert activities that individuals use to alter their experiences and environments to modify behavior change. Decisional balance focuses on the benefits (pros) and costs (cons) of a behavior and is thought to be important in the decision-making process. Self-efficacy is a judgment regarding one's ability to perform a behavior required to achieve a certain outcome. Finally, temptation is the intensity of urges to engage in a specific habit when in the midst of difficulty.

KEY TERMS

decisional balance
processes of change
self-efficacy

stages of change
temptation

REVIEW QUESTIONS

1. List and describe each of the six stages of change of the transtheoretical model.

2. Explain how self-efficacy, decisional balance, and the processes of change are expected to operate across the stages of change, according to Prochaska and DiClemente (1982).

3. Outline some of the potential advantages of the transtheoretical model.

4. Which construct in the transtheoretical model has the most validation? Which construct has received the most criticism?

APPLYING THE CONCEPTS

1. From her first visit to the doctor to her second, what stages of change did Gina progress through?

2. By the end of her story, has Gina arrived at the termination stage of the transtheoretical model? Why or why not?

REFERENCES

Adams, J., & White, M. (2003). Are activity promotion interventions based on the transtheoretical model effective? A critical review. *British Journal of Sports Medicine, 37,* 106–114.

Armitage, C. J. (2009). Is there utility in the transtheoretical model? *British Journal of Health Psychology, 14,* 195–210.

Bandura, A. (1997). *Self-efficacy, the exercise of control.* New York, NY: Freeman.

Bandura, A. (1998). Health promotion from the perspective of social cognitive theory. *Psychology and Health, 13,* 623–649.

Brug, J., Conner, M., Harre, N., Kremers, S., McKellar, S., & Whitelaw, S. (2005). The transtheoretical model and stages of change: A critique. Observations by five commentators on the paper by Adams, J. and White, M. (2004) Why don't stage-based activity promotion interventions work? *Health Education Research, 20,* 244–258.

Canadian Society for Exercise Physiology. (2011). Canadian physical activity guidelines for adults 18–64 years. Available at http://www.csep.ca/english/view.asp?x=804

Cardinal, B. J. (1999). Extended stage model for physical activity behavior. *Journal of Human Movement Sciences, 37,* 37–54.

Courneya, K. S., & Bobick, T. M. (2000). No evidence for a termination stage in exercise behaviour change. *Avante, 6,* 75–85.

DiClemente, C. C., Prochaska, J. O., Velicer, W. F., Fairhurst, S., Rossi, J. S., & Velasquez, M. (1991). The process of smoking cessation: An analysis of precontemplation, contemplation, and preparation states of change. *Journal of Consulting and Clinical Psychology, 9,* 295–304.

Gorely, T., & Gordon, S. (1995). An examination of the transtheoretical model and exercise behavior in older adults. *Journal of Sport & Exercise Psychology, 17,* 312–324.

Grimley, D., Prochaska, J. O., Velicer, W. F., Blais, W. F., & DiClemente, C. C. (1994). The transtheoretical model of change. In T. M. Brinthaupt & R. P. Lipka (Eds.), *Changing the sell: Philosophies, techniques, and experiences* (pp. 201–227). Albany, NY: State University of New York.

Hutchison, A. J., Breckon, J. D., & Johnston, L. H. (2009). Physical activity behavior change interventions based on the transtheoretical model: A systematic review. *Health Education & Behavior, 36,* 829–845.

Janis, I. L., & Mann, L. (1977). *Decision-making: A psychological analysis of conflict, choice, and commitment.* New York, NY: Free Press.

Lewis, B. A., Marcus, B., Pate, R. R., & Dunn, A. L. (2002). Psychosocial mediators of physical activity behavior among adults and children. *American Journal of Preventive Medicine, 23*(2 Suppl), 26–35.

Lubans, D. R., Foster, C., & Biddle, S. J. H. (2008). A review of mediators of behavior in interventions to promote physical activity among children and adolescents. *Preventive Medicine, 47,* 463–470.

Marcus, B. H., Banspach, S. W., Lefebvre, J. S., Rossi, R., Carleton, R. A., & Abrams, D. B. (1992). Using the stages of change model to increase the adoption of physical activity among community participants. *American Journal of Health Promotion, 6,* 424–429.

Marcus, B. H., Dubbert, P. M., Forsyth, L. H., McKenzie, T. L., Stone, E. J., Dunn, A. L., & Blair, S. N. (2000). Physical activity behavior change: Issues in adoption and maintenance. *Health Psychology, 19,* 32–41.

Marcus, B. H., Emmons, K. M., Simkin-Silverman, L. R., Linnan, L. A., Taylor, E. R., Bock, B. C.,… Abrams, D. B. (1998). Evaluation of motivationally tailored vs. standard self-help physical activity interventions at the workplace. *American Journal of Health Promotion, 12,* 246–253.

Marcus, B. H., King, T. K., Clark, M. M., Pinto, B. M., & Bock, B. C. (1996). Theories and techniques for promoting physical activity behaviors. *Sports Medicine, 22,* 321–331.

Marcus, B. H., Selby, V. C., Niaura, R. S., & Rossi, J. S. (1992). Self-efficacy and the stages of exercise behavior change. *Research Quarterly for Exercise and Sport, 63,* 60–66.

Marshall, S. J., & Biddle, S. J. H. (2001). The transtheoretical model of behavior change: A meta-analysis of applications to physical activity and exercise. *Annals of Behavioral Medicine, 23,* 229–246.

Nigg, C. R., Geller, K. S., Motl, R. W., Horwath, C. C., Wertin, K. K., & Dishman, R. K. (2011). A research agenda to examine the efficacy and relevance of the transtheoretical model for physical activity behavior. *Psychology of Sport and Exercise, 12,* 7–12.

Nigg, C. R., Lippke, S., & Maddock, J. E. (2009). Factorial invariance of the theory of planned behavior applied to physical activity across gender, age, and ethnic groups. *Psychology of Sport and Exercise, 10,* 219–225.

Nigg, C. R., McCurdy, D. K., McGee, K. A., Motl, R. W., Paxton, R. J., & Horwath, C. C. (2009). Relations among temptations, self-efficacy, and physical activity. *International Journal of Sport and Exercise Psychology, 7,* 230–243.

Nigg, C. R., Norman, G. J., Rossi, J. S., & Benisovich, S. V. (1999). Processes of exercise behavior change: Redeveloping the scale. *Annals of Behavioral Medicine, 21,* S79.

Prochaska, J. O., & DiClemente, C. C. (1982). Transtheoretical therapy: Toward a more integrative model of change. *Psychotherapy: Theory, Research and Practice, 19,* 276–288.

Prochaska, J. O., & DiClemente, C. C. (1986). Toward a comprehensive model of change. In W. R. Miller & N. Heather (Eds.), *Treating addictive behaviors: Processes of change* (pp. 3–27). New York, NY: Plenum.

Prochaska, J. O., & Velicer, W. F. (1997). The transtheoretical model of health behavior change. *American Journal of Health Promotion, 12,* 38–48.

Reed, G. R. (1999). Adherence to exercise and the transtheoretical model of behavior change. In S. Bull (Ed.), *Adherence issues in sport and exercise* (pp. 19–46). New York, NY: John Wiley & Sons.

Reed, G. R., Velicer, W. F., Prochaska, J. O., Rossi, J. S., & Marcus, B. H. (1997). What makes a good staging algorithm: Examples from regular exercise. *American Journal of Health Promotion, 12,* 57–66.

Rhodes, R. E., Berry, T., Naylor, P. J., & Wharf Higgins, S. J. (2004). Three-step validation of exercise processes of change in an adolescent sample. *Measurement in Physical Education and Exercise Science, 8,* 1–20.

Rhodes, R. E., & Pfaeffli, L. A. (2010). Mediators of physical activity behaviour change among adult nonclinical populations: A review update. *International Journal of Behavioral Nutrition and Physical Activity, 7,* 37.

Sonstroem, R. J. (1987). Stage model of exercise adoption. Paper presented at the American Psychological Association, New York, NY.

Spencer, L., Adams, T. B., Malone, S., Roy, L., & Yost, E. (2006). Applying the transtheoretical model to exercise: A systematic and comprehensive review of the literature. *Health Promotion Practice, 7,* 428–443.

U.S. Department of Health and Human Services. (2010). Physical activity for everyone: Recommendations. Retrieved March 27, 2010, from http://www.cdc.gov/physicalactivity/everyone/guidelines/adults.html

Weinstein, N. D., Rothman, A. J., & Sutton, S. R. (1998). Stage theories of health behavior: Conceptual and methodological issues. *Health Psychology, 17,* 290–299.

SECTION 3

Psychological Health Effects of Exercise and Sedentary Behavior

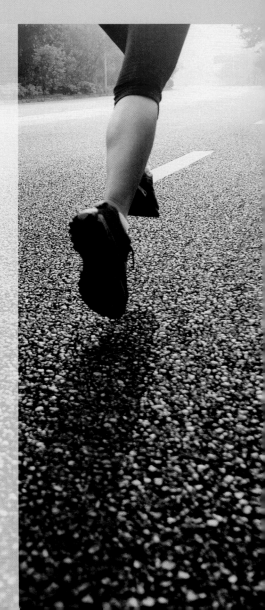

The general purpose of Section 3 is to discuss the antecedents and consequences of physical activity on the individual. In Chapter 7, we discuss the relationship between physical activity and cognitive functioning. In Chapter 8, we examine the effects of physical activity on anxiety and depression. In Chapter 9, the relationship between personality and physical activity is explored. The role of physical activity for self-esteem and body image is reviewed in Chapter 10. Researchers also are interested in the role that physical activity plays in outcomes such as sleep, tolerance for pain, and reactivity to stress, and these topics are discussed in Chapters 11 and 12. Chapter 13 examines the effects of exercise on health-related quality of life and positive psychological variables such as happiness and vigor. Although physical activity is considered almost universally to be a positive behavior, it has become apparent that certain negative behaviors sometimes go hand in hand with exercise. Thus, Chapter 14 outlines the following potential negative effects of exercise: exercise dependence, steroid abuse, muscle dysmorphia, and eating disorders.

Runner: © Izf/Shutterstock

7

Cognition

Runner: © lzf/Shutterstock

Vignette: Mike

Throughout grade school I had trouble focusing. I'm not sure I was alone in this. Most kids in my class were rambunctious and struggled to sit still—more eager to make it to recess than remain inert at an uncomfortable wooden desk. Teachers encouraged my mom to take me to a psychiatrist so that someone could verify whether or not I had ADHD and, potentially, put me on medication. But my mom had a hunch there was a different approach to quelling my excess energy that didn't involve swallowing a pill.

She knew well that the days I had gym class tended to be the ones during which I was able to more easily calm down. She signed me up for an after-school sports program—one where I got to try out everything from basketball to soccer and even roller hockey. I never ended up taking any prescriptions, and mostly was able to do alright as I matured. Once I got to high school it was pretty clear that so long as I could burn off my energy outside of classes I could hold it together while in them.

I think my problems started cropping up in college, when I didn't try out for any teams because I honestly didn't consider myself much of an athlete. Sure, I'd enjoyed sports for most of my adolescent life, but I had no delusions about being any star player. Not having a team to practice with left me little incentive to stay fit. And I wasn't particularly practiced in walking myself through a solo workout at the school's gym.

LEARNING OBJECTIVES

After completing this chapter, you will be able to

- Describe the basic parts of the brain.
- Define *cognition*.
- Describe the relationship between acute and chronic involvement in physical activity and cognitive functioning.
- Describe how physical activity and sedentary behavior are related to cognitive function in children, adults, and older adults.
- Describe how correlational, cross-sectional, and randomized clinical trial designs differ.
- Understand the effects of physical activity on dementia.

159

Needless to say, my time spent exercising dwindled rapidly during my first semester. Shortly after I settled into campus life I picked up the habit of drinking, which further dragged down my fitness. I wanted badly to fit in with my classmates. Looking back, I realize I was seeking a substitute for the camaraderie of being part of a sports team. The surest way to revive that sense of belonging seemed to be chugging beers to the point of blacking out. Exchanging war stories of how many things went wrong during the haze of alcohol-drenched evenings made me feel included and "cool."

I would joke with my college buddies that the so-called freshman 15 would have been preferable. For me, it was more like the freshman 40. By second semester of my freshman year I'd had to buy an entirely new wardrobe—give or take the sweatpants and oversized T-shirts I could still stretch around my newly enlarged waist.

I'll never know if it was the drinking alone or the lack of healthy eating and exercise accompanying it that was to blame, but after my first winter break I felt just like I had in elementary school, when my focus darted around the classroom and I could barely contain my legs from bouncing underneath my desk. Too often, I'd sit through a whole lecture fidgeting madly, biting my nails, and not remembering half of what the professor said because I was too consumed by feelings of restlessness. The only difference was that this time around I was exhausted, often hungover, and increasingly moody.

When I came home for the summer after my first year at college, I was embarrassed when I reconnected with my high school friends. Some of them joked about my weight gain. A few asked me to go for jogs with them but then stopped reaching out to me once I blew them off a couple times.

My mom was the first to swoop in and comment on my laziness. At the time, I felt that she didn't understand and was just being invasive. My dad and her staged what might be likened to an intervention one morning after I'd stumbled home following a late night out on the town. They showed me a picture from my sports playing days and asked me what changed when I left—why I'd decided to completely ignore my health (not to mention my appearance). I was definitely hurt that they were essentially telling me I'd become a really disappointing version of myself. But it was clear that they were more concerned than they were angry.

They decided we should all get a family membership at our local fitness center. The thought of working out alongside my parents was, at first blush, humiliating. But my dad arranged for me to work with a trainer and promised he and my mom wouldn't always be at the gym during the same time as me.

I hated that trainer; in part, because he was so much more fit than I ever could hope to be, even when compared to how I looked during high school, and also because he really took me to task on my drinking—enlightening me to just how many calories a six pack contained—while refusing to let me use being hungover as an excuse to cancel a session.

It took about 3 weeks, if I remember correctly, to actually enjoy the feeling of being physically active again. At first, it was a grueling process filled with self-loathing and anticipation of failure. But after that first week of training I could already feel my mood improving. And by the end of the summer I was even able to join my former high school pals for that previously turned-down jog.

My trainer and I worked to design a fitness plan for when classes started up again. I came back to school armed with some basic body weight exercises to do in my room, and I'd gotten over the intimidation factor of using all that equipment by myself at the school gym.

Being in an environment I associated with drinking made me slip back a bit during the first few weeks of my second year. But I ended up taking advantage of the student health services and seeing a psychologist to deal with the anxiety I had at the prospect of losing friends if I gave up partying. I ended up joining student senate and going to a few student support groups to make some friends who weren't as steeped in the drinking culture as those from my freshman year.

I never gave up drinking entirely. But making fitness a more regular part of my life helped reduce the appeal of alcohol—especially because alcohol interfered with my energy levels and performance. Sure, I'd miss days at the gym and feel worse about myself for it. But I never went back to not going at all. And so long as I was able to make it to the fitness center at least three times a week—or, if not, do some pushups in my room or take a quick jog around campus—my ability to concentrate in class vastly improved.

I ended up graduating with a double major in political science and psychology. And though the job I got out of college working at a congressional research firm is definitely a challenge to being regularly active, I continue to make time for exercise before and after work as well as on weekends. (And I still incorporate the exercises that trainer taught me into my routines.) I've even joined an adult pickup basketball team started by some of my colleagues.

I know that if I cut back on physical activity the concentration I need to get through a workweek won't be there. Plus, not spending enough time moving around makes me sad, depressed, and more inclined to overdo the booze.

These days I work out not because it makes me look good—I've accepted that I'll likely never have the body of a sprinter or a weightlifter—but because it makes me happier and, most importantly, it enables me to get ahead in my career.

■ Introduction

Exercisers will often report that they think better or have less brain fog after they work out. And parents and teachers often report that their students can focus better and are less disruptive following recess and physical education. These anecdotal reports suggest that exercise may have a positive effect on our cognitive abilities. This is evidenced by the vignette on Mike used to introduce this chapter.

This chapter will discuss what cognition is and the science behind how exercise and sedentary behavior affect our cognitive ability. But before we begin to examine this literature, let's take a closer look at the brain.

■ The Brain

The human brain weighs about 1,400 grams, or roughly 3 pounds. It is thought to consist of about 100 billion individual neurons, and it has a texture similar to firm jelly. Despite its small size, the brain is the control center of our nervous system, the storage vault for our memories, and the source of our feelings. The brain is often referred to as the most complex structure in the universe.

Without a brain, we would not be able to think, move, speak, or even breathe. Like any complex machine or computer, the brain contains many parts, each of which has subparts, which themselves have subparts, all the way down to the 100 billion or so neurons. Let's consider the brain's general structure and functions so that we can better understand the impact that exercise and sedentary behavior have on the brain.

The three main parts of the brain are the cerebrum, the brainstem, and the cerebellum (see **FIGURE 7-1**). The biggest part of the brain is the **cerebrum**, or cortex, and it fills up most of the skull. The cerebrum makes up about 80% of the brain's weight. The cerebral cortex is divided into four sections: the frontal lobe, the parietal lobe, the occipital lobe, and the temporal lobe (see **TABLE 7-1**). The cerebrum is involved in remembering, problem solving, thinking, and feeling. This part of the brain also controls movement.

Lying at the back of the brain is the **cerebellum**, which is also known as the *little brain*. Its main function is to maintain balance and coordinate voluntary muscle movement. Damage to the cerebellum results in a loss of muscle tone, tremors, and abnormal posture. The cerebellum contributes to memory and language. Children with dyslexia or **attention deficit hyperactivity disorder (ADHD)**, for example, have either smaller cerebella or reduced activity in this region of the brain.

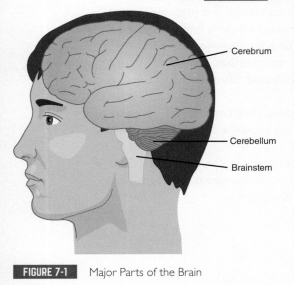

Cerebrum

Cerebellum

Brainstem

FIGURE 7-1 Major Parts of the Brain

TABLE 7-1	Functions of the Four Lobes of the Cerebrum
Lobe	**Function**
Frontal	Associated with reasoning, planning, parts of speech, movement, emotions, and problem solving
Parietal	Associated with movement, orientation, recognition, and perception of stimuli
Occipital	Associated with visual processing
Temporal	Associated with perception and recognition of auditory stimuli, memory, and speech

The **brainstem** sits beneath the cerebrum and in front of the cerebellum. This structure is responsible for basic vital life functions such as breathing, heartbeat, and blood pressure. In other words, it is responsible for the nonthinking actions, and it is in charge of all the functions your body needs to stay alive, such as breathing air, digesting food, and circulating blood.

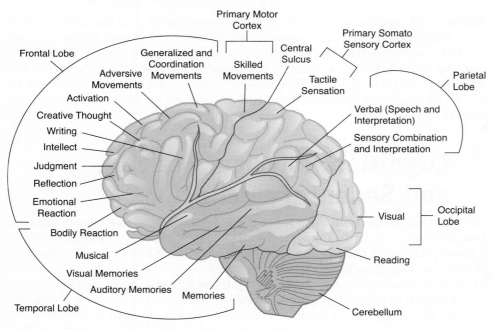

What Is Cognition?

Historically, the term **cognition** comes from the Latin verb *cognoscere*, which is translated to mean "to know," "to conceptualize," or "to recognize." Today, cognition represents a wide group of mental processes that reflect a person's knowledge or awareness. These mental processes interact in a hierarchical fashion and include thinking, knowing, remembering, reasoning, decision making, learning,

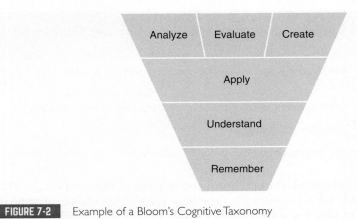

FIGURE 7-2 Example of a Bloom's Cognitive Taxonomy

judging, and problem solving. Mental processes high in the hierarchy include those that are associated with language, imagination, perception, evaluation, and planning. Higher-order cognitive tasks, for example, would include planning to compete in an ironman or choosing to engage in physical activity as opposed to watching television. **FIGURE 7-2** represents a common taxonomy developed by Bloom for classifying learning objectives that is based on higher-order cognitive tasks (Bloom et al., 2013).

■ Cognition, Physical Activity, and Sedentary Behavior

An issue that has long intrigued researchers is contained in Homer's dictum *mens sana in corpore sano*. This Latin aphorism is usually translated as "a sound mind in a sound body" or "a healthy mind in a healthy body." The intended meaning here is that only a healthy body can support a healthy mind, so we should strive to keep our bodies in top condition. However, is this aphorism supported by science?

Hundreds of studies have been carried out to determine if there is a relationship between exercise and the brain; that is, whether **acute** and **chronic physical activity** influence cognitive functioning. Researchers have used a variety of different types of cognitive functioning tasks (e.g., memory, mathematical ability, verbal ability, reasoning creativity, academic achievement, mental age, intelligence quotient, reaction time, and perception) to examine this important research question.

Although research examining the effects of cognition across the lifespan is important, the focus has been on youth and older adults. For youth, the potential for cognitive and academic growth is important, including brain development. For older adults, cognitive decline is a possibility. Thus, we will focus on the research examining the effects of exercise on the cognitive abilities of these two populations.

Exercise and Cognition in Children and Adolescents

A good starting point when examining the effects of exercise on cognition is with youth. Children and adolescents spend most of their day at school learning. Several reviews have found that both acute and chronic physical activity positively influences brain health and cognition in children (Chaddock, Pontifex, Hillman, & Kramer, 2011; Hillman, Kamiho, & Scudder, 2011; Mahar, 2011).

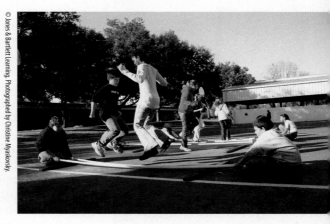

For example, Alicia Fedewa and Soyeon Ahn (2011) undertook a meta-analysis of 59 studies examining the effects of physical activity on cognitive performance of school-age children between the ages of 3 to 18 years. They found that being physically active has a small beneficial effect on children's achievement (ES = .28), with aerobic exercise having the greatest effect.

Fedewa and Ahn (2011) also examined a variety of moderator variables, such as the research paradigm or design. Researchers use a variety of paradigms (approaches) to answer important questions. The research design used often is influenced by such considerations as availability of participants and financial resources. Two of the simplest and easiest to use designs are cross-sectional and correlational. A **cross-sectional design** involves observation of all of a population, or a representative subset, at one specific point in time. With a **correlational design**, a single sample of individuals is tested and a correlation coefficient is computed to assess the degree of relationship between the level of cognitive functioning and the level of fitness.

The researchers found that in studies where either a cross-sectional or correlational design was used, a small positive relationship between physical activity and cognitive functioning was observed (ES = .32), indicating that children with higher levels of physical fitness exhibited higher cognitive functioning and academic achievement.

A major limitation, however, in cross-sectional and correlational designs is that they do not give any insight into the question of whether physical activity directly causes improved cognition. Experimental and quasi-experimental studies do permit inferences about cause and effect. With experimental studies, participants may be randomly assigned to control and treatment groups and the treatment or intervention—physical activity in this case—is then provided over an extended period of time. The 39 experimental/quasi-experimental studies examined by Fedewa and Ahn found that physical activity had a small positive effect (ES = .35) on cognitive functioning. This finding indicates that all physical activity programs had a positive impact on children's cognitive outcomes and academic achievement. Of interest, the physical activity interventions that had a special focus on aerobic exercise yielded the largest impact on children's cognitive outcomes, followed by physical education programs and perceptual motor training.

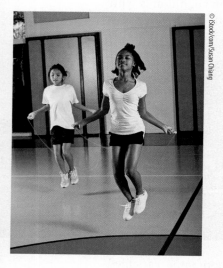

Fedewa and Ahn (2011) also examined the effects of physical activity on cognitive tasks. Cognitive tasks were categorized into intelligence quotient, total achievement, vocabulary/spelling/language arts achievement, reading achievement, mathematics achievement, science achievement, grade point average, and other (e.g., creativity). Among the cognitive outcome measures, the largest effect of physical activity was found to be with regard to children's mathematics achievement, followed by their **intelligence quotient (IQ)** and reading achievement. As the authors pointed out, ironically all three of these areas are critical elements in the standardized testing movement. The authors concluded that not only is physical activity worth the time, but that it appears to benefit those children who need it the most, particularly in the areas of math and reading. For children with learning disabilities who struggle in meeting math and reading benchmarks, physical activity interventions significantly improved their academic performance.

In another study, Charles Hillman and his colleagues (2014) found that running around outside for at least an hour daily helps kid think better. Using a randomized controlled design, 221 children (ages 7 to 9 years old) were assigned to either 9 months of after-school physical activity or a wait-list control. The students

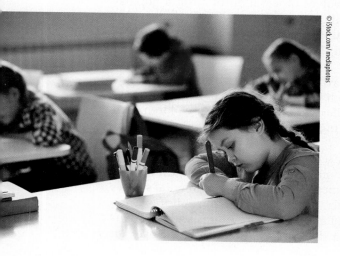

in the physical activity group met after school nearly every day for a snack and a brief lesson on fitness and nutrition. Then the children spent over an hour running around and playing tag, soccer, jump rope, and other games. The focus was not on competition, but rather on playing.

The researchers found that the children who ran around had improved fitness scores compared to the wait-list control group. With regard to cognition, the physical activity group also had improved thinking skills, particularly in multitasking, compared to the wait-list control children at the end of the intervention. The researchers concluded that their study findings demonstrate a causal effect of unstructured physical activity on cognitive abilities for young children and provide further support for physical activity for improving childhood cognition and brain health.

Classroom-Based Physical Activity

Although it may seem logical to consider physical education classes as the target for increasing the physical activity levels of schoolchildren, there are several reasons why this may not be the case. First, time allocated to physical education has steadily declined. Statistics reveal that only 4% of elementary schools, 8% of middle schools, and 2% of high schools in the United States provide daily physical education (Lee, Burgeson, Fulton, & Spain, 2007). Second, there is also a decline in recess, which is an opportunity for students to obtain unstructured physical activity. In fact, it is estimated that only 57% of school districts require regularly scheduled recess for elementary school children (Lee et al., 2007). Third, coupled with the decline in physical education classes is the fact that children often get limited physical activity during physical education classes (Simons-Morton et al., 1993).

Finally, the current emphasis on end-of-grade testing can cause decreased opportunities during school for students to be physically active by inadvertently pressuring administrators and teachers to spend more sedentary time in the classroom and less physically active time in physical education in an effort to improve standardized testing scores. The result is that most youth are not meeting the physical activity guidelines, with 42% of children aged 6 to 11 years and only 8% of adolescents obtaining the recommended 60 minutes per day of moderate- and/or vigorous-intensity physical activity (Troiano et al., 2008). And, not surprisingly, obesity rates have tripled among school-age youth in the last three decades (Singh, Kogan, & Van Dyck, 2008).

If physical activity is to be increased in elementary schools, venues other than physical education need to be developed and evaluated. An alternative to physical education for increased physical activity is the regular classroom where students spend most of their time. Indeed, children are easily accessible in school settings because they spend a large portion of their day at school. In many countries children spend about 6 to 8 hours a day at school. Thus, a practical, although challenging, solution is to promote classroom-based physical activity (Donnelly & Lambourne, 2011). Classroom-based physical activity is either linked to an established curriculum or physical activity is coupled with the teachers' existing lessons. Thus, the physical activity is integrated with the academic lesson and does not take time away from the curriculum.

CRITICAL THINKING ACTIVITY 7-1

© ecco/Shutterstock, Inc.

Excluding recess and physical education classes, how could you increase physical activity for children while they are at school?

One such classroom-based program is the Physical Activity Across the Curriculum (PAAC). This program is guided by the association among physical activity, fitness, fatness, and academic achievement; it provides a unique opportunity to improve both the health (e.g., fitness levels) and cognitive achievement of children during school.

PAAC lessons can be used in a variety of academic areas, including math, language arts, geography, history, spelling, science, and health. An example of a math lesson might consist of students hopping and skipping across the room and counting their own "laps," as well as adding or multiplying laps of groups of children (i.e., 6 children × 6 laps each = 36). Geometry might be taught by having students form different shapes, such as squares or triangles, while either walking or skipping. Geography can be taught by having children run to the appropriate area designated for one of the directions (i.e., north, south, east, west). For example, if the teacher calls the state of Florida, students would run or skip to the south space. A floor mat with alphabet letters printed on it could be used to teach spelling, where the children spell out words by hopping onto the letters. The scope of physically active lessons is almost limitless.

The conceptual framework for PAAC includes no additional teacher preparation time, uses existing academic lessons, has no additional costs, and incorporates activities that are fun for both students and teachers. Additionally, PAAC promotes the concept that physical activity can occur at many times and places without the need to report to a special place (such as a gym or track) and to change into gym clothes.

Specifically, PAAC promotes 90 minutes a week of moderate to vigorous physically active academic lessons that last about 10 minutes each. The lessons are delivered intermittently throughout the school day. Lessons are mostly delivered in the classroom, but can also be delivered in alternate school sites, such as hallways and outdoors.

Joseph Donnelly and his colleagues (2009) conducted a 3-year cluster randomized controlled trial of 24 elementary schools to compare changes in fitness and fatness with changes in academic achievement in schools that either received PAAC or schools that served as controls. A **cluster randomized controlled trial** is a type of randomized controlled trial in which groups of subjects, in this case schools (as opposed to individual subjects), are randomized.

The participants were 665 boys and 677 girls initially in grades 2 and 3 and who progressed to grades 4 and 5. The primary outcome for PAAC was change in body mass index (BMI) from year 1 to year 3. The authors found that the overall change in BMI for PAAC schools compared to control schools was not significantly different. However, the change in BMI from baseline to 3 years was significantly influenced by exposure to PAAC; that is, as minutes of PAAC exposure increased, the change in BMI decreased. More specifically, schools with 75 minutes or more of PAAC a week showed significantly smaller increases in BMI at 3 years compared to schools with fewer than 75 minutes of PAAC each week.

A secondary outcome examined was daily physical activity that was measured by an **accelerometer**. Although accelerometers are objective measures of physical activity, they are expensive, so they were used to measure physical activity in a subsample of the participants. Daily physical activity was measured in 77 PAAC and 90 control students each spring of the 3-year intervention. Accelerometers were used for 4 consecutive days, including 2 weekend days. The researchers found that children in the PAAC schools had significantly greater levels of physical activity during the school day (by 12%) and on the weekends (by 17%) compared to children in the control schools. Children in PAAC schools also had a 27% greater level of moderate to vigorous exercise compared to children in the control schools.

Another secondary outcome assessed by the researchers was academic achievement. Academic achievement was measured with the Wechsler Individual Achievement Test-Second Edition (Wechsler, 2005) by a third party. This test assesses the academic achievement of children in the following four areas: reading, math, oral language, and writing. The researchers found significant improvements in academic achievement from baseline to 3 years in the PAAC schools compared to the control schools for reading, math, oral language, and writing (see **FIGURE 7-3**). Of interest, the teachers who themselves were more physically active had students who were also more physically active. In other words, teacher participation in classroom physical activity was directly related to children's physical activity levels.

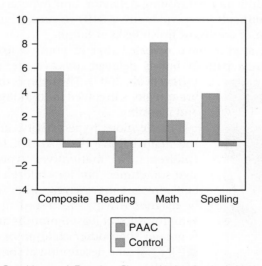

FIGURE 7-3   Youth Cognition and Exercise: Change in Academic Achievement from Baseline to 3 Years

Note: Y-axis represents change in academic score from baseline to 3 years.

Reprinted from Donnelly, J. E., Greene, J. L., Gibson, C. A., Smith, B. K., Washburn, R. A., Sullivan, D. K., Williams, S. L. (2009). Physical Activity Across the Curriculum (PAAC): A randomized controlled trial to promote physical activity and diminish overweight and obesity in elementary school children. *Preventive Medicine*, 49(4), 336–341. With permission from Elsevier.

Other research examining the impact of physically active academic instruction is promising (see Singh, Uijtdewilligen, Twick, van Mechelen, & Chinapaw, 2012) and supports the findings of Donnelly and Lambourne (2011). For example, a recent review by Matthew Mahar (2011) revealed that students who participated in classroom-based physical activities that incorporated academic concepts had better attention-to-task than control students. As well, a review by the Centers for Disease Control and Prevention (2010) found that interventions that combined physical activity and academic lessons resulted in students having improvements in on-task behavior, word recognition, and spatial, reading, and math aptitude. In summary, the literature strongly supports the relationship between physical activity, cognition, and academic performance in youth. There is no scientific evidence to support the argument that increasing the time allotted to physical activity during the school day results in decreased academic performance. In short, schools may be able to address several health issues in conjunction with improving academic performance by delivering academic lessons using physical activity in the classroom (Donnelly & Lambourne, 2011).

Attention Deficit Hyperactivity Disorder

ADHD is one of the most common childhood disorders and can continue through adolescence and into adulthood. Symptoms include difficulty staying focused and paying attention, difficulty controlling behavior, and hyperactivity. These symptoms can make it difficult for a child with ADHD to succeed in school, get along with other children or adults, or finish tasks at home.

Brain imaging studies have revealed that in youth with ADHD the brain matures in a normal pattern but is delayed, on average, by about 3 years

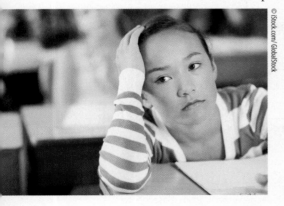

© iStock.com/GlobalStock

(Shaw et al., 2007). The delay is most pronounced in brain regions involved in thinking, paying attention, and planning.

Inattention, hyperactivity, and impulsivity are the main behaviors of ADHD. It is normal for all children to be inattentive, hyperactive, or impulsive sometimes, but for children with ADHD these behaviors are more severe, intense, and frequent. To be diagnosed with this disorder, a child must have symptoms for at least 6 months and to a degree that is greater than other children of the same age. See **TABLE 7-2** for a description of some of the symptoms of ADHD.

Treatments can relieve many symptoms of ADHD, but there is currently no cure for the disorder. With treatment, most people with ADHD can be successful in school, work, and social situations and lead productive lives. The main treatment for ADHD is drug therapy, which uses psychostimulants to help increase attention and focus. However, emerging research continues to identify exercise as a potential "natural" solution in preventing and improving ADHD symptoms.

TABLE 7-2	Symptoms of Attention Deficient Hyperactivity Disorder	
Inattention	**Hyperactivity**	**Impulsivity**
Easily distracted, misses details, forgets things, and frequently switches from one activity to another.	Fidgets and squirms in his or her seat.	Very impatient.
Difficulty focusing on one thing.	Talks nonstop.	Blurts out inappropriate comments, shows emotions without restraint, and acts without regard for consequences.
Becomes bored with a task after only a few minutes, unless doing something enjoyable.	Dashes around, touching or playing with anything and everything in sight.	Has difficulty waiting for things or waiting for turns in games.
Has trouble completing or turning in homework assignments; often loses things (e.g., pencils, toys, assignments) needed to complete tasks or activities.	Has trouble sitting still during dinner, school, or story time.	Often interrupts conversations or others' activities.

Data from the National Institute of Mental Health. (2012). What is attention deficit hyperactivity disorder? Retrieved August, 13, 2015, from http://www.nimh.nih.gov/health/publications/attention-deficit-hyperactivity -disorder/index.shtml?rf=71264\.

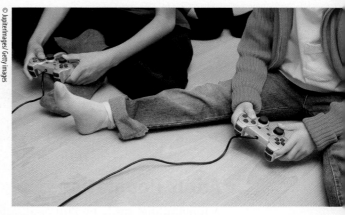

For example, researchers from Brazil examined the effect of physical activity on children's attention using a computer game (Silva et al., 2015). Intense physical activity was promoted by a relay race, which required a 5-minute run without a rest interval. The relay race was performed by 28 children, of which 14 had ADHD and 14 did not have ADHD symptoms. After 5 minutes of rest, the children accessed the computer game to accomplish the tasks in the shortest time possible. The computer game was also accessed by another 28 volunteers who did not exercise: 14 children with ADHD and 14 without these symptoms. The response time to solve the tasks that require attention was recorded.

The researchers found that the children with ADHD who exercised performed about 30% better for the tasks that required attention compared with the children with ADHD who did not exercise. The children with ADHD who exercised performed similarly (2.5% difference) to the children who had no ADHD symptoms and did not exercise (see **FIGURE 7-4**). The researchers concluded that intense

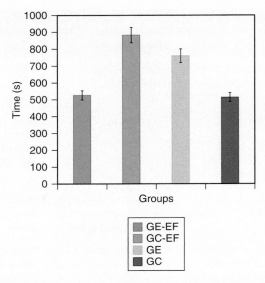

FIGURE 7-4   Graph of the Average Performance of the Four Groups

Note: The group with ADHD that participated in the proposed physical activity (GE-EF) obtained 30.52% better performance than the group with signs of ADHD that did not participate in physical activity (GE), and 40.36% better than the group without characteristics of ADHD that participated in physical activity (GC-EF). The group that more rapidly reached the goal proposed by the assessment game was that group without characteristics of ADHD and not involved in the physical activity proposed (GC), ending the testing game 2.5% faster than the GE-EF group.

Reproduced from Silva, A.P., Prado, S. O. S., Scardovelli, T. A., Silvia, R. M. S., Campos, L. C., & Frere, A. F. (2015). Measurement of the effect of physical exercise on the concentration of individuals with ADHD. *PLoS ONE, 10*(3): e0122119.   doi:10.1371/journal.pone.0122119;   http://127.0.0.1:8081/plosone/article?id=info:doi/10.1371/journal. pone.0122119

exercise can improve the attention of children with ADHD and may help their school performance.

CRITICAL THINKING ACTIVITY 7-2

© ecco/Shutterstock, Inc.

Do you think that moderate and/or mild physical activity can improve the attention and concentration of children with ADHD? Explain why or why not.

Adult Populations

A longitudinal study by Zhu et al. (2014) revealed that physical activity in young healthy adults can benefit brain health when they reach middle age. The researchers recruited 2,747 young adults between the ages of 18 and 30 years in 1985–1986 (baseline year 0) and then followed them for 25 years. The participants' cardiorespiratory fitness via a maximal treadmill test was assessed at year 0 and again at year 20. At year 25 of the study a battery of cognitive tests were administered to assess the participants' verbal memory, psychomotor speed, and executive functioning. The researchers found that better verbal memory and faster psychomotor speed at ages 43 to 55 years were related to better fitness 25 years earlier. In other words, the results revealed that those who ran for longer on the treadmill as young adults performed better at tests of memory and thinking skills in middle age, even after adjusting for factors such as smoking, diabetes, and high cholesterol.

Patrick Smith and his colleagues (2010) conducted a large meta-analysis of randomized controlled trials examining the association between aerobic exercise training on **neurocognitive function** of adults. They reviewed 29 studies with data from 2,049 adults aged 18 or older. The studies reviewed had to incorporate aerobic exercise for at least 1 month, have supervised exercise training, and have incorporated a nonaerobic-exercise control group.

They found that adults who were randomly assigned to receive aerobic exercise training had modest improvements in **attention**, **processing speed**, **executive function**, and **memory** compared to the nonexercise control participants. *Processing speed* refers to the speed at which the brain processes information. Faster processing speed means more efficient thinking and learning. *Executive functioning* is the cognitive process that regulates an individual's ability to organize thoughts and activities, prioritize tasks, manage time efficiently, and make decisions. They found that aerobic exercise did not appear to benefit working memory (i.e., short-term memory). Smith et al. (2010) also found via moderator analyses that studies using combined aerobic exercise and strength training interventions improved attention and processing speed and working memory to a greater extent than aerobic exercise alone.

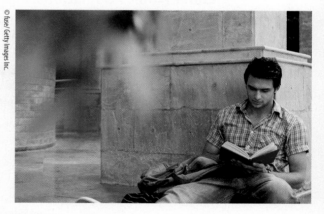
© fuse/Getty Images Inc.

Of importance, Smith et al. (2010) found preliminary evidence that exercise in individuals with mild cognitive impairment may be associated with greater improvements in memory relative to those without cognitive impairment. **Mild cognitive impairment** is an intermediate stage between the expected cognitive decline of normal aging and the more pronounced decline of dementia. It involves problems with memory, language, thinking, and judgment that are greater than typical age-related changes. A person with mild cognitive impairment may be aware that his or her memory or mental function has "slipped," and family and close friends may also notice a change. However, generally these changes are not severe enough to interfere with the person's day-to-day life and usual activities.

Mild cognitive impairment increases a person's risk of later developing dementia, including Alzheimer's disease, especially when the person's main difficulty is with memory. **Dementia** (which literally means "madness from the mind") is a serious loss of global cognitive ability in a previously unimpaired person, beyond what might be expected from normal aging. Although dementia is far more common in older adults, it can occur before the age of 65, in which case it is termed *early onset dementia*. Dementia is not a single disease, but rather a non-specific illness syndrome (i.e., set of signs and symptoms). It can affect memory, attention, language, and problem solving. It is normally required to be present for at least 6 months to be diagnosed. Especially in the later stages of the condition, affected persons may be disoriented in time (not knowing what day of the week, day of the month, or even what year it is), in place (not knowing where they are), and in person (not knowing who they or others around them are). Dementia, though often treatable to some degree, is usually due to causes that are progressive and incurable. There are many specific types (causes) of dementia, often showing slightly different symptoms. One of the most common forms of dementia is **Alzheimer's disease**, a neurodegenerative disease characterized by a progressive deterioration of higher cognitive functioning in the areas of memory, problem solving, and thinking.   **TABLE 7-3**   lists potential signs of Alzheimer's disease.

Older Adult Populations

With age, physical and cognitive functioning decline. It is well-established that as we age both the structure and function of our brain changes. These changes are

TABLE 7-3   Signs of Alzheimer's Disease

Sign	Example
Recent memory loss	Asking the same question repeatedly, forgetting about already asking it.
Difficulty completing familiar tasks	Making a drink or cooking a meal, but forgetting and leaving it.
Problems communicating	Difficulty with language by forgetting simple words or using the wrong ones.
Disorientation	Getting lost on a previously familiar street close to home and forgetting how they got there or would get home again.
Poor judgment	Forgetting all about the child they are watching and just leaving the house for the day.
Problems with abstract thinking	Difficulty with money and finances.
Misplacing things	Putting items in the wrong places and forgetting about doing this.
Mood changes	Swinging quickly through a set of moods.
Personality changes	Becoming irritable, suspicious, or fearful.
Loss of initiative	Showing less interest in starting something or going somewhere.

Adapted from American Academy of Family Physicians. (2001). The signs of dementia (patient information). *American Family Physician, 63,* 717–718.

associated with decreased cognitive function. For example, as we age our reaction time becomes slower, our memory is not as good, and we may have a more difficult time making decisions. We know that physical activity is beneficial for healthy aging, and it may also help maintain good cognitive functioning in older adults. A great deal of research has examined the relationship between physical activity and cognitive functioning in older adults.

A meta-analysis by Sofi and colleagues (2011) sought to examine the association between physical activity and cognitive decline in nondemented participants. Their review included 15 prospective cohort studies with 30,331 nondemented participants (aged 35 and older) who were followed for a period of 1 to 12 years. A **prospective cohort study** is a study that follows a group of similar people (a cohort) over time. Of the 30,331 followed, the researchers found that 3,003 of the participants had developed cognitive decline. Of importance, physically active people at baseline had a significantly reduced rate of developing cognitive decline during the follow-up period. In fact, highly physically active people had a 38% reduced risk of cognitive decline compared to sedentary people. Furthermore, even low to moderate levels of exercise had a protective effect against cognitive impairment, reducing the risk of cognitive decline by 35%. The authors concluded that all levels of physical activity may protect against the occurrence of cognitive decline.

A 35-year longitudinal study found that regular exercise is the most effective lifestyle choice people can make to reduce their risk of dementia. Peter Elwood and his colleagues (2013) conducted a longitudinal study to examine the effects of the following five health behaviors on cognitive function and dementia: non-smoking (including ex-smokers), acceptable BMI (range = 18 to 25), high fruit and vegetable intake (i.e., three or more portions of fruit and vegetables a day), regular exercise (i.e., walking 2 or more miles to work each day, cycling 10 or more miles to work each day, or "vigorous" exercise), and low to moderate alcohol intake (i.e., three or fewer drinks per day, with abstinence not treated as a healthy behavior). Starting in 1979, the five aforementioned healthy behaviors were recorded on a cohort of 2,235 men aged 45 to 49 years who lived in a typical small town in South Wales in the United Kingdom.

The researchers recorded the incidence of diabetes, vascular disease, cancer, and death over a 30-year period. In 2004, they determined the participants' cognitive state. They found that men who followed at least four of the health behaviors had a reduced incidence of diabetes, vascular disease, all-cause mortality, cognitive impairment, and dementia. In fact, consistently following just four out of five key behaviors was found to reduce dementia risk by 60%, while also cutting the chance of heart disease and stroke by 70%. Of the five behaviors—exercise, not smoking, having a low bodyweight, a healthy diet, and low alcohol intake—exercise was found to be the most effective at improving long-term physical and mental health. Unfortunately, less than 1% of the men followed all five health behaviors, and only 5% reported four or more during the study period from 1979 to 2009. The researchers concluded that a healthy lifestyle is associated with increased disease-free survival and reduced cognitive impairment but that the uptake of these behaviors remains low. Healthy behaviors have a far more beneficial effect than any medical treatment or preventive procedure.

A group of Dutch researchers conducted a meta-analysis of 11 randomized controlled trials that examined the effects of physical activity on cognitive function in older adults (age 55 and older) without known cognitive impairment

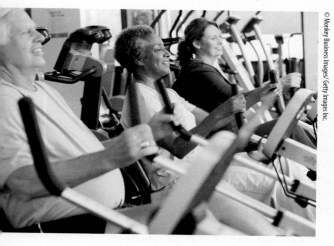

© Monkey Business Images/ Getty Images Inc.

(Angevaren et al., 2008). They found that improvements in fitness (as determined by a **maximum oxygen uptake** test, which is considered the best indicator of cardiorespiratory health) coincided with improvements in cognitive capacity. The largest effect on cognitive function was found on **motor function** (i.e., ability to use and control muscles and movements; ES = 1.17), and then **auditory attention** (i.e., ability to focus on relevant acoustic signals, particularly speech or linguistic stimuli; ES = .50). Moderate effects were observed for cognitive speed (i.e., speed at which information is processed; ES = .26) and visual attention (ES = .26).

Angevaren and his colleagues (2008) concluded that aerobic physical activities that improve cardiorespiratory fitness are beneficial for cognitive function in healthy older adults, with improvements observed in motor function, cognitive speed, auditory attention, and visual attention. They did mention, however, that the data were insufficient to show that the improvements in cognitive function that can be attributed to physical exercise are due to improvements in cardiovascular fitness, although the temporal association suggests that this might be the case.

A very important question is determining the effects of physical activity for people at risk for dementia. Can physical activity be used as a treatment for dementia? Can it improve cognitive function in those at risk for dementia? Small-scale clinical trials are revealing that Alzheimer's patients who engage in exercise have less cognitive deterioration compared to Alzheimer's patients who do not exercise (Nascimento et al., 2012). For example, researchers found that in patients with mild to moderate Alzheimer's disease those who engaged in regular walking over 1 year had attenuations in global cognitive decline. In comparison, sedentary patients (defined as those who did not engage in any activity) over the same time period had a significant decline in cognitive ability (Winchester et al., 2013).

Nicola Lautenschlager and her colleagues (2008) conducted a randomized controlled trial in an attempt to answer the important research question of the effects of physical activity on cognitive function in older adults at risk for Alzheimer's disease. The participants were adults aged 50 and older who had memory problems but did not meet the criteria for dementia. The adults (N = 138) were randomly assigned to an education and usual care group or to a 24-week home-based physical activity program. The researchers found that cognitive function in the physical activity group improved by the end of the intervention. In comparison, the control group had deteriorated in their cognitive function at the end of the intervention. Because of the promising aforementioned results, researchers are currently examining whether physical activity reduces the rate of cognitive decline among individuals with Alzheimer's disease (Cyarto et al. 2010). Of interest, a recent study by a group from Brazil and Spain (Nascimento et al., 2013) found that 6 months of a multimodel physical exercise program resulted in improvements in both daily living activities and sleep in patients with Alzheimer's disease and **Parkinson's disease**.

In a meta-analytical review, Canadian researchers found that physical activity is associated with a reduced risk of Alzheimer's disease in adults older than age 65 years (Beckett, Ardern, & Rotondi, 2015). The researchers concluded that given the limited treatment options, greater emphasis should be paid to primary prevention through physical activity among individuals at high risk of Alzheimer's disease, such as those with a strong genetic and family history.

German researchers examined the effects of a home-based physical activity program on clinical symptoms, functional abilities, and caregiver burden in patients with Alzheimer's disease (Holthoff et al., 2015). Using a randomized controlled trial design, 30 patients (mean age 72 years) with Alzheimer's disease and their family caregivers were allocated to either a home-based 12-week physical activity intervention group or the usual care group. The intervention changed between passive, motor-assisted, or active-resistive leg training and changes in direction on a movement trainer using a chair. Participants were required to train three times a week for 30 minutes at an individually chosen time with at least 1 day without training in between two training days.

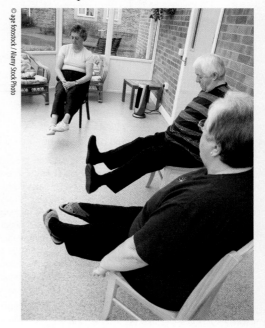

The researchers found that the control group experienced decreases in activities of daily living performance at weeks 12 and 24, whereas patients in the intervention group remained stable. Analyses of executive function and language ability revealed that patients in the intervention group improved during the intervention and returned to initial performance at week 12, whereas the controls revealed continuous worsening. Analyses of reaction time, hand-eye quickness, and attention revealed improvement only in the intervention group. Caregiver burden remained stable in the intervention group but worsened in the control group (see FIGURE 7-5).

Holthoff and colleagues (2015) concluded that physical activity in a home-based setting might be an effective and intrinsically attractive way to promote physical activity training in Alzheimer's patients and modulate caregiver burden.

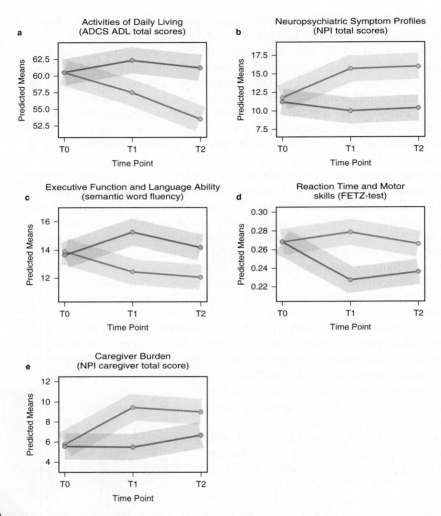

Effects of Physical Activity on Clinical Performance

This figure shows the effects of physical activity on the patients when compared to the control group for the three time points (T0, baseline; T1, 3 months later or after completion of the intervention; and T2, 3-month followup). Activities of daily living (ADCS ADL total scores): Patients in the control group experienced significant decreases in their performance over 12 weeks and at the 3-month follow up, whereas patients in the intervention group remained stable during the study period and followup (a). Neuropsychiatric symptom profiles (NPI total scores): Controls suffered a considerable increase in behavioral changes over 24 weeks, whereas patients in the intervention group remained stable over 24 weeks (b). Executive function and language ability: Patients in the intervention group improved during the intervention period and returned to initial performance after completion but without revealing the continuous worsening over 24 weeks demonstrated in the controls (c). Reaction time, hand-eye quickness, and attention (FETZ-test or Ruler Drop Test): Only patients in the intervention group improved their performance during the study period (d). Caregiver burden (NPI): Burden increased in the control group during the first 3 months whereas caregiver burden remained stable in the intervention group during the study period (e).

Reproduced from Holthoff, V. A., Marschner, K., Scharf, M., Steding, J., Meyer, S., Koch, T., & Donix, M. (2015). Effects of physical activity training in patients with Alzheimer's dementia: Results of a pilot RCT study. *PLoS ONE, 10*(4): e0121478. doi:10.1371/journal.pone.0121478; http://127.0.0.1:8081/plosone/article?id=info:doi/10.1371/journal.pone.0121478

CRITICAL THINKING ACTIVITY 7-3

© ecco/Shutterstock, Inc.

How does exercise affect cognitive abilities across the lifespan?

◼ Cognition and Sedentary Behavior

Emerging research is revealing that sedentary behavior has negative effects on cognition (Loprinzi & Kane, 2015). In school-age children and youth aged 5 to 17 years, watching TV for more than 2 hours per day was associated with increased body mass index, decreased fitness, lower self-esteem and pro-social behaviors (emotional stability, sensitive, outgoing, self-controlled), and decreased academic achievement (school performance, grade point average; Tremblay et al., 2011).

Similar results have been found for older adults, with TV viewing being negatively associated with cognitive ability, including executive functioning (Kesse-Guot et al., 2012). It appears, however, that computer use, which represents a sedentary behavior, may actually be associated with improved cognitive ability, at least in older adults. Computer use of greater than 1 hour a day is associated with better verbal memory and executive functioning compared to nonusers in older adults, after controlling for a number of covariates, including physical activity. Specific sedentary behaviors are differentially associated with cognitive performance. In contrast to TV viewing, regular computer use may help maintain cognitive function during the aging process.

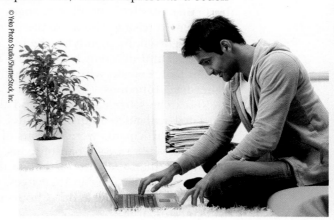

© Yeko Photo Studio/ShutterStock, Inc.

◼ Mechanism of Effect

Relatively little is known about the underlying mechanisms of the associations between physical activity and cognitive functioning in human populations (Brown, Peiffer, & Martins, 2013). Most of the research examining the mechanisms of how exercise affects brain function has been undertaken with animal models. Based on these studies, much of the observed changes in the brain involve neurogenesis (i.e., new nerve cell generation), neurotransmitters (i.e., chemical substances that transmit nerve impulses across a synapse, the tiny communication gap between the neurons in the brain), and vascular adaptations, such as the formation of new blood vessels (van Praag, 2009). In fact, van Praag (2009) stated that animal research reveals that exercise is the strongest neurogenic stimulus. Much of this neurogenesis occurs in the hippocampus of the brain, which is an important area for learning and memory. Charles Hillman and his colleagues (Hillman, Erickson, & Kramer, 2008) stated that this hippocampus cell proliferation is the most consistently observed effect from exercise and that it can occur at all stages of life.

Early brain and exercise research indicated that exercise results in an increase in some brain neurotransmitters that induce a "runner's high" with some endurance exercisers (Hillman, Erickson, & Kramer, 2008). Presently, other neurotransmitters have been shown to increase with exercise and appear to increase the synapse communication capacity in the brain. As well, aerobic exercise induces the formation of new blood vessels in the brain during childhood and adulthood, improving brain circulation (for oxygen and nutrient delivery), function, and health.

Preliminary research is also revealing that exercise can lead to changes in the brain, making it more plastic (i.e., its ability to change physically, functionally, and chemically) and improving memory and motor skill coordination. Using a small sample size, Michael Ridding and his colleagues (2014) had young adults ride a bike vigorously for 30 minutes (Smith et al., 2014). The researchers monitored changes in the brain directly after the exercise session and again 15 minutes later. Results show that even one 30-minute session of physical activity can improve the brain's plasticity. Positive changes in the brain were sustained for 15 minutes after exercising. The more plastic the brain becomes, the better its ability to reorganize itself, by modifying the number and strength of connections between nerve cells and different brain areas. This exercise-related change in the brain may, in part, explain why physical activity has a positive effect on memory and higher-level functions.

Researchers from Finland found that greater levels of physical activity are associated with increased gray matter in the brain (Rottensteiner et al., 2015). The study participants were 10 pairs of identical male twins between the ages of 32 and 36 years. In each pair of twins, one brother had exercised more over the past 3 years than the other, although they reported that they carried out similar levels of exercise earlier in their lives. On average, the more active members of twin pairs were jogging about 3 hours more per week compared to their inactive twin counterparts.

The twins had MRI scans of their brains to determine the effects that physical activity had on the size of their brains. Results revealed that exercise did not affect the size of the brain as a whole. However, there was a connection between more activity and more brain volume in areas related to movement (i.e., balance and coordination). The researchers concluded that these changes in the brain may have long-term health implications, such as reduced risk of falling.

■ Summary

Historically, a longstanding belief has been that being physically active has positive mental as well as physical consequences. This is reflected in Homer's dictum *mens sana in corpore sano*. Research examining the relationship between physical activity and cognitive functioning has found a small relationship between involvement in physical activity and improvements in cognitive functioning. Also, the relationship is greater after chronic physical activity than after acute physical activity.

The dose–response issue is unclear at this point (Singh et al., 2012). Practitioners (and participants) are often interested in what is referred to as the dose–response issue; that is, how much of the dose (physical activity in this case) is necessary to obtain the desirable response (improved cognitive performance). For people engaged in chronic physical activity, a "dose" can represent a number of different considerations. For example, it is possible to vary the duration of each training session, the days of training per week, and/or the total number of weeks of training.

In general, physical activity results in improved cognitive performance across the lifespan. Further research is needed to determine the effects of exercise on older adults with dementia and to elucidate the mechanisms of the effect. As well, emerging research will reveal the effects of sedentary behavior on our cognitive abilities.

KEY TERMS

accelerometer
acute physical activity
Alzheimer's disease
attention
attention deficit hyperactivity disorder (ADHD)
auditory attention
brainstem
cerebellum
cerebrum
chronic physical activity
cluster randomized controlled trial
cognition

correlational design
cross-sectional design
dementia
executive function
intelligence quotient (IQ)
maximum oxygen uptake
memory
mild cognitive impairment
motor function
neurocognitive function
Parkinson's disease
processing speed
prospective cohort study

REVIEW QUESTIONS

1. Define *cognition*? How is cognition measured?

2. Describe the benefits of class-based physical activity over physical education for increasing children's physical activity levels.

3. Develop a geography lesson for elementary schoolchildren that is based on the Physical Activity Across the Curriculum (PAAC) project.

4. Describe the effects of physical activity on cognitive function of adults with noncognitive impairment.

5. Describe dementia, Alzheimer's disease, and Parkinson's disease.

6. Describe some of the effects of physical activity on cognitive function of older adults.

7. What are some of the mechanisms of how exercise may affect brain function?

8. Develop a math lesson for elementary schoolchildren that incorporates physical activity into the lesson.

APPLYING THE CONCEPTS

1. Describe the various ways in which physical activity affected Mike's cognitive abilities.

2. If Mike maintains his physical activity levels well into old age, what cognitive and motor issues might he be less likely to suffer from?

3. What neural mechanisms might explain why exercise affects Mike's cognitive functions?

REFERENCES

Angevaren, M., Aufdemkampe, G., Verhaar, J. J., Aleman, A., & Vanhees, L. (2008). Physical activity enhances fitness to improve cognitive function in older people without known cognitive impairment. *Cochrane Database of Systematic Reviews*, July 16;(3):CD0053181.

American Academy of Family Physicians. (2001). The signs of dementia (patient information). *American Family Physician, 63*, 717–718.

Beckett, M. W., Ardern, C. I., & Rotondi, M. A. (2015). A meta-analysis of prospective studies on the role of physical activity and the prevention of Alzheimer's disease in older adults. *BMC Geriatrics*. doi:10.1186/s12877-015-0007-2

Bloom, B. S., Engelhart, M. D., Furst, E. J., Hill, W. H., & Krathwohl, D. R. (2013). *Taxonomy of educational objectives: The classification of educational goals; Handbook I: Cognitive Domain*. New York, NY: Shortmans, Green.

Brown, B. M., Peiffer, J. J., & Martins, R. (2013). Multiple effects of physical activity on molecular and cognitive signs of brain aging: Can exercise slow neurodegeneration and delay Alzheimer's disease? *Molecule Psychiatry, 18*, 864–874.

Centers for Disease Control and Prevention. (2010). The association between school-based physical activity, including physical education, and academic performance. Retrieved August 17, 2015, from http://www.cdc.gov/healthyyouth/health_and_academics/pdf/pa-pe_paper.pdf

Chaddock, L., Pontifex, M. B., Hillman, C. H., & Kramer, A. F. (2011). A review of the relation of aerobic fitness and physical activity to brain structure and function in children. *Journal of the International Neuropsychological Society, 17*, 975–985.

Cyarto, E. V., Cox, K. L., Almeida, O. P., Flicker, L., Ames, D., Byrne, G.,... Lautenschlager, N. T. (2010). The fitness for the Ageing Brain Study II (FABS II): Protocol for a randomized controlled trial evaluating the effect of physical activity on cognitive function in patients with Alzheimer's disease. *Trials, 11*, 120–128.

Donnelly, J. E., Greene, J. L., Gibson, C. A., Smith, B. K., Washburn, D. K., Sullivan, D. K.,... Williams, S. L. (2009). Physical Activity Across the Curriculum (PAAC): A randomized controlled trial to promote physical activity and diminish overweight and obesity in elementary school children. *Preventive Medicine, 49*, 336–341.

Donnelly, J. E., & Lambourne, K. (2011). Classroom-based physical activity, cognition, and academic achievement. *Preventive Medicine, 52*, S36–S42.

Elwood, P., Galante, J., Pickering, J., Palmer, S., Bayer, A., Ben-Schlomo, Y.,... Gallacher, J. (2013). Healthy lifestyles reduce the incidence of chronic diseases and dementia: Evidence from the Caerphilly cohort study. *PLOS One*, Dec. 09. doi:10.1371/journal.pone.0081877

Fedewa, A. L., & Ahn, S. (2011). The effects of physical activity and physical fitness on children's achievement and cognitive outcomes: A meta-analysis. *Research Quarterly for Exercise and Sport, 82*, 521–535.

Hillman, C. H., Erickson, K. I., & Kramer, A. F. (2008). Be smart, exercise your heart: Exercise effects on brain and cognition. *Nature Reviews Neuroscience, 9*, 58–65.

Hillman, C. H., Kamijo, K., & Scudder, M. (2011). A review of chronic and acute physical activity participation on neuroelectric measures of brain health and cognition during childhood. *Preventive Medicine, 52*, S21–S28.

Hillman, C. H., Pontifex, M. B., Castelli, D. M., Khan, N. A., Raine, L. B., Scudder, M. R.,... Kamijo, K. (2014). Effects of the FITkids randomized controlled trial on executive control and brain function. *Pediatrics, 134*(4): e1063–71.

Holthoff, V. A., Marschner, K., Scharf, M., Steding, J., Meyer, S., Koch, R., & Donix, M. (2015). Effects of physical activity training in patients with Alzheimer's dementia: Results of a pilot RCT study. *PLoS One*, Apr 17;*10*(4):e0121478.

Kesse-Guot, E., Charreire, H., Andreeva, V. A., Touvier, M., Hercberg, S., Galan, P., & Oppert, J. M. (2012). Cross-sectional and longitudinal associations of different sedentary behaviors with cognitive performance in older adults. *PLoS One, 7*(10):e47381. doi:10.1371/journal.pone.0047831

Lautenschlager, N. T., Cox, K. L., Flicker, L., Foster, J. K., van Bockxmeer, F. M., Xiao, J.,... Almeida, O. P. (2008). Effect of physical activity on cognitive function in older adults at risk for Alzheimer disease. A randomized trial. *JAMA, 300*, 1027–1037.

Lee, S. M., Burgeson, C. R., Fulton, J. E., & Spain, C. G. (2007). Physical education and physical activity: Results from the School Health Policies and Programs Study 2006. *Journal of School Health, 77*, 435–463.

Loprinzi, P. D., & Kane, C. J. (2015). Exercise and cognitive function: A randomized controlled trial examining acute exercise and free-living physical activity and sedentary effects. *Mayo Clinic Proceedings*, Apr;*90*(4):450–460. doi:10.1016/j.mayocp.2014.12.023

Mahar, M. T. (2011). Impact of short bouts of physical activity on attention-to-task in elementary school children. *Preventive Medicine*, *52*, S60–S64.

Nascimento, C. M., Ayan, C., Cancela, J. M., Gobbi, L. T., Gobbi, L. T., & Stella, F. (2013). Effect of a multimodal exercise program on sleep disturbances and instrumental activities of daily living performance on Parkinson's and Alzheimer's disease patients. *Geriatrics and Gerontology International*. Epub, May 6.

National Institutes of Mental Health. (2012). What is attention deficit hyperactivity disorder? Retrieved August, 13, 2015, from http://www.nimh.nih.gov/health/publications/attention-deficit-hyper-activity-disorder/index.shtml?rf=71264\.

Rottensteiner, M., Leskinen, T., Niskanen, E., Aaltonen, S., Mutikainen, S., Wikgren, J.,… Kujala, U. M. (2015). Physical activity, fitness, glucose homeostasis, and brain morphology in twins. *Medicine and Science in Sports and Exercise*, 47, 509–518.

Shaw, P., Eckstrand, K., Sharp, W., Blumenthal, J., Lerch, J. P., Greenstein, D.,… Rapoport, J. L. (2007). Attention-deficit/hyperactivity disorder is characterized by a delay in cortical maturation. *Proceedings of the National Academy of Sciences*, *104*, 19649–19654.

Silva, A. P., Prado, S. O., Scardovelli, T. A., Boschi, S. R., Campos, L. C., & Frere, A. F. (2015). Measurement of the effect of physical exercise on concentration of individuals with ADHD. *PLoS One*, Mar 24;*10*(3):e0122119.

Simons-Morton, B. G., Taylor, W. C., Snider, S. A., & Huang, I. W. (1993). The physical activity of fifth-grade students during physical education classes. *American Journal of Public Health*, *83*, 262–264.

Singh, G. K., Kogan, M. D., & van Dyck, P. C. (2008). A multilevel analysis of state and regional disparities in childhood and adolescent obesity in the United States. *Journal of Community Health*, *33*, 90–102.

Singh, G. K., Kogan, M. D., & van Dyck, P. C. (2010). Changes in state-specific childhood obesity and overweight prevalence in the United States from 2003 to 2007. *Archives of Pediatrics and Adolescent Medicine*, *164*, 598–607.

Singh, A., Uijtdewilligen, L., Twick, J. W., van Mechelen, W., & Chinapaw, M. J. (2012). Physical activity and performance at school: A systematic review of the literature including a methodological quality assessment. *Archives of Pediatric and Adolescent Medicine*, *166*, 49–55.

Sofi, F., Valecchi, D., Bacci, D., Abbate, R., Gensini, G. F., Casini, A., & Macchi, C. (2011). Physical activity and risk of cognitive decline: A meta-analysis of prospective studies. *Journal of Internal Medicine*, *269*, 107–117.

Smith, P. J., Blumenthal, J. A., Hoffman, B. M., Cooper, H., Strauman, T. A., Welsh-Bohmer, K.,… Sherwood, A. (2010). Aerobic exercise and neurocognitive performance: A meta-analytic review of randomized controlled trials. *Psychosomantic Medicine*, *72*, 239–252.

Smith, A. E., Goldsworthy, M. R., Garside, T., Wood, F. M., & Ridding, M. C. (2014). The influence of a single bout of aerobic exercise on short-interval intracortical excitability. *Experimental Brain Research*, *232*, 1875–1882.

Tremblay, M. S., LeBlanc, A. G., Kho, M. E., Saunders, T. J., Larouche, R., Colley, R. C., Goldfield, G., & Connor Gorber, S. (2011). Systematic review of sedentary behavior and health indicators in school-age children and youth. *International Journal of Behavioral Nutrition and Physical Activity*. doi: 10.1186/1479-5868-8-98

Troiano, R. P., Berrigan, D., Dodd, K. W., Masse, L. C., Tilert, T., & McDowell, M. (2008). Physical activity in the United States measured by accelerometer. *Medicine and Science in Sports and Exercise, 40*, 181–188.

van Prag, H. (2009). Exercise and the brain: Something to chew on. *Trends in Neuroscience, 32*, 283–290.

Wechsler, D. (2005). Wechsler Individual Achievement Test, 2nd Edition (WIAT II). London: The Psychological Corp.

Winchester, J., Dick, M. B., Gillen, D., Reed, B., Miller, B., Tinklenberg, J.,… Cotman, C. W. (2013). Walking stabilizes cognitive functioning in Alzheimer's disease (AD) across one year. *Archives of Gerontology and Geriatrics, 56*, 96–103.

Zhu, N., Jacobs, D. R. Jr., Schreiner, P. J., Yaffe, K., Bryan, N.,… Sternfeld, B. (2014). Cardiorespiratory fitness and cognitive function in middle age: The CARDIA study. *Neurology, 82*, 1339–1346.

Anxiety and Depression

Runner © Izf/Shutterstock

Vignette: Laura

I'd struggled with untreated depression since adolescence. I have a hunch mental health issues run in my family, though neither my mother nor my father ever sought help for their mood swings and long stretches of sadness that sometimes kept them bedridden for days.

After I got my first job out of college as a real estate broker, I tried therapy. But it just seemed to make me sadder. And I found it too hard to commit to the twice weekly sessions the professional I was seeing recommended. Searching for deals and showing clients apartments took up too much time, and I wanted to be good at my job.

Though my job often required me to be on my feet a lot, I never was one to pursue fitness. Many of my colleagues often referred to the gyms they went to throughout the city I worked in, and there was constant talk in my office of trending yoga classes, Cross Fit, and spin. So that I wouldn't burst into tears during normal business hours, I decided to go on antidepressants. I took them for about 4 years. But after tiring of their accompanying loss of sex drive and weight gain,

LEARNING OBJECTIVES

After completing this chapter, you will be able to

- Understand the difference between clinical and nonclinical anxiety and depression.
- Understand the effects of physical activity on depressive symptoms in people with clinical and nonclinical depression.
- Understand how moods, emotions, and affect differ.
- Describe the effects of physical activity and sedentary behavior on clinical and nonclinical anxiety.

I gradually decreased the milligrams of sertraline I was taking until I was completely drug free at 31.

Throughout the course of my coming off the pills, I didn't feel my mood crash drastically (at least not right away.) But I did feel increasingly anxious—perhaps due to the chemical let down as well as the hesitation that I wouldn't be able to function in the absence of a prescription.

Then my living situation changed. To have some extra income, I decided to rent out the spare bedroom in my apartment. A young woman moved in who taught fitness classes at an upscale gym in our neighborhood. For months she kept beseeching me to drop into one of her yoga or cycling sessions. But I kept telling her, "No, I'll make an idiot of myself."

What made me finally bite the bullet and attend an extremely overcrowded Saturday afternoon spin class wasn't the desire to be healthy, per se, it was a realization that the weight I thought would miraculously fall off after I stopped the antidepressants wasn't budging at all. Wanting to look a bit better, fit into my "skinny" clothes again, and possibly boost my self-esteem in the process, I bought a pair of exercise pants, a sports bra, and found the most secluded bike in the classroom.

I can honestly say that my first spin class was the most brutal, unenjoyable 45 minutes of my life. I would even go so far as to place it on par with the depressions I fell into that left me listless; hopeless; and, in my worst hours, suicidal. But after I got off that bike, every inch of my flesh dripping with sweat, I felt that I'd accomplished something as rewarding as closing a real estate deal. I guess you could call it my first exercise high.

I came back the following weekend. (I needed about 7 days to get over the insane amount of soreness in my leg muscles, lower back, and even my arms.) And though it was just as hard as the first time, once I got to the end I still felt that same rush.

I must say, it was addicting—but in a good way. My depressions tend to come in waves, often during the colder seasons or when my sleep schedule gets off track. Getting a membership at a cycling studio—which I finally did last March as a little birthday present to myself—made me feel that in order to get my money's worth I should really commit to at least three classes a week. Often—due to the constraints of my work schedule—this required me to be on a bike around 6:30 in the morning. Having this obligation helped me get to bed at an earlier hour and keep to a more regular routine.

It would be too far reaching to say that my new exercise habits have cured my depression for good. I still experience really low moods when I encounter setbacks at work, or when my new attempts to date don't go well. But I will say that despite my desire on some days to stay in bed until the afternoon or itemize all the things I hate about the world, I know if I just make it to an exercise class—even if I sit in the back and pedal slowly—I'll feel a little bit better.

Introduction

Considerable anecdotal testimony supports the popular belief that physical activity contributes to a "feel good" state in people. The following quote by Wilhelm von Humboldt, a famous Prussian philosopher, is consistent with this popular belief: "True enjoyment comes from activity of the mind and exercise of the body; the two are ever united" (Edwards, 1908). von Humboldt suggested that physical exercise contributes to positive feelings. However, science seldom relies on popular beliefs. As a consequence, researchers have concentrated their efforts for a number of years on examining the impact of physical activity on people's mood.

What does that research tell us? There exists a large body of scientific literature suggesting that regular exercise can improve someone's mood and help decrease anxiety and depression. In this chapter, we will provide definitional clarity to mood and other related constructs. We will also describe the literature examining the effects of physical activity on both clinical and nonclinical mood issues, with a focus on anxiety and depression.

Affect, Emotion, and Mood

A great deal of debate has taken place on the effects physical activity has on a person's mood. One reason that there is such debate is that mood is a complex construct to operationally define; it is closely related to other constructs, such as emotion and affect; and different authors have used the term in different ways. Before we begin to examine the literature, it is necessary to define just what we are talking about when we discuss affect, mood, and emotion.

Affect is a generic term that covers a broad range of feelings that people can experience. It is an umbrella concept that encompasses both people's emotions and moods (Ekkekakis, 2008). **Emotions** are intense feelings that are either directed at a specific person or event. Examples of emotions are reacting with anger immediately when another driver cuts you off, being nervous right before you give a presentation, or being happy when you receive a compliment.

Moods are feelings that tend to be less intense than emotions and are usually not directed at either a person or an event. In other words, moods differ from emotions in that they are less specific, less intense, and less likely to be triggered by either a particular person or an event. For example, if someone is rude to you, you may feel anger right

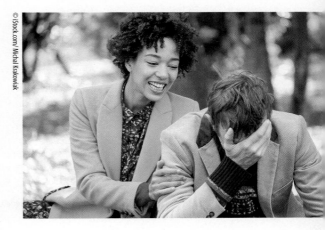
© iStock.com/Michal Krakowiak

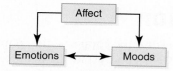

FIGURE 8-1 Relationship Among Affect, Mood, and Emotion

away. That intense feeling of anger usually comes and goes quickly, even in a matter of seconds. In comparison, when you are in a good mood, you can feel good for several hours. **FIGURE 8-1** presents an illustration that describes the distinction among emotion, mood, and affect. See **TABLE 8-1** for a more detailed description of the differences between emotions and moods.

CRITICAL THINKING ACTIVITY 8-1

© ecco/Shutterstock, Inc.

Describe how affect, mood, and emotion differ. How do you think physical activity can influence each of these constructs?

TABLE 8-1 Differences Between Emotions and Moods

Characteristic	Emotions	Moods
Duration	Short-lived	Longer lasting
Cause	Clear cause	Less likely to be triggered by a particular stimulus or event
Intensity	High	Lower
Facial expressions	Usually indicated by distinct facial expressions	Generally not indicated by distinct facial expressions
Nature	Action oriented	Cognitive
Generality	Specific	General
Number	Many types of emotions (e.g., anger, fear, sadness, happiness, disgust, surprise)	Typically two main mood dimensions (i.e., positive and negative) that are composed of many specific emotions

Retrieved February 2015, from http://catalogue.pearsoned.co.uk/samplechapter/0132431564.pdf

■ Depression, Physical Activity, and Sedentary Behavior

Mood disorders include disorders that influence mood regulation (American Psychiatric Association, 2013). In this section, we will examine the effects of physical activity and sedentary behavior on people who have both clinical and nonclinical mood disorders. A good starting point is with the best known and most researched mood—depression.

In the health sciences, a distinction is made between **clinical** and **nonclinical depression**. The latter is viewed as a transient mental state characterized by feeling unhappy, sad, miserable, down in the dumps, or blue. Most of us feel this way at one time or another for short periods. Nonclinical depression arises because of many circumstances, such as the result of a loss of some type, such as a death, family breakup, poor grade, or negative change in job status. However, depression can also arise following positive events, such as a birth, graduation, holiday period, or completion of a major assignment.

In comparison, major depression (also known as clinical depression disorder, major depressive disorder, unipolar depression, or unipolar disorder) is a psychiatric disorder in which feelings of sadness, loss, anger, or frustration interfere with everyday life for weeks, months, or years. With major depression, it may be difficult to work, study, sleep, eat, and enjoy friends and activities. Some people have clinical depression only once in their life, while others have it several times over the course of their lifetime. The exact cause of depression is not known. We do know that around 50% of the cause of depression is genetic, and around 50% is unrelated to genes and is therefore caused by psychological factors (such as triggered by a stressful event) or physical factors. Research on the heredity of depression within families shows that some people are more likely to develop the illness than others. For example, if you have a parent or sibling that has had major depression, you may be 1.5 to 3 times more likely to develop depression than those who do not have a close relative with the disorder (Lohoff, 2010).

Clinical depression is marked by a depressed mood most of the day, particularly in the morning, and a loss of interest in normal activities and relationships. To be diagnosed with clinical depression, a person must have at least five of the symptoms outlined in **TABLE 8-2** , one of which must include depressed mood or loss of interest or pleasure. These symptoms must be present every day for at least 2 weeks (APA, 2013).

Researchers have long been interested in exploring the potential benefits of physical activity as an intervention strategy for the treatment of depression (e.g., Franz & Hamilton, 1905). As a consequence, numerous studies have been undertaken examining the effects of physical activity on depressive symptoms. Some of those studies, however, suffer from poor research design, and others from small or nonrepresentative samples. Therefore, it is difficult for readers unfamiliar with the area to make sense out of this body of research. Fortunately, several meta-analyses have been carried out over the past 30 years examining the effects

TABLE 8-2	Symptoms of Clinical Depression
Category	**Symptom**
Behavior	Fatigue or loss of energy almost every day.
	Insomnia or hypersomnia (excessive sleeping) almost every day.
	Restlessness or feeling slowed down.
Affective	Feelings of worthlessness or guilt almost every day.
	Markedly diminished interest or pleasure in almost all activities nearly every day (i.e., anhedonia).
Cognitive	Impaired concentration, indecisiveness.
	Recurring thoughts of death or suicide.
Physical	Significant weight loss or gain (a change of more than 5% of body weight in a month).

American Psychiatric Association. (2013). *Diagnostic and statistical manual of mental disorders* (5th ed.). Washington, DC: Author.

of physical activity on both clinical and nonclinical depression (Lawlor & Hopker, 2001; Mead et al., 2009; North, McCullagh, & Vu Tran, 1991; Rimer et al., 2012). These reviews provide an opportunity to examine the effects of physical activity on both nonclinical and clinical depression.

CRITICAL THINKING ACTIVITY 8-2

© ecco/Shutterstock, Inc.

What is the difference between clinical and nonclinical depression? Provide examples of both types of depression. How does physical activity affect clinical and nonclinical depression?

Nonclinical Depression

Some depressive symptoms are common among people without clinical depression, such as feeling sad, blue, or down in the dumps. Everyone occasionally feels blue or sad, but these feelings are usually fleeting and pass within a few hours or a couple of days. Many physical activity interventions conducted with healthy adults have measured depressive symptoms because these symptoms are an important component of mental health and quality of life.

Adult Populations

Both meta-analytic and epidemiological studies have revealed that regular physical activity reduces the likelihood of depressive symptoms in healthy adults

(Conn, 2010b; Mammen & Faulkner, 2013; Sieverdes et al., 2012). For example, an epidemiological study that included 9,580 men aged 20 to 87 years found an inverse relationship between physical activity and depressive symptoms (Sieverdes et al., 2012). In other words, in healthy adults physical activity may prevent the onset of depression in the future.

A relationship has also been found between sitting time (i.e., sedentary behavior) and current depressive symptoms. For example, greater depression symptoms are related with greater time spent sitting in U.S. veterans, a population that faces a disproportionate chronic disease burden (Millstein et al., 2015). As further support, Steven Blair and his colleagues (Sui et al., 2015) examined the longitudinal association between sedentary behaviors and the risk of developing depressive symptoms. The study participants were 4,802 men and women aged 18 to 80 years in the Aerobics Center Longitudinal Study who did not report depressive moods when they completed a health survey in 1982. The participants also reported their time spent watching television and riding in a car each week. Approximately 9 years later the participants completed a depression scale.

The researchers found that among the 4,802 participants, 568 reported depressive symptoms during the follow-up assessment. After adjusting for the baseline moderate- and vigorous-intensity physical activity, time spent riding in a car, time spent watching television, and the combined time spent in the two, sedentary behaviors were positively associated with depressive symptoms at the follow-up assessment. More specifically, adults who reported 9 hours a week or more riding in a car, more than 10 hours a week of watching television, or 19 hours a week or more of the combined sedentary behavior had a 28%, 52%, and 74% greater risk of development of depressive symptoms than those who reported less than 5 hours a week of riding in a car, less than 5 hours a week of watching television, or less than 12 hours a week of the combined sedentary behavior, after adjusting for baseline covariates and moderate- and vigorous-intensity physical activity (see **FIGURE 8-2**). In other words, the positive association between time riding in a car or time watching television and depressive symptoms was only observed among individuals who did not meet the current physical activity guidelines. The researchers concluded that more time reported in these two sedentary behaviors was positively associated with depressive symptoms. However, the direct associations between time spent in car riding and television viewing and depressive symptoms were only significant among those who did not meet the current physical activity recommendations.

In another study, van Uffelen and colleagues (2013) examined both concurrent and prospective associations of time spent sitting and physical activity with depressive symptoms in 8,950 middle-aged women

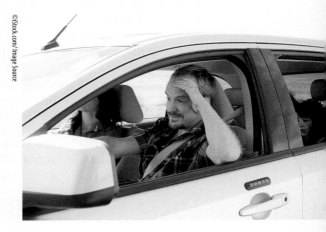
©iStock.com/Image Source

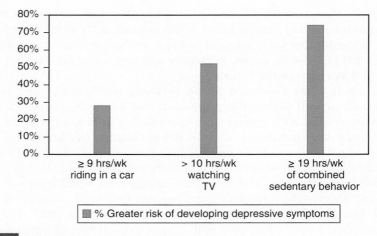

FIGURE 8-2 Risk of Developing Depressive Symptoms

Adults who reported 9 hours a week or more riding in a car, more than 10 hours a week watching TV, or 19 hours a week or more of the combined two sedentary behaviors had 28%, 52%, and 74% greater risk of development of depressive symptoms than those who reported less than 5 hours a week of riding in a car, less than 5 hours per week of watching TV, or less than 12 hours a week of the combined sedentary behaviors, respectively, after adjusting for baseline covariates and moderate- and vigorous-intensity physical activity.

Reprinted from Sui, X., Brown, W. J., Lavie, C. J., West, D. S., Pate, R. R., Payne, J. P., & Blair, S. N. (2015). Association between television watching and car riding behaviors and development of depressive symptoms: A prospective study. *Mayo Clinic Proceedings*, Feb;90(2):184–193. doi:10.1016/j.mayocp.2014.12.006. With permission from Elsevier.

(50 to 55 years). For the concurrent associations, women who sat more than 7 hours a day and women who did no physical activity were more likely to have depressive symptoms than women who sat less than or equal to 4 hours a day and who met the physical activity guidelines. In fact, the likelihood of depressive symptoms in women who sat more than 7 hours a day and did no physical activity was triple that of women who sat less than or equal to 4 hours a day and met the physical activity guidelines. For the prospective associations, sitting-time was not related with depressive symptoms, but women who did no physical activity were more likely than those who met physical activity guidelines to have future depressive symptoms. These study findings showed that engaging in at least 150 minutes a week of moderate physical activity can alleviate current depression symptoms and prevent future depressive symptoms. In comparison, reducing sitting-time may reduce current depressive symptoms. Other researchers have also found that sedentary behavior may not predict subsequent depressive symptoms but can predict current depression symptoms (Hamer & Stamatakis, 2014; Teychenne, Abbott, Ball, & Salmon, 2014). Thus, limiting sedentary behaviors such as TV viewing and video games may reduce current depressive symptoms (Carli et al., 2014).

Youth and Adolescents

What about younger populations? Depression in childhood and adolescence is similar to adult major depressive disorder, although young sufferers may exhibit increased irritability or aggressive and self-destructive behavior. Children who are under stress, who experience loss, or who have attention, learning, behavioral, or anxiety disorders are at a higher risk for depression. About 8% of children and adolescents suffer from depression (Eapan, 2012). It is recommended that treatment with medication with young populations should only be given acutely, and thus other "safer" forms of childhood depression treatment are needed.

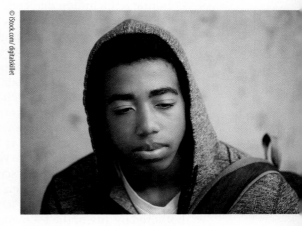

Ian Janssen and Allana LeBlanc (2010) conducted a systematic review of the health benefits of physical activity in school-age children (ages 5 to 7 years). They found that physical activity was associated with many health benefits for youth, including improvements in depression symptoms. The researchers thus concluded that children should accumulate at least 60 minutes of daily moderate physical activity for mental and physical health.

As well, childhood physical activity reduces the risk of depression in young adulthood, with larger effects found for men than women (McKercher et al., 2014). Compared with those who were persistently inactive, males who were increasingly and persistently active had about a 67% reduced risk of depression in adulthood. In comparison, females who were persistently active had a 51% reduced risk of depression in adulthood.

What about patients with chronic illnesses? Both physical inactivity and comorbid depressive symptoms are prevalent among patients with a chronic illness. Matthew Herring and his colleagues (2012) conducted a meta-analysis examining whether exercise training affected depressive symptoms among patients with chronic illnesses. Their meta-analysis included 90 articles and 10,534 sedentary patients with chronic illnesses such as cardiovascular disease, fibromyalgia, obesity, multiple sclerosis, and **cardiometabolic disease**. They found that exercise reduces depressive symptoms among patients with a chronic illness. They also found that patients with mild to moderate depressive symptoms and for whom exercise training improved function-related outcomes achieved the largest antidepressant effects. The researchers concluded that their findings provide evidence to recommend exercise training to patients as a potential low-risk, adjuvant treatment for depressive symptoms that may develop during chronic illness.

In summary, the results of the aforementioned reviews, taken as a whole, provide strong evidence that physical activity is beneficial for healthy adults, adults with chronic illnesses, and young children in improving depression symptoms.

Clinical Depression

Major Depressive Disorder

The global lifetime prevalence of major depression ranges from 3% in Japan to 17% in the United States (Kessler et al., 2003). Almost twice as many women as men have major depression. Depression also often co-occurs with many medical conditions, including diabetes, obesity, stroke, multiple sclerosis, and cardiovascular disease.

Major depression is diagnosed by a psychiatric interview. In addition to psychiatric interviews, a number of self-report questionnaires have been developed to assess the severity of depressive symptoms. It should be noted that although questionnaires may have established "cut-points" to identify persons who may be clinically depressed, such assessments are not diagnostic tools but rather measures of the presence and severity of depressive symptoms.

One of the most widely used self-report instruments to identify if a person may be clinically depressed is the Patient Health Questionnaire-9 (Lichtman et al., 2009; Spitzer, Kroenke, & Williams, 1999). The two-item Patient Health Questionnaire-2 is used as a brief screen, followed by the full Patient Health Questionnaire-9 for people who screen positive on the two-item questionnaire. For each question people are asked: "Over the past 2 weeks, how often have you been bothered by any of the following problems?" Questions are scored on a scale from 0 indicating "Not at all" to 3 indicating "Nearly every day." See **TABLE 8-3** for a description of these Patient Health Questionnaire items.

TABLE 8-3	**The Patient Health Questionnaire: PHQ-2 and PHQ-9**
PHQ Items	**Question**
2	1. Little interest or pleasure in doing things. 2. Feeling down, depressed, or hopeless.
9	1. Little interest or pleasure in doing things. 2. Feeling down, depressed, or hopeless. 3. Trouble falling asleep, staying asleep, or sleeping too much. 4. Feeling tired or having little energy. 5. Poor appetite or overeating. 6. Feeling bad about yourself, feeling that you are a failure, or feeling that you have let yourself or your family down. 7. Trouble concentrating on things such as reading the newspaper or watching television. 8. Moving or speaking so slowly that other people could have noticed; or being so fidgety or restless that you have been moving around a lot more than usual. 9. Thinking that you would be better off dead or that you want to hurt yourself in some way.

Conventional treatments for depression typically include psychotherapy and pharmacotherapy. Psychotherapy (also called talk therapy) involves either individual or group counseling of 4 months or longer, and it is an effective long-term treatment for depression. In comparison, pharmacotherapy involves taking an antidepressant medication, and it is the most commonly used treatment for major depression. About 50% of patients taking an antidepressant will have a clinical response to treatment, meaning that they have at least a 50% reduction in depressive symptoms. Many people, however, will require augmented treatment with more than one antidepressant. Although a variety of pharmaceutical agents are available for the treatment of depression, psychiatrists find than many patients cannot tolerate the side effects, do not respond adequately, or finally lose their response to the prescribed antidepressant medication (Fournier et al., 2010). Thus, there is a need for more effective and less toxic treatments for major depression. Let's take a closer look at the research that has examined the effects of exercise as an alternative treatment for depression.

The effects of exercise on people with major depression have been examined in over 35 randomized controlled trials (Mead et al., 2009). In a large-scale review, Gary Cooney and his colleagues (2013) conducted a meta-analysis that included 39 trials examining the effects of exercise on people suffering with depression ($N = 2,326$ total patients). They found that when compared with no treatment or with the control interventions, exercise was associated with a moderate to high treatment effect (ES = −.62). Many of the trials reviewed, however, had either biases or other faults. Thus, the researchers examined the effects of the exercise on depressive symptoms with only well-designed trials.

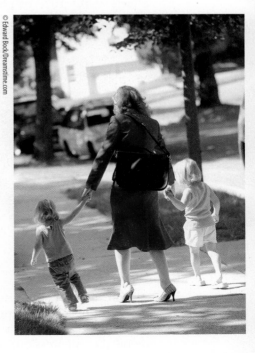

When the analyses were limited to these higher-quality trials that used **intention-to-treat analyses** and blinded outcome assessment, the effect was slightly weaker, suggesting only a small antidepressant effect associated with exercise. These later findings highlight that although multiple trials have been conducted among adults with major depression, few studies have used high-quality methods in which treatment allocation is concealed, intention-to-treat analyses are used, a control group is included in the design, and depression is assessed by clinical interview in which the assessor is blinded to the treatment group (Blumenthal, Smith, & Hoffman, 2012). In fact, many trials included in the review used participant self-report rating as a method for postintervention analysis. Of importance, exercise was as effective as psychological therapy and pharmacological treatment, and more effective than bright light therapy in treating depressive symptoms.

CRITICAL THINKING ACTIVITY 8-3

© ecco/Shutterstock, Inc.

Why do you think that childhood physical activity reduces the risk of depression in young adulthood, with larger effects found for men than women? What are the possible explanations for this gender difference?

Sedentary behavior is also related to major depressive disorder (de Wit, van Straten, Lamers, Cuijpers, & Penninx, 2011). After controlling for physical activity level, people with major depressive disorder spend significantly more leisure time using the computer compared to healthy people. As well, people with **dysthymia** (most recently renamed to *persistent depressive disorder*) spend significantly more hours a day watching television compared to healthy people. These findings reveal that sedentary behavior is an independent correlate of depressive disorders.

Postpartum Depression

Postpartum depression is not recognized as a separate depressive disorder, but rather women must meet the criteria for a major depressive episode with onset either during pregnancy or within 4 weeks of delivery. Postpartum depression affects about 10% of postpartum women. Symptoms include sadness, fatigue,

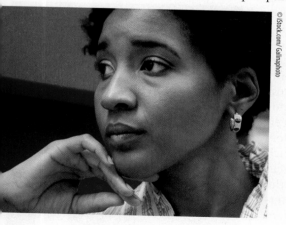

© iStock.com/ Galinaphoto

changes in sleeping and eating patterns, reduced libido, crying episodes, anxiety, and irritability.

Emerging research reveals that leisure-time physical activity prior to, during, and after pregnancy may be important for reducing the risk of postnatal depression and improving the overall mental well-being of the mother (Bahadoran, Tirkesh, & Oreizi, 2014). There is a dose–response effect, with moderate and vigorous activities more likely to be associated with maternal well-being than mild physical activities. As well, a positive relationship between sedentary behavior and the presence of postnatal depressive symptoms has also been found (Teychenne & York, 2013).

Bipolar Disorder

Bipolar disorder was historically classified as a depressive disorder; however, in the current *DSM-5* it appears in the section with bipolar and related disorders (APA, 2013). **Bipolar disorder** is a condition in which a person has periods of low mood (i.e., depression) and periods of high mood (i.e., mania). The symptoms of bipolar disorder are severe, and they differ from the normal ups and downs that everyone goes through from time to time. During mania, an individual feels abnormally happy, energetic, or excitable, but often makes poor decisions due to either unrealistic ideas or poor regard of consequences. Manic and depressive episodes can impair the individual's ability to function in ordinary life.

Little is known about the effects of physical activity and sedentary behavior on adults with bipolar disorder; however, a recent study by Janney et al. (2014) has shed some light on the topic. The purpose of their study was to objectively measure physical activity and sedentary behavior among adult outpatients with bipolar disorder. To accomplish their purpose, the researchers had 60 adults with bipolar disorder wear an accelerometer for 7 consecutive days. On average, the adults wore the accelerometers more than 17 hours a days (i.e., the monitoring time).

The researchers found that for most of the monitoring time these patients were sedentary (i.e., about 13.5 hours a day, or 78% of the monitoring time). With regard to physical activity, they found that these bipolar patients spent only 21% (or 215 minutes) of the monitoring time each day engaged in light activity, and no patients achieved the physical activity guidelines of accumulating 150 minutes a week of at least moderate physical activity or 75 minutes of vigorous physical activity. In other words, bipolar patients spent 78% of their waking hours engaged in sedentary activities, about 21% engaged in light activities, and 1% (14 minutes a day) in at least moderate physical activities (see **FIGURE 8-3**). In short, adults with bipolar disorder are less active and more sedentary than mentally healthy individuals.

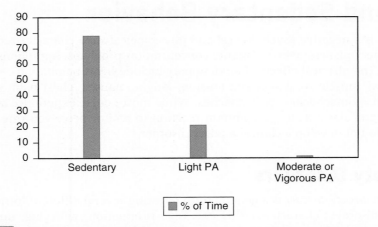

FIGURE 8-3   Percentage of Time/Day Bipolar Patients Spend in Sedentary Behavior and Physical Activity

Reprinted from Janney, C. A., Fagiolini, A., Swartz, H. A., Jakicic, J. M., Holleman, R. G., & Richardson, D. R. (2014). Are adults with bipolar disorder active? Objectively measured physical activity and sedentary behavior using accelerometry. *Journal of Affective Disorders*, 498–504. With permission from Elsevier.

In summary, physical activity seems to be an effective treatment for depression, improving depression symptoms to a comparable extent as pharmacotherapy and psychotherapy. While the optimal dose of exercise is unknown, any exercise is better than no exercise. Although physical activity is a useful treatment for individuals suffering from depression, adherence to a plan for physical activity is often low. Patients with major depression often find it difficult to initiate and sustain an exercise routine. Motivation for exercise may be affected by depressive symptoms such as fatigue, low self-esteem, and poor sleep. Also, depressed people with higher levels of anxiety and lower levels of fitness are at even higher risk for exercise nonadherence (DiMatteo, Lepper, & Croghan, 2000). Thus, exercise professionals working with depressed individuals should become familiar with applying the motivational theories such as the theory of planned behavior and social cognitive theory in an attempt to increase adherence.

CRITICAL THINKING ACTIVITY 8-4

© ecco/Shutterstock, Inc.

Why does the quality of the trial have an effect on the strength of the results for the research examining the effects of exercise on depression? How would you design a high-quality trial to examine the effects of exercise on patients with clinical depression?

Anxiety, Physical Activity, and Sedentary Behavior

Anxiety is a negative psychological and physiological state characterized by feelings of nervousness, worry, fatigue, concentration problems, apprehension, and arousal. The physical effects of anxiety may include heart palpitations, sweating, trembling, muscle weakness and tension, fatigue, nausea, chest pain, shortness of breath, stomachaches, or headaches. While most people experience anxiety to some degree daily, as it is a common reaction to real or perceived threats, most people do not develop a clinical anxiety disorder.

Anxiety Disorders

The term *anxiety disorder* is a general term covering several different forms of psychiatric disorders characterized by excessive rumination, worrying, uneasiness, and fear about future uncertainties that are either based on real or imagined events. The global prevalence of people who suffer from an anxiety disorder is estimated to be 7.3% (Baxter, Scott, Vox, & Whiteford, 2013). Anxiety disorders are pervasive and include the following disorders of generalized anxiety disorder, **specific phobias**, social phobia, agoraphobia, panic disorder, and **separation**

TABLE 8-4	Clinical Anxiety Disorders
Anxiety Disorder	**Description**
Generalized anxiety disorder	Long-lasting anxiety that is not focused on any one object or situation. Nonspecific persistent fear and worry and becoming overly concerned with everyday matters.
Specific phobias	Fear and anxiety is triggered by a specific stimulus or situation.
Panic disorder	Brief attacks of intense terror and apprehension, often marked by trembling, shaking, confusion, dizziness, nausea, and difficulty breathing.
Social anxiety disorder	Intense fear and avoidance of negative public scrutiny, public embarrassment, humiliation, or social interaction.
Separation anxiety disorder	Excessive anxiety regarding separation from home or from people to whom the person has a strong emotional attachment such as a parent, grandparents, or siblings.
Panic attack	Sudden onset periods of intense fear that range from minutes to hours.
Agoraphobia	Anxiety in situations where the person perceives certain environments as dangerous or uncomfortable (e.g., bridges, shopping malls, airports).

anxiety disorder (APA, 2013). See **TABLE 8-4** for descriptions of these clinical anxiety disorders.

About 75% of people who suffer with clinical depression are also affected by an anxiety disorder (Myers et al., 1984). Not surprisingly, common treatments of psychotherapy and antidepressants for clinical depression are similar to those for anxiety disorders. Despite their modest effectiveness, the use of antidepressants and psychotherapy to treat anxiety disorders, however, has drawn criticism. Common criticisms include a slow onset of action and time to maximal effect and a number of side effects, such as increased anxiety in the short term (which often leads to lower compliance) and sexual issues (Schweitzer, Maguire, & Ng, 2009). New treatments for anxiety disorders that are effective, widely accessible, and have minimal negative side effects are needed. One such potential method of treatment for anxiety disorders that has generated a great deal of research is physical activity.

State and Trait Anxiety

Besides understanding the distinction between clinical and nonclinical anxiety, it is important to differentiate between *state* and *trait anxiety*. **State anxiety** is characterized by a state of heightened emotions that develop in response to either a fear or danger of a particular situation. State anxiety is what we experience, for example, when we are doing a presentation, writing an exam, and watching a closely matched sporting event; that is, state anxiety is a reaction that produces a number of anxiety symptoms associated with the respiratory system (e.g., increased breathing rate), digestive system (e.g., butterflies in the stomach), and circulatory system (e.g., increased heart rate) to an immediate threat. After the "threat" has subsided, the anxiety state lessens until we feel "normal" again.

In comparison, **trait anxiety** refers to a general level of anxiety that is characteristic of an individual. Thus, trait anxiety is often referred to as a personality characteristic. Trait anxiety varies according to how people have conditioned themselves to respond to and manage their stress. What may cause anxiety in one person may not generate any emotion in another. People with high levels of trait anxiety are often quite easily stressed and anxious in many different types of situations.

CRITICAL THINKING ACTIVITY 8-5

© ecco/Shutterstock, Inc.

What are the differences between clinical and nonclinical anxiety and state and trait anxiety? Can exercise affect these four distinct types of anxiety? Provide support for your answer.

The State-Trait Anxiety Inventory (STAI) (Spielberger, Gorssuch, Lushene, Vagg, & Jacobs, 1983) is a self-report psychological questionnaire that is commonly used to assess state and trait anxiety. It can be used in clinical settings to diagnose anxiety and to distinguish anxiety from depression. The STAI has 20 items for assessing trait anxiety (i.e., how you generally feel) and 20 items for assessing state anxiety (i.e., how you feel right now, at this moment). See **TABLE 8-5** for sample items from the STAI. Each item is answered on a Likert-type scale of 1 (almost never), 2 (sometimes), 3 (often), and 4 (almost always). Higher scores indicate greater anxiety.

State Anxiety

A number of meta-analyses have been conducted to summarize the research on physical activity and anxiety (e.g., Conn, 2010a; Kugler, Seelback, & Krüskemper, 1994; Long & van Stavel, 1995; Petruzzello, Landers, Hatfield, Kubitz, & Salazar, 1991; Sarris et al., 2012; Wipfli et al., 2008). The number and types of studies included in these meta-analyses have varied widely. Nonetheless, the overriding conclusion reached in these reviews is that physical activity is associated with small to moderate reductions in anxiety.

For example, in the Petruzzello et al. (1991) study, dependent measures of anxiety were divided into three categories: self-reported state anxiety, self-reported

TABLE 8-5	Sample Items from the State–Trait Anxiety Inventory
State Anxiety Items	I am tense.
	I am worried.
	I feel anxious.
	I feel jittery.
Trait Anxiety Items	I worry too much over something that really doesn't matter.
	I feel nervous and restless.
	I lack confidence.
	I feel like a failure.

Data from Spielberger, C. D., Gorssuch, R. L., Lushene, P. R., Vagg, P. R., & Jacobs, G. A. (1983). *Manual for the State-Trait Anxiety Inventory.* Palo Alto, CA: Consulting Psychologists Press.

trait anxiety, and psychophysiological measures of anxiety. While the effect sizes for all three categories indicated that exercise was associated with a reduction in anxiety, effect sizes ranged from .24 for state anxiety and .34 for trait anxiety to .56 for psychophysiological measures of anxiety.

The beneficial effect that physical activity has on state anxiety begins within 5 minutes following an acute bout of exercise. Although there is some research that shows that this beneficial effect could last for up to 6 hours, it is generally accepted that the duration is substantially less, typically lasting up to about 2 hours (Landers & Petruzzello, 1994). Therefore, the effects of exercise on anxiety levels is almost immediate (i.e., 5 minutes following exercise) and typically lasts up to 2 hours.

Nonclinical Anxiety

Vicki Conn (2010a) conducted a meta-analysis to examine the effects of physical activity interventions ($N = 19$ reports) on anxiety levels of 3,289 healthy adults without anxiety disorders. The overall effect size was small (ES = .22) but showed that physical activity interventions resulted in decreased anxiety scores for healthy adults. Exploratory moderator analyses revealed larger anxiety improvement among studies that included larger samples, used random allocation of participants to treatment and control conditions, targeted only physical activity behavior instead of multiple health behaviors, included supervised exercise (vs. home-based physical activity), used moderate- or high-intensity instead of low-intensity physical activity, and suggested participants exercise at a fitness facility (vs. home) following the interventions. Conn concluded that even healthy adults experience reduced anxiety following diverse unsupervised and supervised physical activity interventions. She also noted that the clinical importance of her meta-analytic findings are difficult to assess given the absence of either gold standard measures or criterion values for anxiety in the studies she reviewed.

In an effort to overcome the issue of study quality, Bradley Wipfli and his colleagues (2008) examined the anxioltyic (i.e., anxiety reducing) effects of exercise with studies that used randomized controlled trial designs. The trials had to include a self-report measure of anxiety (e.g., the STAI) and an independent exercise intervention (i.e., trials that did not include additional interventions). The groups included either exercise compared with a no-treatment control or exercise compared with another form of anxiety-reducing treatment (such as cognitive behavioral therapy, group therapy, light exercise, relaxation/mediation, stress management, pharmacotherapy, or music therapy).

The researchers also reviewed studies that assessed people with both clinical (n = 3 studies) and nonclinical (n = 46 studies) anxiety. Thus, most of the trials included participants who were either not clinically diagnosed with an anxiety disorder or not receiving treatment for anxiety. They found an overall effect size of −.48, indicating larger reductions in anxiety among people in the exercise groups than people in the no-treatment control groups. The exercise groups also had equal or slightly greater reductions in anxiety in all the comparison groups, except for pharmacotherapy. The authors concluded that exercise alone can be effective at reducing anxiety because none of the studies included in their meta-analysis combined exercise with some other form of treatment. In addition, the comparison of exercise to other forms of treatment revealed that exercise is as effective, and nearly as effective as the two most common treatments for anxiety disorders—psychotherapy and pharmacotherapy, respectively. This finding supports the use of exercise as a promising treatment for anxiety.

Researchers have also found that exercise interventions are effective in reducing anxiety levels in several special populations, including cancer patients undergoing treatment, cancer survivors (Mishra et al., 2012a, 2012b), and patients with systemic lupus erythematosus (Zhange, Wei, & Wang, 2012).

Clinical Anxiety

Only recently have researchers begun to examine the effects of exercise on people with a clinical anxiety disorder. This emerging body of research is revealing that exercise may be an effective treatment for some anxiety disorders. Epidemiological surveys have found that regular physical activity is associated with reduced anxiety symptoms in people with a clinical anxiety disorder (Goodwin, 2003). For example, using cross-sectional data from the U.S. national comorbidity study of 8,098 adults aged 15 to 54, Renee Goodwin (2003) found that regular exercise was associated with reduced prevalence of an anxiety disorder. A limitation, however, with cross-sectional studies is their inability to explain the direction of the physical activity and anxiety relationship; that is, are people who exercise less likely to have anxiety disorders or does regular exercise result in the reduction of anxiety disorders? Regardless, anxiety disorders (similar to major depression) are associated with many symptoms that are related to low physical activity adherence (e.g., fatigue, poor motivation, and social isolation; de Assis et al., 2008).

Emerging research is revealing that physical activity may be an effective treatment for anxiety disorders (Sarris et al., 2012; Zschucke, Gauditz, & Strohle, 2013). For example, physical activity shows initial promise as a treatment for patients with **social anxiety disorder** (Jazaieri, Goldin, Werner, Ziv, & Gross, 2012), **generalized anxiety disorder** (Herring, Jacob, Suveg, Dishman, & O'Conner, 2012), and **panic disorder** (Broocks et al., 1998; Hovland et al., 2013). More research is needed with larger sample sizes with control conditions before firm conclusions can be made regarding the efficacy of exercise for the treatment of anxiety disorders (Asmundson et al., 2013; Bartley, Hay, & Bloch, 2013).

Sedentary behaviors are also related to panic disorder and agoraphobia (de Wit et al., 2011); that is, independent of physical activity, people suffering with panic disorder and **agoraphobia** spend more daily hours watching television compared to healthy people.

In summary, meta-analyses clearly reveal that exercise has an acute anxiolytic effect in nonclinical populations. Preliminary research reveals that exercise may be an effective therapy for treating anxiety disorders. Rigorously controlled trials, however, are needed to provide stronger support of the use of physical activity as an effective therapy for anxiety disorders (Sarris et al., 2012).

Optimal Amount of Exercise Needed

Unfortunately, the optimal dose of physical activity needed to improve or sustain mental health and mood is not known (Kim et al., 2012). In other words, how much exercise is needed to reduce anxiety and depressive symptoms. A recent study by Yeon Soo Kim and colleagues (2012) sheds some light on this important question. It appears that an optimal range of 2.5 to 7.5 hours (approximately 150 to 450 minutes) per week of physical activity is ideal for mental health. Kim et al. found that study participants who engaged in 2.5 to 7.5 hours per week of physical activity had better mental health than those who exercised either below or above this range. The authors note that the upper end (i.e., > 7.5 hours a week) could be attained, for example, by running about an hour a day. The idea that there may be an upper limit for mental health benefits of exercise is intriguing, and provides some support for the research on the negative health effects of excessive exercise and exercise dependence. The relationship between physical activity and general mental health findings of Kim et al. (2012) may have important implications from a public health perspective, because mental health disorders such as anxiety and depression are common. If physical activity can either prevent or improve mental health, the public health impact of promoting regular physical activity, although a challenge, could be great.

Potential Mechanisms

Science proceeds from description to explanation and then from prediction to intervention. Investigations of the link between acute and chronic bouts of physical activity and anxiety and depression have produced a substantial body of descriptive research. That research shows that the link is often small, but nevertheless positive. Acute and chronic physical activity is associated with positive psychological benefits, with the latter being more beneficial than the former. A question that now arises is, why is this the case? What are the underlying reasons for these benefits? In other words, what are the mechanisms causing these effects? A number of explanations have been advanced (Asmundson et al., 2013; Landers & Arent, 2007). The therapeutic effect of physical activity in improving mood is likely the result of complex interactions between physiological and psychological processes.

Physiological hypotheses that have been developed to explain the anxiolytic and antidepressive effects of exercise include the brain-derived neurotrophic factor hypothesis, the endorphin hypothesis, the endocannabinoid hypothesis, the hypothalamic-pituitary-adrenal axis hypothesis, and the norepinephrine hypothesis. These hypotheses remain tenable and are supported primarily by animal models, and only a paucity of research has examined these hypotheses in humans (Landers & Arent, 2007).

Many psychological theories are still under investigation, including improvements in sleep, self-esteem, and self-efficacy as a means of reducing depression and anxiety (Landers & Arent, 2007). Understanding this association and the manner in which physical activity contributes to enhanced positive feelings in everyday life may help to answer whether people can manage their mood through their physical activities.

Summary

Scientists have had a long-standing interest in the association between physical activity and moods such as anxiety and depression. The results from this body of research are unequivocal. For male and female populations across the age spectrum, physical activity is related to improvements in anxiety and depression. This effect is found in both people suffering with clinical anxiety and depression disorders as well as individuals without clinical anxiety disorders. There is no doubt that physical activity is effective as an intervention strategy to reduce depression. And preliminary research reveals that exercise shows promise as a treatment for clinical anxiety disorders. The challenge with these special populations is adherence to physical activity.

KEY TERMS

affect
agoraphobia
anxiety
bipolar disorder
cardiometabolic disease
clinical depression
dysthymia
emotions
generalized anxiety disorder
intention-to-treat analyses

moods
nonclinical depression
panic disorder
postpartum depression
separation anxiety disorder
social anxiety disorder
specific phobia
state anxiety
trait anxiety

REVIEW QUESTIONS

1. Define *affect*, *mood*, and *emotion*. How do these three terms differ from each other?

2. What is the difference between clinical and nonclinical depression?

3. Describe the symptoms of clinical depression (major depression). Is physical activity an effective treatment for clinical depression? Explain.

4. What is the difference between clinical and nonclinical anxiety?

5. Identify three clinical anxiety disorders and describe their symptoms.

6. What is the difference between state and trait anxiety?

7. What does preliminary research reveal regarding physical activity as an effective therapy for treating anxiety disorders?

8. How is sedentary behavior related to both current depressive symptoms and future depressive symptoms?

9. What is postpartum depression? What role do both sedentary behavior and physical activity have with this type of depression?

APPLYING THE CONCEPTS

1. What type of anxiety (state or trait) did Laura likely experience when she went off her antidepressants? Was it clinical?

2. What might explain the positive effects becoming regularly active has had on Laura's depression?

3. What factors explain why many people suffering from depression are reluctant to exercise, despite the improvements physical activity can confer to their symptoms?

REFERENCES

American Psychiatric Association. (2013). *Diagnostic and statistical manual of mental disorders* (5th ed.). Washington, DC: Author.

Asmundson, G. J., Fetzner, M. G., Deboer, L. B., Powers, M. B., Otto, M. W., & Smits, J. A. (2013). Let's get physical: A contemporary review of the anxiolytic effects of exercise for anxiety and its disorders. *Depression and Anxiety, 30*, 362–373.

Bahadoran, P., Tirkesh, F., & Oreizi, H. R. (2014). Association between physical activity 3–12 months after delivery and postpartum well-being. *Iran Journal of Nursing and Midwifery Research, 19*, 82–87.

Bartley, C. A., Hay, M., & Bloch, M. H. (2013). Meta-analysis: Aerobic exercise for the treatment of anxiety disorders. *Progress in Neuro-Psychopharmacology and Biological Psychiatry, 45*, 34–39.

Baxter, A. J., Scott, K. M., Vos, T., & Whiteford, H. A. (2013). Global prevalence of anxiety disorders: A systematic review and meta-regression. *Psychological Medicine, 45*, 897–910.

Blumenthal, J. A., Smith, P. J., & Hoffman, B. M. (2012). Opinion and evidence: Is exercise a viable treatment for depression? *ACSM's Health & Fitness Journal, 16*, 14–21.

Broocks, A., Bandelow, B., Pekrun, G., George, A., Meyer, T., Bartmann, U., . . . Ruther, E. (1998). Comparison of aerobic exercise, clomipramine, and placebo in the treatment of panic disorder. *American Journal of Psychiatry, 155*, 603–609.

Carli, V., Hoven, C. W., Wasserman, C., Chiesa, F., Guffanti, G., Sarchiapone, M., . . . Wasserman, D. (2014). A newly identified group of adolescents at "invisible" risk for psychopathology and suicidal behavior: Findings from the SEYLE study. *World Psychiatry, 13*, 78–86.

Conn, V. S. (2010a). Anxiety outcomes after physical activity interventions: Meta-analysis findings *Nursing Research, 59*, 224–231.

Conn, V. S. (2010b). Depressive symptom outcomes of physical activity interventions: Meta-analysis findings. *Annals of Behavioral Medicine, 39*, 128–138.

Cooney, G. M., Dwan, K., Greig, C. A., Lawlor, D. A., Rimer, J., Waugh, F. R., . . . Mead, G. E. (2013). Exercise for depression. *Cochrane Database of Systematic Reviews.* Sept. 12;9:CD004366.

de Assis, M. A., de Mello, M. F., Scorza, F. A., Cadrobbi, M. P., Schooedl, A. F., da Silva, S., . . . Arida, R. M. (2008). Evaluation of physical activity habits in patients with posttraumatic stress disorder. *Clinics, 63*, 473–478.

de Wit, L., van Straten, A., Lamers, F., Cuijpers, P., & Penninx, B. (2011). Are sedentary television watching and computer use behaviors associated with anxiety and depressive disorders? *Psychiatry Research, 186*, 239–243.

DiMatteo, M. R., Lepper, H. S., & Croghan, T. W. (2000). Depression is a risk factor for noncompliance with medical treatment: Meta-analysis of the effects of anxiety and depression on patient adherence. *Archives in Internal Medicine, 160*, 2101–2107.

Eapen, V. (2012). Strategies and challenges in the management of adolescent depression. *Current Opinion in Psychiatry, 25*, 7–13.

Edwards, T. (1908). *A dictionary of thoughts: Being a cyclopedia of laconic quotations from the best authors of the world, both ancient and modern.* Whitefish, MT: Kessinger Publishing.

Ekkekakis, P. (2008). Affect, mood, and emotion. In G. Tenenbaum, R. C. Eklund, & A. Kamata (Eds.). *Measurement in sport and exercise psychology* (pp. 321–332). Champaign, IL: Human Kinetics.

Fournier, J. C., DeRubeis, R. J., Hollon, S. D., Dimidjian, S., Amsterdam, J. D., Shelton, R. C., & Fawcett, J. (2010). Antidepressant drug effects and depression severity: A patient-level meta-analysis. *JAMA, 303*, 47–53.

Franz, S. I., & Hamilton, G. V. (1905). The effect of exercise upon retardation in conditions of depression. *American Journal of Insanity, 62*, 239–256.

Goodwin, R. D. (2003). Association between physical activity and mental disorders among adults in the United States. *Preventive Medicine, 36*, 698–703.

Hamer, M., & Stamatakis, E. (2014). Prospective study of sedentary behavior, risk of depression, and cognitive impairment. *Medicine and Science in Sports and Exercise, 46*, 718–723.

Herring, M. P., Jacob, M. L., Suveg, C., Dishman, R. K., & O'Connor, P. J. (2012). Feasibility of exercise training for the short-term treatment of generalized anxiety disorder: A randomized controlled trial. *Psychotherapy and Psychosomatics, 81*, 21–28.

Herring, M. P., Puetz, T. W., O'Connor, P. J., & Dishman, R. K. (2012). Effect of exercise training on depressive symptoms among patients with a chronic illness: A systematic review and meta-analysis of randomized controlled trials. *Archives of Internal Medicine, 172*, 101–111.

Hovland, A., Nordhus, I. H., Sjobo, T., Giestad, B. A., Birknes, B., Martinsen, E. W., . . . Pallesen, S. (2013). Comparing physical exercise in groups to group cognitive behaviour therapy for the treatment of panic disorder in a randomized controlled trial. *Behavioural and Cognitive Psychotherapy, 41*, 408–432.

Janney, C. A., Fagiolini, A., Swartz, H. A., Jakicic, J. M., Holleman, R. G., & Richardson, D. R. (2014). Are adults with bipolar disorder active? Objectively measured physical activity and sedentary behavior using accelerometry. *Journal of Affective Disorders, 152–154*, 498–504.

Janssen, I., & Leblanc, A. G. (2010). Systematic review of the health benefits of physical activity and fitness in school-age children and youth. *International Journal of Behavioral Nutrition and Physical Activity.* May 11;7:40. doi: 10.1186/1479-5868-7-40

Jazaieri, H., Goldin, P. R., Werner, K., Ziv, M., & Gross, J. J. (2012). A randomized trial of MBSR versus aerobic exercise for social anxiety disorder. *Journal of Clinical Psychology, 68*, 715–731.

Kessler, R. C., Berglund, P., Demler, O., Jin, R., Koretz, D., Merkangas, K. R., . . . Wang, P. S. (2003). The epidemiology of major depressive disorder: Results from the National Comorbidity Survey Replication (NCS-R). *JAMA, 18*, 3095–3105.

Kim, Y, S., Park, Y. S., Allegrante, J. P., Marks, R., Ok, H., Cho, K. O., & Garber, C. E. (2012). Relationship between physical activity and general mental health. *Preventive Medicine, 55*, 458–463.

Kugler, J., Seelback, H., & Kruskemper, G. M. (1994). Effects of rehabilitative exercise programmes on anxiety and depression in coronary patients: A meta-analysis. *British Journal of Clinical Psychology, 33*, 401–410.

Landers, D. M., & Arent, S. M. (2007). Physical activity and mental health. In G. Tenenbaum, & R. C. Eklund (Eds.), *Handbook of sport psychology* (3rd ed.) (pp. 469–491). New York, NY: Wiley & Sons.

Lawlor, D. A., & Hopker, S. W. (2001). The effectiveness of exercise as an intervention in the management of depression: Systematic review and meta-regression analysis of randomized controlled trials. *BMJ, 322,* 763–767.

Lichtman, J. H., Bigger, J. T. Jr., Blumenthal, J. A., Frasure-Smith, N., Kaufmann, P. G., Lesperance, F., . . . Froelicher, E. S. (2009). AHA science advisory. Depression and coronary heart disease. Recommendations for screening, referral, and treatment. A science advisory from the American Heart Association Prevention Committee to the Council on Cardiovascular Nursing, Council on Clinical Cardiology, Council on Epidemiology and Prevention, and Interdisciplinary Council on Quality of Care Outcomes Research. Endorsed by the American Psychiatric Association. *Progressive Cardiovascular Nursing, 24,* 19–26.

Long, B. C., & van Stavel, R. (1995). Effects of exercise training on anxiety: A meta-analysis. *Journal of Applied Sport Psychology, 7,* 167–189.

Lohoff, F. W. (2010). Overview of the genetics of major depressive disorder. *Current Psychiatry Reports, 12,* 539–546.

Mammen, G., & Faullkner, G. (2013). Physical activity and the prevention of depression: A systematic review of prospective studies. *American Journal of Preventive Medicine, 45,* 649–657.

McKercher, C., Sanderson, K., Schmidt, M. D., Otahal, P., Patton, G. C., Dwyer, T., & Venn, A. J. (2014). Physical activity patterns and risk of depression in young adulthood: A 20-year cohort study since childhood. *Social Psychiatry and Psychiatric Epidemiology,* epub.

Mead, G. E., Morley, W., Campbell, P., Greig, C. A., McMurdo, M., & Lawlor, D. A. (2009). Exercise for depression. *Cochrane Database Systematic Review, 3:*CD004366.

Millstein, R. A., Hoerster, K. D., Rosenberg, D. E., Nelson, K. M., Reiber, G., & Saelens, B. E. (2015). Individual, social, and neighborhood associations with sitting time among veterans. *Journal of Physical Activity and Health,* Nov.;49(11):1823–1834. doi:10.1007/s00127-014-0863-7

Mishra, S. I., Scherer, R. W., Snyder, C., Geigle, P. M., Berlanstein, D. R., & Topaloglu, O. (2012a). Exercise interventions on health-related quality of life for people with cancer during active treatment. *Cochrane Database of Systematic Reviews, 8:*CD008465.

Mishra, S. I., Scherer, R. W., Geigle, P. M., Berlanstein, D. R., Topaloglu, O., Gotay, C. C., & Snyder, C. (2012b). Exercise interventions on health-related quality of life for cancer survivors. *Cochrane Database Systematic Review,* Aug. 15;8:CD007566.

Myers, J. K., Weissman, M. M., Tischler, G. L., Holzer, C. E., Leaf, P. J. et al. (1984). Six-month prevalence of psychiatric disorders in three communities 1980 to 1982. *Archives of General Psychiatry, 41,* 959–967.

North, T. C., McCullagh, P., & Tran, Z. V. (1990). Effect of exercise on depression. *Exercise and Sport Science Reviews, 18,* 379–415.

Petruzzello, S. J., Landers, D. M., Hatfield, B. D., Kubitz, K. A., & Salazar, W. (1991). A meta-analysis on the anxiety-reducing effects of acute and chronic exercise. *Sports Medicine, 11,* 143–182.

Rimer, J., Dwan, K., Lawlor, D. A., Greig, C. A., McMurdo, M., Morley, W., & Mead, G. E. (2012). Exercise for depression. *Cochrane Database Systematic Reviews, 11:*CD004366.

Sarris, J., Moylan, S., Camfield, D. A., Camfeld, D. A., Pase, M. P., Mischoulon, D., . . . Schweitzer, I. (2012). Complementary medicine, exercise meditation, diet, and lifestyle modification for anxiety disorders: A review of current evidence. *Evidence-Based Complementary and Alternative Medicine,* 2012:809653. doi:10.1155/2012/809653

Schweitzer, I., Maguire, K., & Ng, C. (2009). Sexual side-effects of contemporary antidepressants: Review. *Australian and New Zealand Journal of Psychiatry, 43,* 795–808.

Sieverdes, J. C., Ray, B. M., Sui, X., Lee, D. C., Hand, G. A., Baruth, M., & Blair, S. N. (2012). Association between leisure time physical activity and depressive symptoms in men. *Medicine and Science in Sports and Exercise, 44,* 260–265.

Spielberger, C.D., Gorssuch, R.L., Lushene, P.R., Vagg, P.R., & Jacobs, G.A (1983). *Manual for the State-Trait Anxiety Inventory.* Santa Clara, CA: Consulting Psychologists Press.

Spitzer, R. L., Kroenke, K., & Williams, J. B. (1999). Patient Health Questionnaire Primary Care Study Group, 1999. Validation and utility of a self-report version of PRIME-MD: the PHQ Primary Care Study. *JAMA, 282,* 1737–1744.

Sui, X., Brown, W. J., Lavie, C. J., West, D. S., Pate, R. R., Payne, J. P., & Blair, S. N. (2015). Association between television watching and car riding behaviors and development of depressive symptoms: A prospective study. *Mayo Clinics Proceedings,* Feb;*90*(2):184–93. doi:10.1016/j.mayocp.2014.12.006

Teychenne, M., Abbott, G., Ball, K., & Salmon, J. (2014). Prospective associations between sedentary behaviour and risk of depression in socio-economically disadvantaged women. *Preventive Medicine,* May 5. *pii:*S0091-7435(14)00156-X. doi:10.1016/j.ypmed.2014.04.025

Teychenne, M., & York, R. (2013). Physical activity, sedentary behavior, and postnatal depressive symptoms: A review. *American Journal of Preventive Medicine, 45,* 217–227.

van Uffelen, J. G., van Gellecum, Y. R., Burton, N. W., Peeters, G., Heesch, K. C., & Brown, W. J. (2013). Sitting-time, physical activity, and depressive symptoms in mid-aged women. *American Journal of Preventive Medicine, 45,* 276–281.

Wipfli, B. M., Rethorst, C. D., & Landers, D. M. (2008). The anxiolytic effects of exercise: A meta-analysis of randomized trials and dose-response analysis. *Journal of Sport and Exercise Psychology, 30,* 392–410.

Zhang, J., Wei, W., & Wang, C. M. (2012). Effects of psychological interventions for patients with systemic lupus erythematosus: A systematic review and meta-analysis. *Lupus, 21,* 1077–1087.

Zschucke, E., Gauditz, K., & Strohle, A. (2013). Exercise and physical activity in mental disorders: Clinical and experimental evidence. *Journal of Preventive Medicine and Public Health, 46,* S12–S21.

Personality Traits

Runner: © lzf/Shutterstock

Vignette: Lauren

There is no way you'll ever get me to go to a gym unless it's a few months before a wedding or a summer event where I need to wear a swimsuit. Even then, I need to be screamed at by a personal trainer or fitness instructor to actually break a sweat.

I hate working out. I always have. I use the excuse that my bone structure doesn't allow me to move as fluidly as some of my friends who are more sports and activity oriented. But that's a lie I came up with in high school in a failed attempt to get an exemption from P.E. class. The truth is, I'm just not a fan of exercise.

I was the younger sister of two very active older brothers—both of whom went on to play sports in college. And I was intimidated by their involvement in athletics. I far preferred to camp out in my room (or on the sidelines of their games) and read than attempt to keep up with them. In this regard, I took after my mother—who was perfectly content staying at home to garden while my father went rock climbing, hiking, and biking with my brothers.

I wouldn't exactly call myself lazy. I have a lot on my plate between work, a 9-year-old and a 6-year-old at home, and a mother who is exhibiting the early stages of Alzheimer's and isn't adjusting well to her new senior living establishment. On

LEARNING OBJECTIVES

After completing this chapter, you will be able to

- Describe the history of trait psychology and the main personality traits used to understand human behavior.
- Discuss the physical activity research that has applied the five-factor and three-factor models of personality.
- Discuss the advantages and limitations of using personality traits to customize interventions to increase physical activity.

many occasions, I've made plans to hit a yoga, spin, or Zumba class with a friend of mine. But at the last minute I end up cancelling, often because I get anxious about how much time the class will take out of my day and I feel guilty because I think I should be doing other things.

I'm also incredibly wary about the germs slathered on the walls of gyms and on exercise equipment. I imagine every inch of a space in which people work out to be teeming with bacteria in the wake of hundreds of strangers' sweat. (Gross!) What's more, I already shower at least twice a day as it is. Working myself to perspiration makes me feel disgusting.

I know I should be more active—especially because I sit at a desk all day for work and commute to and from it via car. But there's nothing that makes me excited about forcing myself to move.

My husband is a different story entirely. He wakes up around 5:30 each morning to go for a bike ride before heading to work. After work hours he does yoga, while I come home to cook, clean around the house, and (if there's time) catch an episode of one of my favorite television shows after we put the kids to bed.

He's tried for about 5 years now to get me to bike with him. But I'm not interested. I've fallen off. I don't like the dirt that accumulates on my calves. (I can barely stand the mud his shoes are covered in when he gets home from an extended ride. I make him remove his socks and shoes and wipe his legs and feet off before he even *thinks* of entering our house—but that's another story.)

We have been incredibly fortunate between my job and his to afford to outfit our basement with a home gym. It's nothing impressive. But we've managed to squeeze in a stationary bike, a treadmill, a squat rack, and a full rack of free weights. And for Christmas this past year my husband bought me a series of way too many sessions with a personal trainer who comes to our apartment twice a week to walk me through a basic weight-training regimen. I've been following this program somewhat against my will for several months now, and I enjoy the changes I'm seeing in my body. But I wish I could just achieve them through diet alone.

I've been diagnosed in the past with generalized anxiety disorder. And my husband has, on more than one occasion, suggested I may be a bit of a hypochondriac. (Again, here, I take after my mother.) I know about the health benefits of physical activity. I'm reminded of them ad nauseam by the personal trainer I work with and by my husband. But for me to stick with any program is just too much to deal with on top of everything I do at work and home.

My being active is completely dependent on the fitness professional who comes to my house two times a week and barks orders at me no matter how much I protest. I'm not sure how long this new weight program will even last. (I could quit tomorrow, were it not for the slight relief seeing myself in the mirror affords me from my anxiety over aging.) But I guess one does what one has to in order to remain healthy.

Introduction

Have you ever tried to characterize yourself or another person in terms of a general disposition? Do you consider yourself sociable or upbeat? Have you ever suggested that someone is a kind or gentle person? Are there other times where you have suggested that someone is generally mean-spirited or selfish? If you have made these characterizations, then you may be operating on the underlying assumption that people behave in stable and enduring patterns of behavior, thoughts, and feelings. You are describing *personality trait psychology*. In this chapter, we will outline the history of trait psychology, overview the structure of the most popular personality models, discuss the relationship between personality and physical activity, and conclude with the contemporary evidence for how personality may be used in physical activity interventions.

Despite the frequent application of personality trait psychology in our everyday lives, personality research was the source of several spirited debates over the 20th century (Digman, 1990; McCrae & Costa, 1995; Wiggins, 1997). These debates focused on whether people are influenced by the situation and not individual personality differences (Mischel, 1968) and whether **personality traits** are actually mechanisms/causes of behavior (Costa & McCrae, 2009). Some scientists believe that personality is a reflection of a person's neurology or physiology, and is thus controlled by a person's genes. They refer to personality traits as being *genotypic*. In contrast, others suggest that personality merely describes behavior, and thus refer to personality traits as being *phenotypic*. They do not describe how the behavior is caused. In the last 30 years, however, personality researchers have amassed a considerable body of evidence to support the importance of personality traits as mechanisms of behavior. This research has provided evidence that personality is structured similarly across over 50 cultures, is extremely heritable, has high stability across time, and does not relate strongly to parental rearing style (Costa & McCrae, 2009; McCrae et al., 2000).

CRITICAL THINKING ACTIVITY 9-1

© ecco/Shutterstock, Inc.

Although personality is thought to be immutable and consistent, it is thought to stabilize in early adulthood and show some minor variability across adult life (Costa & McCrae, 2009). Think of your own personality. Have you changed in sociability, conscientiousness, or openness since the beginning of high school?

Another difficulty when understanding personality is the lack of agreement over its basic definition. In this chapter, we use the definition provided by Paul Costa and Robert McCrae (McCrae et al., 2000) that traits are enduring and consistent individual-level differences in tendencies to show consistent patterns of thoughts, feelings, and actions. Many researchers further theorize that personality has a biological/genetic basis but that the expression of a trait is still culturally and environmentally conditioned (Eysenck, 1970; Funder, 2001; McCrae et al., 2000). For example, a student with high extraversion may choose to socialize a lot more with friends in leisure time than a student lower on extraversion, but both individuals will choose not to talk during class because this is a cultural standard of respect for one's teacher and fellow students. This has direct implications for how personality integrates with social cognitive and environmental models to explain physical activity, and we will discuss this later in the chapter.

Structure of Personality

Another major area of debate and active scholarship over the last 80 years has been on the creation of working models of personality. Researchers have asked and attempted to answer questions like: How many personality traits do we have?

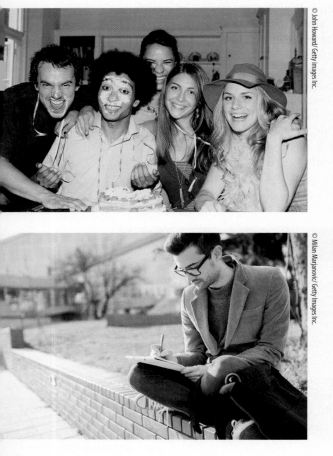

© John Howard/ Getty Images Inc.

© Milan Marjanović/ Getty Images Inc.

Which traits are the most important? How do traits relate to each other? The person who started this process—the proverbial grandfather of all personality trait research—was Gordon Allport. Allport (1937) surmised that the best way to start answering these questions was through the use of language. This was based on the premise that all important human feelings, characteristics, and behaviors would be present in our language. Basically, if something was important, he assumed we would have created a word for it. His assumption became known as the *fundamental lexical hypothesis*. Allport and his colleagues identified 18,000 potential human traits by looking up these descriptions in English dictionaries (Allport & Odbert, 1936).

Of course, 18,000 traits does not make for a very parsimonious theory of personality! Certainly some of these words are synonyms for each other, and other words may be representations of a collection of other words. In order to make sense of all of these potential descriptors, researchers began to reduce these data with the use of analytical techniques called *factor analysis* (Guilford & Guilford, 1934). Factor analysis reduces data to common elements. With the use of factor analysis and careful scrutiny of the English terms, Raymond Cattell (1947) identified 16 traits that he felt characterized the larger collection of traits. This 16PF (i.e., personality factors) became the dominant trait framework of the 1950s and 1960s. These traits include warmth, reasoning, emotional stability, dominance, liveliness, rule-consciousness, social boldness, sensitivity, vigilance, abstractness, privateness, apprehension, openness to change, self-reliance, perfectionism, and tension (see **TABLE 9-1**). Cattell also developed 5 supertraits that encompass these 16 more specific traits. These included extraversion, anxiety, tough-mindedness, independence, and self-control.

Taking the supertrait approach to understanding personality, Eysenck developed his theory with two factors: (1) extraversion-introversion (i.e., the tendency to be sociable, assertive, energetic, seek excitement, and experience positive

TABLE 9-1 Primary Factor Scale Descriptions for the 16PF

Factor	From	To
Warmth	Reserved, impersonal, distant	Warm, outgoing, attentive to others
Reasoning	Concrete	Abstract
Emotional stability	Reactive, emotionally changeable	Emotionally stable, adaptive, mature
Dominance	Differential, cooperative, avoids conflict	Dominant, forceful, assertive
Liveliness	Serious, restrained, careful	Lively, animated, spontaneous
Rule-consciousness	Expedient, nonconforming	Rule-conscious, dutiful
Social boldness	Shy, threat sensitive, timid	Socially bold, venturesome, thick-skinned
Sensitivity	Utilitarian, objective, unsentimental	Sensitive, aesthetic, sentimental
Vigilance	Trusting, unsuspecting, accepting	Vigilant, suspicious, skeptical, wary
Abstractedness	Grounded, practical, solution oriented	Abstracted, imaginative, idea oriented
Privateness	Forthright, genuine, artless	Private, discreet, nondisclosing
Apprehension	Self-assured, unworried, complacent	Apprehensive, self-doubting, worried
Openness to change	Traditional, attached to familiar	Open to change, experimenting
Self-reliance	Group-oriented, affiliative	Self-reliant, solitary, individualistic
Perfectionism	Tolerates disorder, unexacting, flexible	Perfectionistic, organized, self-disciplined
Tension	Relaxed, placid, patient	Tense, high energy, impatient, driven

Adapted from Russell, M. T., & Karol, D. L. (1994). *The 16PF Fifth Edition Administrator's Manual.* Champaign, IL: Institute for Personality and Ability Testing.

affect) and (2) neuroticism-emotional stability (i.e., the tendency to be emotionally unstable, anxious, self-conscious, and vulnerable) (Eysenck & Eysenck, 1963). More than his predecessors, Eysenck also theorized that personality traits had a biological and genetic basis. He suggested that extraversion and **neuroticism** could be linked to biological systems and brain chemistry. He later added a third trait called **psychoticism** (i.e., risk taking, impulsiveness, irresponsibility, manipulativeness, sensation-seeking, tough-mindedness, nonpragmatism) to his model (Eysenck, 1970). This model serves as one of the dominant frameworks of personality to the present day.

Still, during the mid-20th century, personality trait psychology suffered from an abundance of investigator-created traits and independent research agendas (Digman, 1990). Because of this, it was difficult for research to advance with any common theoretical model. A move toward a common trait taxonomy has helped bridge this gap. The most popular personality model at present is a five-factor taxonomy. This model suggests that neuroticism (i.e., the tendency to be emotionally unstable, anxious, self-conscious, and vulnerable); extraversion (i.e., the tendency to be sociable, assertive, energetic, seek excitement, and experience positive affect); **openness to experience/intellect** (i.e., the tendency to be perceptive, creative, reflective, and appreciate fantasy and aesthetics); **agreeableness** (i.e., tendency to be kind, cooperative, altruistic, trustworthy, and generous); and **conscientiousness** (i.e., the tendency to be ordered, dutiful, self-disciplined, and achievement oriented) are the basic factors of personality structure.

CRITICAL THINKING ACTIVITY 9-2

© ecco/Shutterstock, Inc.

For some people, all of the subtrait descriptions explain them very well. For example, some extraverts are active, social, positive, and adventurous. Other people may express one particular facet more than others. For example, someone may be super orderly but not score as high on self-discipline, although both are facet traits of conscientiousness. The difference highlights why some researchers prefer the specific facet traits to understand people, whereas others prefer the more general supertraits. Look at the descriptors for each of the five factors. Is there one facet that best describes you, or do they all describe you about the same?

Similar to the work of both Cattell and Eysenck, these common-factor taxonomies are thought to represent the basic building blocks of personality, and subsequently cause the expression of more specific subtraits (Costa & McCrae, 2009). Thus, individuals high in extraversion may express this higher-order trait through excitement seeking, sociability, a positive outlook, and energetic activity (see **FIGURE 9-1**).

Mixtures of these five factors of personality may also produce traits of interest. For example, type A behavior (Jenkins, 1976) may be a combination of high extraversion, high neuroticism, low agreeableness, and high conscientiousness. Although it is important to continue with a higher-order supertrait understanding

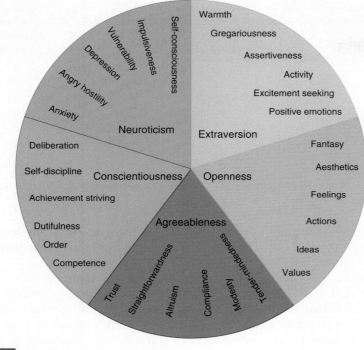

FIGURE 9-1 Five-Factor Model of Personality

of personality and behavior, these facets or specific traits may help define the relationship between personality and specific behaviors such as physical activity (Costa & McCrae, 1992). The greater specificity provided by these facet traits allows for a more precise understanding of personality relationships with an outcome variable; indeed, it is this higher level of specificity and its applied value in understanding traits and behavior that defines the facet approach (Costa & McCrae, 1995). In the next section, we review the research conducted on both supertraits and their more specific facet traits and physical activity.

Personality and Physical Activity

Although several pathways for how personality interacts with health have been postulated, the focus in this chapter is the evidence that personality traits influence physical activity through a health behavior model (Wiebe & Smith, 1997). This position suggests that the principle impact of personality on health-oriented behaviors is through the quality of one's health practices. More specifically, personality is hypothesized to affect social cognitions (e.g., perceptions, attitudes, norms, self-efficacy) toward a behavior, which, in turn, influence the health behavior itself (Ajzen, 1991; McCrae & Costa, 1995; Rhodes, 2006). We overview

TABLE 9-2 Relationship Between the Five-Factor Model and Personality		
Personality Trait	Number of Studies	Correlation with Physical Activity
Neuroticism	21	–.11
Extraversion	23	.23
Openness to Experience	12	.08
Agreeableness	11	.01
Conscientiousness	12	.20

Reproduced from Rhodes, R. E., & Smith, N. E. I. (2006). Personality correlates of physical activity: A review and meta-analysis. *British Journal of Sports Medicine, 40,* 958–965.

the evidence for this chain of personality to social cognition to physical activity later in the chapter; still, the first consideration should be whether there is any evidence for an exercising personality.

Research on personality and physical activity has spanned over 40 years. While early work considered sport performance and the potential impact of physical activity on personality (Eysenck, Nias, & Cox, 1982), more recent approaches have focused on physical activity and the health behavior model. In 2006, Rhodes and Smith reviewed and systematically appraised the relationship between personality and physical activity for Eysenck's (1970) three-factor model, the five-factor model, and Cattel's (1947) 16 personality factors. A meta-analysis of the five-factor model was conducted, and the results can be found in **TABLE 9-2** .

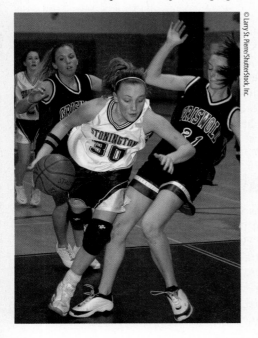

© Larry St. Pierre/ShutterStock, Inc.

Overall, neuroticism showed a small negative relationship with physical activity, while extraversion and conscientiousness had positive correlations. The most compelling evidence is from a 40-year longitudinal trial that showed that neuroticism and extraversion were predictive of physical activity changes across time (Kern, Reynolds, & Friedman, 2010). Agreeableness and openness to experience did not have a relationship with physical activity. Eysenck's third construct of psychoticism also had no evidence of a relationship with physical activity. Several trait differences emerged for the 16 personality factors, but the studies were too limited to form any generalizations of these effects.

When taken together, it appears that neuroticism, extraversion, and conscientiousness are the most reliable, yet small, correlates of physical activity. Extraversion concerns the differences in preference for social interaction and lively activity (Eysenck, 1970; McCrae & Costa,

1995). The seeking out of physical activity behaviors appears a logical extension for people high in this trait, whereas the disinterest in physical activity seems likely for those low in extraversion (Eysenck et al., 1982). Individuals high in neuroticism represent those people with less emotional stability and more distress, anxiety, and depression than those with lower neuroticism. Avoidance of physical activity or cancellation of physical activity plans is a logical extension of this trait. The relationship between conscientiousness and health behaviors more generally also has been established (Booth-Kewley & Vickers, 1994; O'Connor, Conner, Jones, McMillan, & Ferguson, 2009). High scores on conscientiousness represent a purposeful, self-disciplined individual (Digman, 1990; McCrae & Costa, 1995), suggesting that this factor may be important in terms of adherence behavior. The predisposition to maintain physical activity behavior appears to be logical for individuals who possess higher conscientiousness than their low conscientiousness counterparts.

Moderators of Personality and Physical Activity

Rhodes and Smith (2006) and a follow-up review (Rhodes & Pfaeffli, 2012) also examined whether other variables interacted with the relationship between personality and physical activity. The stability of personality suggests that it should be relatively invariant to most factors across demographics and cultures, and this is generally what has been found. The researchers concluded that no reliable differences by gender, age, and study design or instrumentation were evident. They did notice a potential trend by country, where extraversion had a smaller correlation with physical activity in the United Kingdom than in Canada and the United States. Although Rhodes and colleagues noted that research was limited, they also found that strenuous and moderate-intensity modalities of physical activity may be associated with personality factors of neuroticism, extraversion, and conscientiousness more than lower-intensity activities. For example, Howard, Cunningham, and Rechnitzer (1987) found that high-extraversion individuals were more likely to engage in swimming, aerobic conditioning, dancing, and tennis. By contrast, less extraverted individuals were more inclined to engage in gardening and home improvement, while no differences were identified for walking, jogging, golf, and cycling.

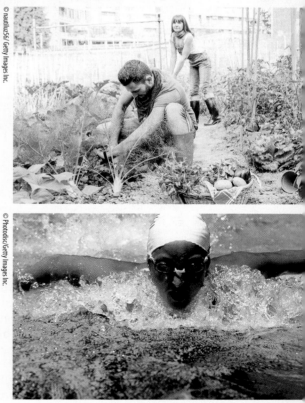

© nautiluz56/ Getty Images Inc.

© Photodisc/Getty Images Inc.

Lower-Order Traits

As mentioned earlier in the chapter, the supertraits featured in the five- and three-factor models are very useful for understanding the basic building blocks of personality structure, but more specific underlying traits may describe exercise behavior and physical activity better. Rhodes and Pfaeffli (2012) reviewed the evidence for several of these more specific traits and their relationship with physical activity.

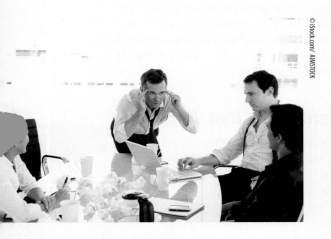

© iStock.com/ AIMSTOCK

One of the most popular traits applied to health behavior is **type A personality**. Type A personality gained popularity from its association with coronary heart disease (Jenkins, 1976). It is marked by a blend of competitiveness and hostility with agitated behavior and continual movement patterns; thus, physical activity could conceivably be a natural extension of type A individuals. Rhodes and Pfaeffli reviewed six studies that appraised the relationship between type A personality and physical activity. Overall, five of the six studies showed some significant positive association between type A personality and physical activity in the small to medium effect size range.

CRITICAL THINKING ACTIVITY 9-3

© ecco/Shutterstock, Inc.

Type A behavior is most well-known for its link to heart disease. It is interesting that the trait also is linked to positive health behaviors, such as physical activity, when physical activity is linked to decreased risk of developing heart disease. Given the type A profile of high neuroticism, high extraversion, low agreeableness, and high conscientiousness, what factors may be associated with physical activity and what factors may not?

Another trait that has received some research attention in the physical activity domain is optimism. Dispositional optimism is defined as generalized expectations of positive outcomes. It stands to reason that individuals with high optimism would conceivably hold higher regard for the positive health benefits of physical activity, and perhaps participate more than their more pessimistic (or less optimistic) counterparts. Rhodes and Pfaeffli (2012), however, found no support for optimism as a correlate.

Extraversion's **activity trait** represents a disposition toward a fast lifestyle and being high energy, fast talking, and keeping busy, as opposed to a more laissez-faire disposition. These properties could conceivably make regular physical activity a behavior of choice given its energy demands. Rhodes and Pfaeffli's (2012) literature review identified six studies that have applied the activity trait of extraversion with physical activity. In all cases, the activity trait showed a medium to large effect-size correlation with behavior ($r = .24$ to $r = .52$). More compelling, the three direct tests that compared the predictive capacity of activity against the supertrait of extraversion showed the superiority of the activity trait. Overall, the results suggest that extraversion's activity trait is a reliable and strong predictor of physical activity.

Extraversion's sociability facet trait is often considered its cornerstone (Costa & McCrae, 1995). People high in sociability prefer the company of others and gravitate to social situations with people. The social component that accompanies many physical activities could therefore make for a logical outlet among highly sociable people. To this end, sociability has been assessed for its relationship with physical activity in six studies (Rhodes & Pfaeffli, 2012). Only two of these studies supported a relationship between sociability and physical activity, suggesting that it may not be a reliable correlate.

Complementary to the examination of extraversion's facet traits, conscientiousness's facet of **industriousness-ambition** has also received attention in four studies (Rhodes & Pfaeffli, 2012). The trait comprises aspects of achievement-striving and self-discipline, and a natural extension of this type of disposition could be regular exercise given its challenge, impact on health and appearance, and self-regulatory barriers. Three of the four studies found a significant relationship between this trait and behavior, suggesting that it may be the critical link between conscientiousness and physical activity.

How Does Personality Affect Physical Activity?

Personality theorists and social psychologists generally agree that behavioral action is unlikely to arise directly from personality (Ajzen, 1991; Bandura, 1998; Eysenck, 1970; McCrae & Costa, 1995; McCrae et al., 2000; Rhodes, 2006). Instead, personality is thought to influence behavioral perceptions, expectations, and cognitions. The theory of planned behavior (TPB; Ajzen, 1991) has been the leading model to test this assumption in the physical activity domain, with 16 such studies (Davies, Mummery, & Steele, 2010; McEachan, Sutton, & Myers, 2010; Rhodes & Pfaeffli, 2012). The relationship between personality and the TPB is specific. According to Ajzen (1991), personality should affect behavior through the constructs of attitude, subjective norm, and perceived behavioral control. Thus, TPB should mediate personality and physical activity relations. However, this was only supported in three of the 16 studies. The remaining studies showed evidence for only partial mediation. Overall, the results suggest that the TPB may not always fully mediate personality.

Another way that personality may affect behavior is by interacting with physical activity motivation. A recent review of factors that interact with the intention–behavior relationship found convincing evidence that conscientiousness may

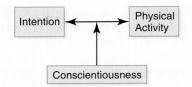

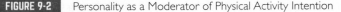

FIGURE 9-2 Personality as a Moderator of Physical Activity Intention

alter this relationship (Rhodes & Dickau, 2013). The basic premise for this finding is that people who are more conscientious are more likely to act on their good intentions than their less conscientious counterparts. It may be that the disposition toward achievement keeps high-conscientiousness individuals from slipping in their original physical activity plans (see **FIGURE 9-2**). Some evidence suggests that extraversion may interact with intention (Rhodes & Dickau, 2013). The theory behind this proposed relationship is that individuals high on extraversion may facilitate their intentions by gravitating toward more active environments than do more introverted individuals.

Personality and Intervention

One of the struggles as a health educator interested in promoting physical activity is what to do with personality traits. Based on their enduring and stable nature, it seems like a difficult enterprise to plan an intervention to change a person's personality! Personality traits have been shown to change, particularly in adolescence, but change among adults generally unfolds very slowly across the life cycle (McCrae et al., 2000). Unlike self-efficacy or attitudes, a strong correlation of personality and physical activity represents a potential obstacle and not a target for change. We believe that the approach taken with personality should resemble other intractable correlates of physical activity, such as age, disability, or gender. For example, the negative correlation of physical activity and advancing age does not signal an intervention to reverse time! Instead, health promoters need to consider age and target effective interventions for older adults. Similarly, introverts or less conscientious individuals may need targeted interventions to help them increase physical activity despite a natural inclination to be less active.

The proposal for personality-matched interventions has appeal, but the research on this approach is very limited at present. Rhodes and Matheson (2008) examined whether a planning intervention among low-conscientiousness individuals could help improve physical activity over a control group. The effects were null, but it may have been from an ineffective intervention, as most of the participants reported that they did not even complete the planning worksheet. In contrast, Why and colleagues (Why, Huang, & Sandhu, 2010) examined the effects of a walking intervention and found that messages were more effective in increasing walking behavior among conscientious individuals than their less conscientious counterparts. The results here underscore that personality traits may need to be targeted to help less conscientious individuals.

CRITICAL THINKING ACTIVITY 9-4

If personality is enduring and immutable, how can one use it to promote physical activity intervention? What might you do to screen and promote physical activity for those low on extraversion and conscientiousness?

Personality and Sedentary Behavior

Given the new focus on sedentary behavior and health, it is not surprising that far less is known about the association between personality traits and TV watching, video game play, and computer use than for moderate and vigorous physical activity. Still, it stands to reason that some of the associations with physical activity and personality may be the opposite for sedentary behavior. For example, whereas the high-energy extravert may seek out activity, the introvert may be motivated to stay home and watch screens from the relative quiet of one's home. At present, there is some evidence for this line of thinking. Introversion has been associated with more overall Internet use in college samples (Landers & Lounsbury, 2006; Servidio, 2014), and extraverts strongly reject that TV can replace socialization as a viable pastime (Weaver, 2003). Low social extraversion also predicted sedentary behavior across 29 years in women (Uijtdewilligen et al., 2011).

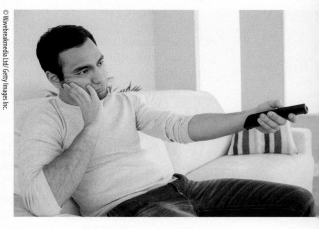

© Wavebreakmedia Ltd/ Getty Images Inc.

High neuroticism has also predicted motivation to watch high levels of TV (Weaver, 2003) and sedentary behavior among men (Uijtdewilligen et al., 2011). Sedentary behaviors may represent a safe and easy behavior for neurotics who tend to be high in anxiety, depressive tendencies, and self-reproach. Unlike the physical activity domain, early evidence also suggests that high Internet use is associated with decreased agreeableness (Landers & Lounsbury, 2006; Servidio, 2014), yet those who use the Internet a lot also tend to be more open to new experiences (Servidio, 2014). This is an interesting trait profile, and it suggests many trait factors can describe different sedentary behaviors. More research is needed to confirm these early findings.

■ Summary

Personality trait psychology has a rich and spirited history, but contemporary research has supported the premise that people have enduring and stable individual differences in how they express thoughts, feelings, and actions. Personality traits are typically organized by supertraits, and then more specific facet traits that are a consequence of the supertrait. The most popular personality supertrait model is the five-factor model composed of neuroticism, extraversion, openness to experience, agreeableness, and conscientiousness.

A review by Rhodes and Smith (2006) identified extraversion ($r = .23$), neuroticism ($r = -.11$), and conscientiousness ($r = .20$) as the key supertraits related to physical activity. A subsequent review of the more specific traits suggested that extraversion's trait of activity/adventurousness and conscientiousness's trait of achievement striving/ambition may be the critical components that are related to physical activity (Rhodes & Pfaeffli, 2012). Type A personality, which includes components of both the activity and achievement-striving traits (as well as hostility), has also been shown as a reliable predictor of physical activity.

These traits are hypothesized to affect a behavior such as physical activity through social cognitive constructs such as attitudes, norms, and self-efficacy. For example, your level of extraversion may affect your perceptions of confidence, your appraisal of how much fun it may be to perform a physical activity, the assessment of whether physical activity is beneficial, or your feeling/shyness about how others will perceive you doing physical activity. Personality may also affect the success of holding to positive physical activity intentions. Research has been quite convincing in demonstrating that people low on conscientiousness have more difficulty holding to their initial physical activity intentions than those who are high on conscientiousness.

Sedentary behaviors also have personality correlates that tend to be the opposite of physical activity, such as low extraversion and high neuroticism. Still, the type of sedentary behavior appears to have slightly different trait makeups, and research in this area is in its infancy.

The findings suggest that understanding "at risk" personalities may be important when creating interventions. Interventions that consider a person's introversion, for example, and that target physical activity behaviors accordingly (e.g., home based, solo or with one friend, low intensity) may have utility. This topic has not yet received much attention from researchers. Future research is needed to examine this personality-matching strategy.

KEY TERMS

activity trait
agreeableness
conscientiousness
extraversion
industriousness-ambition

neuroticism
openness to experience/intellect
personality traits
psychoticism
type A personality

REVIEW QUESTIONS

1. Describe how personality traits are structured.

2. What are the five supertraits in the five-factor model?

3. What supertraits have been linked with physical activity?

4. What traits may determine whether good physical activity intentions translate into behavior?

5. Describe the current evidence for lower-order personality traits and physical activity. What key specific traits may be important?

APPLYING THE CONCEPTS

1. What personality factors might account for Lauren's lack of enthusiasm for and commitment to fitness?

2. What personality traits might account for the enthusiasm and regularity with which Lauren's husband exercises?

REFERENCES

Ajzen, I. (1991). The theory of planned behavior. *Organizational Behavior and Human Decision Processes, 50,* 179–211.

Allport, G. W. (1937). *Personality*. New York, NY: Henry Holt.

Allport, G. W., & Odbert, H. S. (1936). Trait names: A psycho-lexical study. *Psychological Monographs, 47,* 1.

Bandura, A. (1998). Health promotion from the perspective of social cognitive theory. *Psychology and Health, 13,* 623–649.

Booth-Kewley, S., & Vickers, R. R. (1994). Associations between major domains of personality and health behavior. *Journal of Personality, 62,* 281–298.

Cattell, R. B. (1947). Confirmation and clarification of primary personality factors. *Psychometrica, 12,* 197–220.

Cervone, D. (2004). Personality assessment: Tapping the social cognitive architecture of personality. *Behavior Therapy, 35,* 113–129.

Costa, P. T., & McCrae, R. R. (1992). *Revised NEO Personality Inventory (NEO-PI-R) and NEO Five-Factor Inventory (NEO-FFI) Professional Manual*. Odessa, FL: Psychological Assessment Resources.

Costa, P. T., & McCrae, R. R. (1995). Domains and facets: Hierarchical personality assessment using the revised NEO Personality Inventory. *Journal of Personality Assessment, 64,* 21–50.

Costa, P. T., & McCrae, R. R. (2009). The five-factor model and the NEO Inventories. In J. N. Butcher (Ed.), *Oxford handbook of personality assessment*. New York, NY: Oxford University Press.

Davies, C. A., Mummery, K., & Steele, R. M. (2010). The relationship between personality, theory of planned behavior, and physical activity in individuals with type II diabetes. *British Journal of Sports Medicine, 44,* 979–984.

Digman, J. M. (1990). Personality structure: Emergence of the five-factor model. *Annual Review of Psychology, 41,* 417–440.

Eysenck, H. J. (1970). *The structure of human personality*. (3rd ed.). London: Methuen.

Eysenck, H. J., & Eysenck, S. B. J. (1963). *Manual for the Eysenck Personality Inventory*. San Diego, CA: Educational and Industrial Testing Service.

Eysenck, H. J., Nias, D. K. B., & Cox, D. N. (1982). Sport and personality. *Advances in Behavior Research and Therapy, 4,* 1–56.

Funder, D. C. (2001). Personality. *Annual Review of Psychology, 52,* 197–221.

Guilford, J. P., & Guilford, R. B. (1934). An analysis of the factors in a typical test of introversion-extroversion. *Journal of Abnormal and Social Psychology, 28,* 377–399.

Howard, J. H., Cunningham, D. A., & Rechnitzer, P. A. (1987). Personality and fitness decline in middle-aged men. *International Journal of Sport Psychology, 18,* 100–111.

Jenkins, C. D. (1976). Recent evidence supporting psychologic and social risk factors for coronary disease. *New England Journal of Medicine, 294,* 987–1033.

Kern, M. L., Reynolds, C. A., & Friedman, H. S. (2010). Predictors of physical activity patterns across adulthood: A growth curve analysis. *Personality and Social Psychology Bulletin, 36,* 1058–1072.

Landers, R. N., & Lounsbury, J. W. (2006). An investigation of Big Five and narrow personality traits in relation to Internet usage. *Computers in Human Behavior, 22,* 283–293.

McCrae, R. R., & Costa, P. T. (1995). Trait explanations in personality psychology. *European Journal of Personality, 9,* 231–252.

McCrae, R. R., Costa, P. T., Ostendorf, F., Angleitner, A., Hrebickova, M., Avia, M. D., . . . Smith, P. B. (2000). Nature over nurture: Temperament, personality, and life-span development. *Journal of Personality & Social Psychology, 78,* 173–186.

McEachan, R., Sutton, S., & Myers, L. (2010). Mediation of personality influences on physical activity within the theory of planned behavior. *Journal of Health Psychology, 15,* 1170–1180.

Mischel, W. (1968). *Personality and assessment*. New York, NY: John Wiley & Sons.

O'Connor, D. B., Conner, M., Jones, F., McMillan, B., & Ferguson, E. (2009). Exploring the benefits of conscientiousness: An investigation of the role of daily stressors and health behaviors. *Annals of Behavioral Medicine*, *37*, 184–196.

Rhodes, R. E. (2006). The built-in environment: The role of personality with physical activity. *Exercise and Sport Sciences Reviews*, *34*, 83–88.

Rhodes, R. E., & Dickau, L. (2013). Moderators of the intention-behavior relationship in physical activity: A systematic review. *British Journal of Sports Medicine*, *47*(4), 215–225. doi:10.1136 bjsports-2011-090411

Rhodes, R. E., & Matheson, D. H. (2008). Does personality moderate the effect of implementation intentions on physical activity? *Annals of Behavioral Medicine*, *35*, S209.

Rhodes, R. E., & Pfaeffli, L. A. (2012). Personality and physical activity. In E. O. Acevedo (Ed.), *Oxford handbook of exercise psychology* (pp. 195–223). New York, NY: Oxford University Press.

Rhodes, R. E., & Smith, N. E. I. (2006). Personality correlates of physical activity: A review and meta-analysis. *British Journal of Sports Medicine*, *40*, 958–965.

Servidio, R. (2014). Exploring the effects of demographic factors, Internet usage, and personality traits on Internet addiction in a sample of Italian university students. *Computers in Human Behavior*, *35*, 85–92.

Uijtdewilligen, L., Singh, A. S., Twisk, J. W. R., Koppes, L. L. J., van Mechelen, W., & Chinapaw, M. J. M. (2011). Adolescent predictors of objectively measured physical activity and sedentary behavior at age 42: The Amsterdam Growth and Health Longitudinal Study (AGAHLS). *International Journal of Behavioral Nutrition and Physical Activity*, *8*, 107.

Weaver, J. B. (2003). Individual differences in television viewing motives. *Personality and Individual Differences*, *35*, 1427–1437.

Why, Y. P., Huang, R. Z., & Sandhu, P. K. (2010). Affective messages increase leisure walking only among conscientious individuals. *Personality and Individual Differences*, *48*, 752–756.

Wiebe, D. J., & Smith, T. W. (1997). Personality and health: Progress and problems in psychosomatics. In R. Hogan, J. Johnson & S. Briggs (Eds.), *Handbook of personality psychology*. San Diego, CA: Academic Press.

Wiggins, J. S. (1997). In defense of traits. In R. Hogan, J. A. Johnson, & S. R. Briggs (Eds.), *Handbook of personality psychology* (pp. 95–115). San Diego, CA: Academic Press.

CHAPTER 10

Self-Esteem and Body Image

Runner: © Izf/Shutterstock

Vignette: Divya

During adolescence, I stopped fitting in with the other girls in my grade. I was a late bloomer whose body remained boxy and flat while the rest of my former friends' physiques grew shapely. Their newly feminine forms garnered more attention from the boys in our school. I don't recall getting that type of attention at all. I was repeatedly teased for not having a womanly figure. During recess, one of the popular girls at the time even accused me of being a boy because I wouldn't show the rest of the girls my bra. It wasn't unusual for my female classmates to showcase their new purchases from lingerie stores, as if flaunting their need for underwire support in my face. (I didn't wear one at the time because I had no need, so I refused to lift up my shirt out of shame.)

Whereas the rest of the girls in my class wore tight-fitting tank tops to school, I opted for baggier shirts to hide my lack of shapeliness. By the time we all entered high school, I was convinced I was physically unattractive and destined to be forever excluded because I didn't look ladylike, like everyone else.

Once I did begin to fill out—rapidly during the summer after eighth grade—I put on more weight than the other girls. And to top it all off, I had acne.

LEARNING OBJECTIVES

After completing this chapter, you will be able to

- Better understand the meaning of the term *body image*.
- Examine the role that exercise and sedentary behavior plays in changing body image.
- Differentiate among terms used to describe the self, such as self-esteem and self-concept.
- Discuss the role of exercise and sedentary behavior in modifying self-esteem.
- Understand the relationship between exercise and individual attitudes and beliefs about the body.
- Describe the relationship between social physique anxiety and exercise.

I was too afraid to be seen in shorts or even to change in front of my peers in any locker room. So I'd hug the walls in gym class, avoid trying out for sports teams, and rarely do anything physical after school. I took to myself to read and watch television—sometimes zoning out in front of the screen for hours just to take my mind off the agony involved in being such an outsider at school.

I felt increasingly worse throughout high school, and I eventually found refuge in dark rock and metal music, vibrantly unnatural hair colors, and a group of friends who held a very dismal view of humanity. All of us dressed to express this. Our clothing was all black, all the time—and grungy.

I'd say that the most exercise I got before college was the rock concerts I'd go to with my new friends. Lost in a crowd of equally angry, disaffected teens and young adults, I could jump around, thrash my arms, and dance without the anxiety-provoking apprehension that everyone was watching and judging my body.

When it came time to prepare for college, I specifically pinpointed my top choices based on location. I didn't want to be in a warm area, where the weather would call for shorts rather than long pants and jackets. I was accepted early decision to a school in the Northeast. And for the next 4 years I hid my body under layers and layers of sweatshirts, sweatpants, and a parka.

Unexpectedly, I lost a great deal of weight once I began classes, in part, because I had been given a prescription to help me focus for long stretches of time. Also, the food at the college I ended up attending wasn't very palatable. And as far as drinking went, I never developed a taste for alcohol—especially not beer or hard liquor, which were popular among my college peers. So the dreaded freshman 15 didn't end up applying to me.

I became heavily involved in theater during my sophomore year—but mostly from the tech and production end, not the stage. By junior year I was trying my hand at directing and writing scripts. And in between meeting the rest of my requirements, I was trying to hide a burgeoning crush on the supporting actor I casted in the play I wrote for my senior thesis.

He had no idea I was falling in love with him, even if I did gush about his allure to my fellow theater friends. It had been suggested to me—as kindly as possible—that I try to catch his eye by pulling myself together a bit. Buying some nicer, tighter-fitting clothes, possibly toning up my arms, thighs, and abdomen at the campus gym. But I had no idea where to start. I was horrified at the idea of wearing anything smaller than a large, even though I'd come to realize that some medium-sized tops were still loose on my frame.

A friend of mine attempted to drag me to the campus gym and teach me how to use the elliptical several times over the years but to no avail. I hated being seen in exercise clothes. I was convinced the entire gym was judging me. (I could barely stand how I looked in them, and so I just assumed everyone else would agree, if not think even lower of me than I did of myself.) Even worse, I feared I'd run into my crush and risk being seen by him at my worst. Often, I'd put makeup on and then get worried about sweating it off. It always ended up being futile.

There was an alternative, however. And that was a women's-only fitness studio that I could walk to from campus in under a half hour. Sure, the trudge was trying during the colder days of the winter. But I thought at least the walking would shape me up in some way and contribute to the body I wanted to have in order to be more attractive.

The woman's gym was different than my campus fitness center. It didn't have too many mirrors. And during yoga classes—as well as the other class I'd later take involving huge straps hanging from the ceiling, called TRX—the lights in the workout room were dim. Plus, the bodies I was surrounded by weren't obnoxiously slim or insanely muscular, as I'd feared going in. They were average. In fact, I'd say I was on the skinner side of the class gamut.

But a strange thing happened as my muscles grew accustomed to the motions in the classroom. The more able I was to do the yoga postures—and, later, to move my limbs through various rotations on that TRX—the less concerned I became with how I looked while in motion. Gradually, my focus was increasingly absorbed by how it felt to master those movements. And the more of them I could figure out and repeat without flailing, the better I started to feel about myself.

In terms of weight loss, I didn't notice any drastic changes. But I did start to see the muscles in my arms and legs become a bit more prominent. Most of all, I felt my spine elongate during the days, and the way I walked became more confident. After a couple months of classes, I decided to take a risk and buy a slim-fitting pair of jeans alongside a form-fitting V-neck.

"Divya!" My theater friends exclaimed when I tried to keep my chin up as I strode into rehearsal dressed like this for the first time. I was worried they might finish that sentence with a line like, "What did you do to yourself?" or "What on earth are you wearing!?" But instead, holding my breath, I heard "My god, you look amazing!"

That social validation helped motivate me so much to persist in my efforts at the fitness center. And before I graduated I was able to get over my fears of exercising in the campus gym. Sure, it was extremely intimidating to see girls in there who were completely comfortable inhabiting skin-tight yoga pants and stretchy workout tees. But I tried my best to just stick to what I knew I could do, inhabit my own strength, and keep my head up.

In fact, it was after one of those campus gym sessions that the lead actor in my play ended up asking me out for the first time. (I banked on the fact that he'd attribute the flush in my cheeks and the thump in my chest while we were talking to the set of jump squats I'd just done, rather than as a reaction to him acknowledging my presence with so much enthusiasm!)

We ended up dating until the end of school, after which we parted ways to return to our respective home towns and lead separate lives. But until this day, years since I've gone on to work at a small theater company in upstate New York and remain active at my local community fitness center, I've never forgotten something he said to me during our third or fourth date. "Divya, I always noticed you; even before you started changing your wardrobe. I just don't think you were aware of my interest until you learned how to notice yourself."

■ Introduction

Few psychological constructs have received as much research attention as **self-esteem**, and for good reason. High self-esteem is associated with emotional stability, happiness, and resilience to stress. In contrast, low self-esteem is related to mental illnesses such as depression, anxiety, and eating disorders. Thus, self-esteem is a critical component of human functioning and performance. Not surprisingly, researchers have examined various components of self-esteem and how it affects overall health.

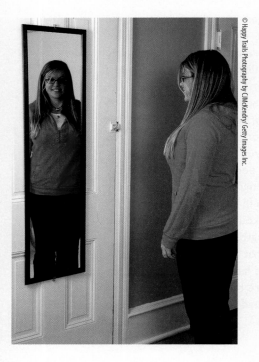

Body image is one such component of self-esteem. Body image represents the mental picture you have of your body; that is, what your body looks like, what you believe about your body, and how you feel about your body. Self-esteem and body image influence each other. For example, it is hard to feel good about yourself if you hate your body. In this chapter, we examine the complex relationship between self-esteem and body image and exercise and sedentary behavior.

■ Self-Esteem

Self-esteem represents a stable global positive or negative evaluative of a person's own self-worth; that is, the degree to which a person possesses positive and negative self-perceptions. Positive self-perceptions include the ability to make statements like "I am competent" or "I am a good person." In comparison, negative self-perceptions would be reflected in statements such as "I am incompetent" or "I am worthless."

The terms *self-esteem* and *self-concept* are often used interchangeably, but they have distinct meanings. The statement "I am a good person" is evaluative in nature, and thus it is a manifestation of the person's self-esteem. In comparison, **self-concept** refers to the many attributes and the roles that people use to evaluate themselves to establish their self-esteem judgments (Fox, 2000). In other words, one's self-concept is a collection of beliefs about oneself that includes such things as academic performance, athletic performance, age, and racial identity. Generally, self-concept embodies the answer to "Who am I?" Thus, the statement "I am a regular exerciser," because it is self-descriptive in nature, would reflect the individual's self-concept.

Self-esteem has received a great deal of research attention largely because it is positively related to psychological health, physical health, and overall quality of life (Fox, 2000). As well, self-esteem is associated with many positive achievements and socially related behaviors, including leadership ability, satisfaction, decreased anxiety, and improved academic and physical performance (Fox, 2000; Trzesniewski, Donnellan, & Robins, 2003).

Historically, the conception and measurement of self-esteem was unidimensional. Self-esteem was considered, and thus was measured, as one overall global index. The implicit assumption made with a unidimensional self-esteem approach was that a single measure would provide insight into a person's evaluative self-worth in a wide range of settings. This approach to measurement was imprecise because it assessed a general sense of self-worth without considering the role of other contributors to self-esteem (Fox, 2000).

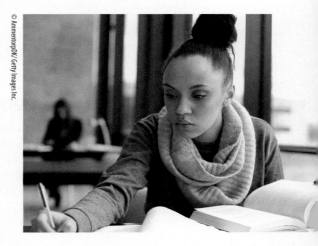

More recently, however, the approach taken by researchers acknowledges that self-esteem should be viewed in both a multidimensional and hierarchical manner. Today, researchers state that at least the following four separate domains contribute to a person's global self-esteem: (1) academic, (2) social, (3) physical, and (4) emotional (Shavelson, Hubner, & Stanton, 1976). Thus, your perceptions of your physical self may be dramatically different from your perceptions of your academic self. Consistent with a multidimensional approach, theoreticians now suggest that perceptions of the self can be organized into a hierarchical structure (Fox, 2000; Sonstroem, Harlow, & Josephs, 1994).

The top of the hierarchy is global self-esteem. In turn, global self-esteem develops as a result of evaluative perceptions arising from a number of life areas such as the physical self, the social self, the spiritual self, and the academic self. Therefore, changes in global self-esteem will be the result of prior changes that have occurred in the facets of self-esteem, because these are at the bottom of the multidimensional hierarchical model, whereas global self-esteem is at the top of this model. As a result, when changes in the facets of self-esteem are not significant, no significant changes will occur in global self-esteem (Sonstroem & Morgan, 1989).

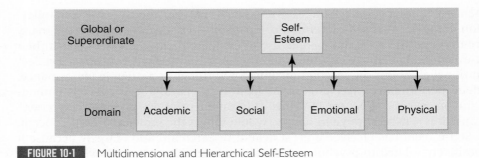

FIGURE 10-1 Multidimensional and Hierarchical Self-Esteem

Furthermore, the aspects of self-esteem that are considered important by the person will have a significant impact on global self-esteem. For example, an adolescent girl may perform well in school (i.e., her academic self), but at the same time feel socially isolated from her peers (i.e., her social self). Because she wants to be popular among her peers, her low social self-esteem will have a greater influence on her global self-esteem. See **FIGURE 10-1** for a hierarchical model of self-esteem.

CRITICAL THINKING ACTIVITY 10-1

© ecco/Shutterstock, Inc.

What domains of self-esteem have the greatest influence on your global self-esteem? Describe these in detail.

Physical Self-Esteem

Based on this hierarchical model of self-esteem, the physical self has the most implications for exercise and sedentary behavior. Fox and Corbin (1989) developed the Physical Self-Perception Profile, which enabled the physical component of self-esteem to be examined in more detail. See **FIGURES 10-2** and **10-3** for more detailed descriptions of physical self-esteem.

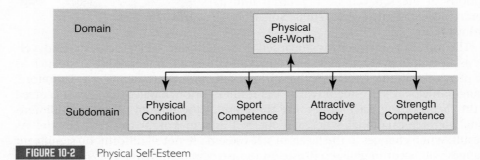

FIGURE 10-2 Physical Self-Esteem

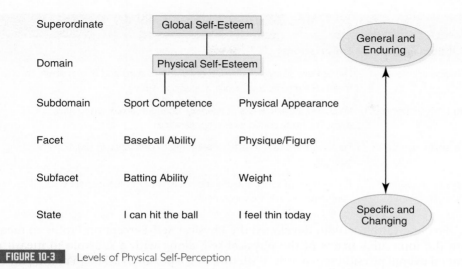

Superordinate	Global Self-Esteem	
Domain	Physical Self-Esteem	
Subdomain	Sport Competence	Physical Appearance
Facet	Baseball Ability	Physique/Figure
Subfacet	Batting Ability	Weight
State	I can hit the ball	I feel thin today

General and Enduring

Specific and Changing

FIGURE 10-3   Levels of Physical Self-Perception

The **Physical Self-Perception Profile** (Fox & Corbin, 1989; Lindwall, Asci, Palmeira, Fox, & Hagger, 2011) is based on a hierarchical, multidimensional theoretical model of self-esteem, in which self-perceptions are categorized as superordinate (i.e., global self-esteem), domain (e.g., physical self-worth), subdomain (e.g., body attractiveness), facet (e.g., figure/physique), subfacet (e.g., slim waistline), and state (e.g., "I feel lean today"). Self-perceptions are general and enduring at the top of the hierarchy. At lower levels, self-perceptions become increasingly specific and unstable. The model holds that the extent to which we feel good about ourselves physically will contribute to how we feel about ourselves in general.

More specifically, the Physical Self-Perception Profile Model states that physical self-worth (i.e., general feelings of pride, satisfaction, happiness, and confidence in the physical self) is formed through the contribution of the following four subdomains of physical self-perceptions: (1) physical conditioning, (2) body attractiveness, (3) physical strength, and (4) sport competence. A detailed description of these subdomains can be found in **TABLE 10-1** . These four subdomains are subordinate to global physical self-esteem and global general self-esteem. Fox (1990) argued that self-perceptions can vary from one level to another, for example, from the superordinate (global self-esteem), domain (physical), subdomain (sport competence), facet (soccer ability), subfacet (shooting ability), and state ("I can score this penalty").

Thus, for example, total weight may contribute to feelings of being fat, which, in turn, may contribute to social physique anxiety and, subsequently, to poor body image. That poor body image, in turn, would influence the individual's physical self-esteem, which, in turn, would influence the individual's overall self-esteem. Although all dimensions (e.g., social self-esteem, academic self-esteem) contribute to global self-esteem, physical self-esteem plays a preeminent role.

TABLE 10-1	Physical Self-Perception Profile Subdomains
Subdomain	**Description**
Physical condition	Perceptions of level of physical condition, stamina and fitness, ability to maintain exercise, confidence in exercise setting
Body attractiveness	Perceived attractiveness of figure or physique, ability to maintain an attractive body, confidence in appearance
Physical strength	Perceived strength, muscle development, confidence in situations requiring strength
Sport competence	Perceptions of sport and athletic ability, ability to learn sport skills, confidence in sport environment

Fox and Corbin (1989) developed the Physical Self-Perception Profile to measure the four subdomains of the physical self, along with a subscale to measure general overall physical self-worth. With this tool, a person is asked to read a pair of contrasting statements and decide which of the two statements is most characteristic of him- or herself. The person then checks a box denoting the extent to which the statement is characteristic of him- or herself by indicating whether the item is "Sort of true for me" or "Really true for me." The Physical Self-Perception Profile has been successfully applied to a variety of populations and cultures (Lindwall et al., 2011). Sample items of each of the subscales can be found in TABLE 10-2 .

TABLE 10-2	Sample Items from the Physical Self-Perception Profile
Subdomain	**Sample Item**
Physical condition	Some people make certain they take part in some form of regular vigorous physical exercise BUT others don't often manage to keep up regular vigorous physical exercise.
Body attractiveness	Some people feel that compared to most, they have attractive bodies BUT others feel that compared to most, their bodies are not quite so attractive.
Physical strength	Some people feel that their muscles are much stronger than most others of their sex BUT others feel that on the whole their muscles are not quite as strong as most others of their sex.
Sport competence	Some people feel that they are among the best when it comes to athletic ability BUT others feel that they are not among the most able when it comes to athletics.
Physical self-worth	Some people feel extremely satisfied with the kind of persons they are physically BUT others sometimes feel a little dissatisfied with their physical selves.

Adapted from Fox, K. R., & Corbin, C. B. (1989). The physical self-perception profile: Development and preliminary validation. *Journal of Sport and Exercise Psychology, 11,* 408–430.

Let's now take a closer look at the research examining the effects of exercise and sedentary behavior on self-esteem.

Effects of Exercise and Sedentary Behavior on Self-Esteem

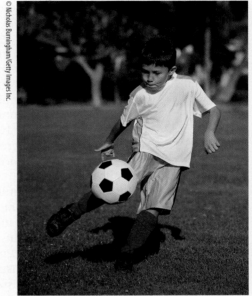

Self-esteem is a predictor of many psychosocial well-being constructs. For example, self-esteem is positively related to self-efficacy, body satisfaction, and leadership; it is negatively related to levels of anxiety and depression (Trzesniewski et al., 2003). Not surprisingly, a large body of research has examined the relationship between self-esteem and exercise. In particular, researchers have focused on the effects of exercise on children's self-esteem. Typically, these studies involve a comparison of the self-esteem of young people before and then after a physical activity intervention program.

For example, Bob Ekeland and his colleagues (Ekelund, Heian, & Hagen, 2005) published a systematic review of 23 randomized controlled trials to determine if exercise alone or as part of a comprehensive intervention could improve the self-esteem of children and young people ages 3 to 20 years. Consistent with other reviews (Fox, 2000; Gruber, 1986; McDonald & Hodgdon, 1991), the authors concluded that exercise can improve self-esteem. They found a moderate effect size of .49 in favor of the exercise intervention. In other words, exercise had a small positive short-term effect on the self-esteem of children and young people. They noted, however, that the results of their review were limited because of the small number of children in the studies reviewed and the low quality of these studies. Despite these methodological issues, the results indicate that exercise may be effective in improving self-esteem in children and young people, at least in the short term. The researchers concluded that because exercise has no known negative effects, and many positive effects on overall health, it is an important construct for improving children's self-esteem. They also noted that they could not identify from the studies reviewed what type of exercise and in what setting resulted in these positive effects of physical activity on self-esteem.

John Spence and his colleagues (Spence, McGannon, & Poon, 2005) conducted a meta-analysis of 113 studies that examined the effects of exercise on global self-esteem in adults. They found that participation in exercise brought about a small change in global self-esteem (mean ES = .23). They also found that change in physical fitness and type of program were significant moderators of the effect of exercise on global self-esteem, such that larger effect sizes were observed for those who experienced significant changes in physical fitness and those participating in either exercise or lifestyle programs as opposed to skills training.

Can physical activity improve self-esteem of cancer patients? Yes. A meta-analysis of 82 controlled trials revealed that physical activity during and following cancer treatment results in positive improvements in self-esteem (Speck, Courneya, Mâsse, Duval, & Schmitz, 2010).

It is important to note that most of the aforementioned research has focused on the effects of aerobic fitness on self-esteem. A recent systematic and meta-analytic review found that muscular fitness shows a positive association with self-esteem for children and adolescents (Smith et al., 2014).

Sedentary behavior is also related to self-esteem. Watching television for more than 2 hours per day is associated with lower self-esteem in school-age children and youth (Tremblay et al., 2011).

It is important to note that the aforementioned reviews focused on global self-esteem. As Figures 10-1 and 10-2 illustrate, physical self-esteem develops as a result of evaluative perceptions arising from a number of dimensions, including sport competence, physical strength, physical condition, and body image. Indeed, within the context of physical activity, researchers have revealed that self-esteem should be considered multidimensional and hierarchical (Sonstroem et al., 1994); that is, exercise can promote positive changes in physical self-perceptions that can manifest as an increase in global self-esteem (McAuley et al., 2005).

Justin Moore and his colleagues (Moore, Mitchell, Bibeau, & Bartholomew, 2011) assessed self-esteem using the hierarchical framework of the exercise and self-esteem model (Sonstroem & Morgan, 1989). The aim of their study was to determine whether resistance training could cause changes in global (i.e., physical self-worth) and subdomain levels (e.g., aerobic condition, attractive body, sport competence, strength) of self-esteem. They had 120 college students complete measures of the physical subdomains (i.e., strength, endurance, physical attractiveness, and sport competence) and global self-esteem before and after a 12-week resistance exercise training program.

They found that the students had significant improvements in their self-perception constructs at all levels of the exercise and self-esteem model. The hierarchical structure of self-esteem was partially supported because successively smaller improvements at each level of the model were found. For example, global self-esteem showed lesser improvements than physical self-worth.

Based on the research we have discussed thus far, it is not clear whether increasing self-esteem leads to higher physical activity or whether increasing physical activity leads to higher self-esteem. To address the direction of the self-esteem and physical activity relationship, Dorothy Schmalz and her colleagues (Schmalz, Deane, Birch, & Krahnstoever Davison, 2007) used data from a longitudinal study to explore the relationship between exercise and global self-esteem among 197 girls from childhood into early adolescence. The girls' physical activity and self-esteem were assessed when they were 9, 11, and 13 years old.

The researchers found that higher physical activity at ages 9 and 11 years predicted higher self-esteem at ages 11 and 13 years. Of importance, the effects of physical activity on self-esteem were most apparent at age 11 and for girls with higher body mass index (BMI). The authors concluded that participating in physical activity can lead to positive self-esteem among adolescent girls, particularly for younger girls and those at greatest risk of being overweight. Their findings support other longitudinal research conducted in older populations that physical activity has positive effects on both global and subdomain self-esteem levels of physical condition and body attractiveness (Elavsky, 2010; McAuley et al., 2005).

Is physical activity related to self-esteem for both genders? Yes, increased levels of physical activity are beneficial for global self-esteem by enhancing both girls' and boys' perceptions of physical self-esteem. However, the influence of physical appearance on global self-worth is stronger for female than for male populations (Haugen, Safvenborn, & Ommundsen, 2011).

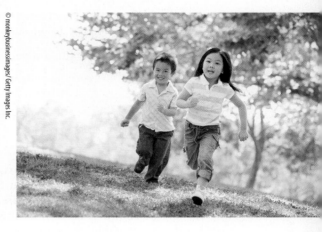

© monkeybusinessimages/ Getty Images Inc.

■ Body Image

As shown in Figure 10-2, one integral component contributing to a person's physical self-esteem (which, in turn, has a major impact on global self-esteem) is body image. As the term suggests, body image refers to the self-perceptions, attitudes, feelings, and behaviors an individual holds with respect to his or her body and physical appearance. Body image is defined as the internal representation of a person's outer appearance (Thompson, Heinberg, Altabe, & Tantleff-Dunn, 1999). Increasingly, the lean and fit body for women and the lean and muscular body for men have been endorsed as ideal body types in the media. Males and females who deviate from the sometimes impossible "ideal" and internalize this ideal may experience body image problems.

Body image is a multidimensional subjective experience composed of five dimensions: perceptual, cognitive, affective, subjective, and behavioral (see **TABLE 10-3**). These dimensions interact with and influence each other. Our body image perception is based on the mental images we have of our appearance, as well as the sensations of being in our bodies. Sometimes our perception is accurate—our mental image matches up with the reality of our appearance and how others perceive our appearance—but sometimes it is distorted, and we see something very different from what others see. When our perception is distorted, we may overestimate our overall body size, size of specific body parts, or evaluate our bodies differently than others—usually more harshly or with a magnified focus.

The affective dimension represents feelings associated with body image and can cover the emotional spectrum. In body image disturbance, these feelings tend

TABLE 10-3	Dimensions of Body Image
Dimension	**Description**
Perceptual	Mental images we have of our appearance and the sensations of being in our bodies.
Cognitive	Beliefs about our appearance.
Affective	Feelings associated with body image.
Subjective	General evaluate form of body image. Often assessed via body satisfaction/dissatisfaction.
Behavioral	Behaviors people engage in with regard to their body image, such as excessive checking and body avoidance.

to take the form of shame, disgust, fear, or sadness. Such feelings may be a constant backdrop, causing significant distress and preoccupation.

The cognitive dimension represents beliefs about our appearance (e.g., "being too big or round"), as well as the meaning of our appearance (e.g., "therefore, I am unacceptable or worthless"). In body image disturbance, people tend to equate appearance with overall self-worth. Thus, if these individuals are dissatisfied with their appearance, they are dissatisfied with themselves as a whole. Research shows that when young women think about their appearance while taking a math test, their performance is markedly worse than young women who do not think about their appearance. For individuals with body image disturbance, thoughts about appearance persist throughout the day and detract from concentration and enjoyment of everyday activities.

The subjective evaluation dimension is more general in nature and tends to encompass body dissatisfaction, for example, a person being satisfied (or dissatisfied) with his or her body as a whole or with specific body parts (e.g., arms, legs, buttocks).

Finally, the behavioral aspect of body image involves behaviors people engage in with regard to their body image, such as excessive checking and body avoidance. Body checking can take many forms, such as weighing, measuring, pinching, or looking in the mirror. Body checking is driven by the desire to get information or reassurance about one's appearance or body size in an attempt to alleviate anxiety. On the opposite end of the spectrum is body avoidance, which involves avoiding exposure (of the self or others) to one's appearance. Examples of body avoidance behaviors include wearing baggy clothes, avoiding mirrors, and preferring not to be touched. The purpose is to avoid upsetting information about one's appearance or body size, and it is fueled by dissatisfaction and the sense that one's body is unacceptable. Someone who is highly body dissatisfied may avoid going to the beach because he or she does not want to be seen in public in a bathing suit. As well, people who are body dissatisfied may not work out at the gym for fear that others are looking at their bodies negatively.

CRITICAL THINKING ACTIVITY 10-2

© ecco/Shutterstock, Inc.

How are body image and self-esteem related? Is one of these constructs more important than the other?

Scope and Significance of Body Image

Several large-scale studies and reviews have revealed that although body dissatisfaction is common in both male and female populations, women and girls tend to be more body dissatisfied than men and boys. A recent online survey among a nationally representative sample of 2,059 American adults (18 years and older) and 200 teens (aged 16 to 17 years) found that 67% of adult women, 52% of adult men, 85% of teen girls, and 56% of teen boys worry regularly about their appearance (defined as worrying at least once a week; Bellomy Research, 2014). In fact, adult women worry more regularly about their appearance than they do about their finances (62%), health (49%), family/relationships (46%), or professional success (40%). Men are not far behind, with only finances, at 59%, ranking higher among weekly worries for men (see **FIGURE 10-4**). In other words, we tend to worry more about our appearance than our health, family, or professional success.

The good news is that when it comes to appearance, with age we become more accepting of our bodies. People who are 55 years or older are half as likely to worry about their appearance as those under the age of 25, and as people get older they spend less time overall on their appearance every day. Also, older people are less likely to worry about being judged by others on their appearance.

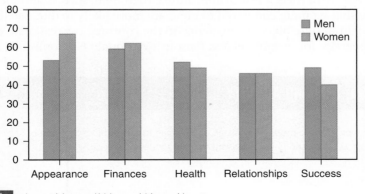

 FIGURE 10-4   Issues Men and Women Worry About

Adapted from Bellomy Research. (2014). TODAY/AOL 'Ideal to Real' body image survey. Retrieved March 12, 2014, from http://www.aol.com/article/2014/02/24/loveyourselfie/20836450/.

Finally, worrying less about appearance may make life better for everyone else. In other words, as people age and worry less about their own appearance, they also complain about it less to others.

This survey also found that the average woman worries about six body parts, while the average man worries about three. For women, the list of common worries are the stomach (69%), skin (40%), thighs (39%), hair (32%), cellulite (29%), and butt (29%). For men, stomach came first (52%), followed by thinning hair (24%), and skin issues (23%).

Indeed, boys generally display less overall body concern than girls (Cochane & Pope, 2001). The survey results revealed that boys' and girls' body dissatisfaction is often associated with reduced self-esteem. Consistent with the ideal physique portrayed in the media of a thin and toned physique for women and a lean and muscular body for men, girls typically wanted to be thinner and boys frequently wanted to be more muscular.

There is nothing wrong with people caring about their appearance. However, for some people the investment in their appearance may become all-consuming, and it may have negative health outcomes. For both genders, negative body image has detrimental physical, social, psychological, and economic consequences. More specifically, negative body image is related to emotional distress (Johnson & Wardle, 2005), higher body mass index (Slevec & Tiggemann, 2011), smoking (Croghan et al., 2006), dramatic measures to alter appearance (e.g., steroid use; Raevuori et al., 2006), social anxiety (Cash & Fleming, 2002), impaired sexual functioning (Wiederman, 2002), depression (Stice & Bearman, 2001), and eating disorders (Stice, Presnell, & Spangler, 2002). In short, body dissatisfaction is common, and it can adversely affect a person's psychosocial functioning and quality of life.

The differences in the prevalence of body dissatisfaction shown by women and men in the studies presented is not atypical. Generally, across a wide variety of studies with participants who varied in age, women were found to have greater dissatisfaction with their physical appearance than men. Also, additional research has shown that women, compared to men, are more likely to diet, see themselves as overweight despite objective evidence to the contrary, overestimate their body size, and exercise for weight-related reasons (McDonald & Thompson, 1992).

CRITICAL THINKING ACTIVITY 10-3

© ecco/Shutterstock, Inc.

Why do women have more body image disturbance than men? Describe the possible psychological, social, and physical reasons for this gender difference.

In contrast to women, who experience pressure to be slender, men often experience pressure to maintain an athletic and muscular body type. For example, men represented as prestigious in popular magazines are often lean and muscular

(Frederick, Fessler, & Haselton, 2005). Although women report more body dissatisfaction than men, it is still common in men. For example, a large-scale survey of 52,677 visitors to a popular U.S. news website found that 48% of men reported that they felt dissatisfied with their weight, 11% felt physically unattractive, and 16% were so uncomfortable with their bodies that they avoided wearing a bathing suit in public (Frederick, Peplau, & Lever, 2006).

Failure to achieve a lean and muscular build, a prominent characteristic of masculinity for many men, may lead to body dissatisfaction. David Frederick and his colleagues (2007) used a figure-rating scale—a tool used to measure body dissatisfaction—to determine men's satisfaction with their muscularity and body fat in a series of international studies conducted in the United States, Ukraine, and Ghana. The researchers found widespread desire for increased muscularity among men, with over half of the U.S. men surveyed (range = 51% to 71%) reporting that they were not satisfied with their body fat level. They also found that over 90% of U.S. undergraduate men wanted to be more muscular, as did many Ukrainian (69%) and Ghanaian (49%) men. In the United States, men's ratings of their current and ideal muscularity were associated with endorsement of the male role, and many men desired increased muscularity for reasons related to increased dominance and attractiveness to women.

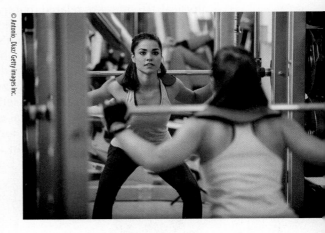

© Antonio_Diaz/Getty Images Inc.

Widespread body image disturbance for both men and women is associated with consumers spending billions of dollars annually for products aimed at changing their body size and shape, such as diet pills, unnecessary cosmetic surgery, beauty products, and fitness products. Because of the detrimental outcomes associated with negative body image and its malleable and subjective nature, society could benefit from a better understanding of the efficacy of interventions aimed at improving body image.

Body image interventions typically consist of psychoeducational, cognitive behavioral, or drug therapies (e.g., weight loss pills/programs; Gollings & Paxton, 2006). Because many of these interventions are expensive, in short supply, and often not suitable for young populations, other, more practical strategies should be examined and promoted. One promising alternative mode of intervention for negative body image is exercise (Hausenblas & Fallon, 2006). Let's take a look at the research examining the effects of physical activity on body image.

Body Image and Physical Activity

A meta-analysis by Anna Campbell and Heather Hausenblas (2009) provides support for the suggestion that physical activity improves body image. In their meta-analysis, they examined the impact that exercise interventions had on people's body image. They reviewed 57 interventions and found a small effect size (.29) that indicated that exercise resulted in improved body image from pre- to postintervention for the physical activity group compared to the nonexercise control group.

Campbell and Hausenblas (2009) concluded that exercise represents a practical and widely accessible intervention for negative body image. Although the effect size was small, exercise has advantages over other types of therapy, such as cognitive behavioral therapy. For example, exercise has the ability to reach and benefit many people. Other practical advantages of exercise are that, compared to other interventions, it is low cost, has minimal side-effects, and is a socially acceptable behavior. These benefits may result in exercise receiving greater acceptance as a treatment. Finally, exercise is self-sustaining because it can be maintained once the basic skills are learned.

In their meta-analysis, Campbell and Hausenblas (2009) found that both aerobic and resistance types of exercise resulted in improvements in body image. However, an important research question is to examine what specific types of physical activities are related to improved body image. Kelly Arbour and Kathleen Martin Ginis (2008) examined the effects of the most common type of physical activity—walking—on women's body image. Using a randomized controlled trial, they sought to determine whether the number of steps walked during an 11-week action planning intervention would effect change in sedentary women's body image. Seventy-five healthy women were assigned to either a control group, where they were required to self-monitor their daily pedometer-determined step count, or to an experimental group, where they were asked to self-monitor and form specific action plans for walking. Of the 75 participants who were randomized, 41 were included in the analyses. Arbour and Martin Ginis found

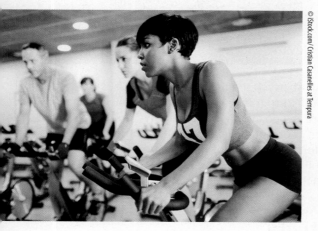

© iStock.com/ Cristian Casanelles at Tempura

greater satisfaction with physical functioning and higher step counts for the experimental group compared to the control group. Moreover, the total number of steps walked over weeks 2 to 11 of the intervention was shown to partially mediate the effect of the intervention on satisfaction with physical functioning. These findings suggest that walking greater distances is associated with greater improvement in women's body image. Other studies have found that moderate to vigorous physical activity has stronger effects on body image than lifestyle physical activity (Rote, Swartz, & Klos, 2013).

Another question is whether a person's body image acts as either a motivator or barrier to exercise participation. A recent study by Laura Brudzynski and William Ebben (2013) sheds light on the relationship between motivations and barriers to exercise and body image. They examined 1,044 university students' self-reported relationships between motivations and barriers to exercise, frequency of exercise, and location of exercise on body image. They found that 78.6% of the students in their study could be classified as exercisers. They also found that body image was related to increased exercise amounts for the exercisers, with 58% of exercisers reporting that body image influenced the amount of physical activity they engaged in.

In particular, negative body image was a primary motive for exercise participation with students when they felt overweight, when they wanted to improve appearance, and when they wanted to change a specific body area. Body image was also identified as a barrier to exercise location, with most exercisers reporting a preference for private locations. The nonexercisers (34.2%) were satisfied with their overall appearance and did not identify body image as a significant barrier to exercise participation. The researchers concluded that body image is a motivator for exercise amount and a barrier to exercise location for exercisers, but that it is not a barrier to exercise for nonexercisers.

CRITICAL THINKING ACTIVITY 10-4

© ecco/Shutterstock, Inc.

How can physical activity be both a motivator and demotivator for exercise behavior?

An interesting question is what happens to regular exercisers' body dissatisfaction during brief periods of nonexercise. Regular exercisers who take even 3 days off of exercise report increases in body dissatisfaction (Niven, Rendell, & Chisholm, 2008). This finding reveals the transient nature of body image, and indicates that body image may be an important motivator for regular exercise.

Appearance-based exercise motivation (i.e., the extent that exercise is pursued to influence weight or shape) affects both body image and exercise frequency in women (Lepage & Crowther, 2010). Exercise frequency has been shown to be related to higher positive body image, but high levels of appearance-based exercise motivation weakened these relationships (Homan & Tylka, 2014). Thus, messages promoting exercise need to deemphasize weight loss and appearance and promote positive body image. For example, **fitspiration** is any message (usually in the form of an image with a quote included) designed to inspire people to attain a fitness goal. The results of the aforementioned study suggest that fitspiration messages should not focus on appearance-related images, such as six-pack abs.

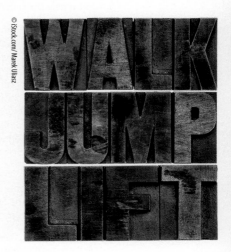
© iStock.com/ Marek Uliasz

Self-Presentational Anxiety

Self-presentation is an important determinant of physical activity because self-presentation affects people's exercise cognitions, attitudes, and behaviors (Hausenblas, Brewer, & van Raalte, 2004). **Self-presentation** is the process by which people attempt to control and monitor how they are perceived and evaluated by others (Leary, 1992). People generally want others to view them in desirable ways. Thus, they attempt to control the inferences made by others by only presenting information about themselves that will bring about the desired impression, while hiding things that would be inconsistent with this desired image. The impressions that we make on other individuals affect how they treat us; therefore, self-presentation underlies most of our social interactions. Some people, however, are more apprehensive about incurring negative evaluation, and thus are more prone to self-presentational concerns than their less apprehensive counterparts.

When the individual doubts that he or she will be unable to generate positive impression or forestall an undesirable impression, social anxiety results (Leary, 1992). Because physical appearance is such an important component of both physical self-esteem and global self-esteem, social anxiety can arise as a result of concerns about the self-presentation of one's body. In fact, Elizabeth Hart, Mark Leary, and Jack Rejeski (1989) proposed the presence of a trait (i.e., a stable personal disposition) that they called **social physique anxiety**. TABLE 10-4 provides

TABLE 10-4   Social Physique Anxiety Scale

1 = Not at all characteristic
2 = Slightly characteristic
3 = Moderately characteristic
4 = Very characteristic
5 = Extremely characteristic

1. I wish I wasn't so uptight about my physique/figure. _____
2. I am bothered by thoughts that other people are evaluating my weight or muscular development negatively. _____
3. Unattractive features of my physique/figure make me nervous in this social settings. _____
4. In the presence of others, I feel apprehensive about my physique/figure. _____
5. I am comfortable with how fit my body appears to others. _____
6. It would make me uncomfortable to know others are evaluating my physique/figure. _____
7. When it comes to displaying my physique/figure to others, I am a shy person. _____
8. I usually feel relaxed when it is obvious that others are looking at my physique/figure. _____
9. When in exercise clothes, I often feel nervous about the shape of my body. _____

Scoring

1. Reverse score: Items 5 and 8.
2. Add up the 9 items. Score range = 9 to 45.
3. High score = high social physique anxiety.

Data from Martin, K. A., Rejeski, W. J., Leary, M. R., McAuley, E., & Bain, S. (1997). Is the Social Physique Anxiety Scale really multidimensional? Conceptual and statistical arguments for a unidimensional model. *Journal of Sport and Exercise Psychology, 19*, 359–367.

the items from the Social Physique Anxiety Scale (Martin et al., 1997), which can be used to assess for this trait.

Hart and her colleagues (1989) found that women who score high on the social physique anxiety trait also have more stress and discomfort during physique evaluations and more negative thoughts about their body's appearance. Also, Sally Crawford and Robert Eklund (1994) noted that women who are higher in the trait of social physique anxiety also reported a greater tendency to exercise for self-presentation reasons such as weight control, body tone, and physical attractiveness. Conversely, women lower in the trait of social physique anxiety were more likely to exercise for motives generally unrelated to self-presentation, such as fitness, mood enhancement, health, and enjoyment.

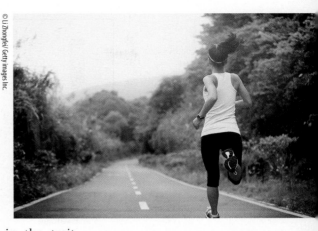

A similar result was found when Heather Hausenblas and Kathleen Martin (2000) measured levels of social physique anxiety and exercise behavior in 286 female aerobics instructors. Instructors who were involved in leading classes primarily for self-presentation reasons (e.g., weight loss, improved body tone) had higher levels of social physique anxiety. In comparison, instructors who were involved in leading classes for leadership opportunities (i.e., to educate or to lead) or to affect enhancement (i.e., to have fun or to reduce stress) possessed a lower degree of social physique anxiety.

Brian Focht and Heather Hausenblas (2003, 2004) found that social physique anxiety can also affect how women feel during and after exercise. They examined the influence of different exercise environments upon state anxiety and positive feeling states in women with high social physique anxiety. The study participants completed the following three conditions: (1) exercise in a self-presentational environment that involved exercising in a coed gym in front of mirrors, (2) exercise in a laboratory alone, and (3) quiet rest in a laboratory alone. Participants completed task assessments of their state anxiety and feeling states before, during, and after each condition.

Focht and Hausenblas (2003, 2004) found that only the exercise environment perceived to be high in evaluative threat (i.e., self-presentational environment) was associated with elevated in-task state anxiety (see **FIGURE 10-5**). Also, significant reductions in state anxiety were observed from pre-exercise to 5 minutes post-exercise in both the self-representational and laboratory exercise environments.

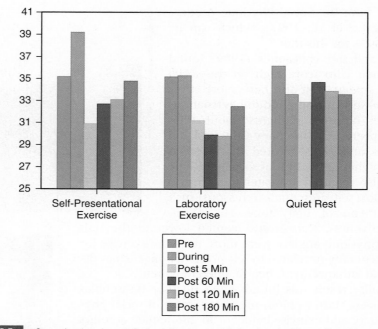

FIGURE 10-5 State Anxiety Levels Before, During, and Following the Three Conditions

Data from Focht, B. C., & Hausenblas, H. A. (2004). Perceived evaluative threat and state anxiety during exercise in women with high social physique anxiety. *Journal of Applied Sport Psychology*, *16*, 361–368; Focht B. C., & Hausenblas, H. A. (2006). Exercising in public and private environments: Effects on feeling states in women with social physique anxiety. *Journal of Applied Behavioral Research*, *11*, 147–165.

The reduction in state anxiety, however, was significantly larger in the self-presentational environment. Also, whereas the anxiolytic response persisted through the 120-minute postexercise assessment following the laboratory environment, state anxiety did not differ significantly from baseline at any of the remaining assessments following exercise in the self-presentational exercise environment. No significant changes in state anxiety were detected following quiet rest. In summary, state anxiety increased during exercise in the self-presentational environment, and the anxiolytic effect observed 5 minutes after both exercise conditions only persisted following exercise in the laboratory environment.

Focht and Hausenblas (2003, 2004) also found that increases in positive feeling states emerged following exercise, but not following quiet rest. Finally, they reported that whereas feeling states returned to baseline within 1 hour following the self-presentational exercise condition, improvements in feeling states persisted for 2 hours following exercise in the lab condition.

Focht and Hausenblas (2003, 2004) concluded that the psychological benefits of acute exercise may not generalize to women with high social physique anxiety, meaning that the negative feeling states that emerged during exercise in the self-presentational environment support the idea that psychological distress experienced with public exercise settings may deter women with social physique anxiety from exercising (McAuley et al., 1995). Thus, given that negative in-task feeling states only emerged during the self-presentational environment, exercising in settings where evaluative threatening aspects of the environment can be modified (e.g., locations of mirrors, privacy) would be advantageous for women with social physique anxiety, particularly during the adoption phase of a physical activity program (Focht & Hausenblas, 2006). Initiating physical activity in settings that minimize evaluative threat may allow women with social physique anxiety to avoid self-presentational anxiety, while providing them with the opportunity to enhance their perceptions of their exercise abilities and body image.

CRITICAL THINKING ACTIVITY 10-5

© ecco/Shutterstock, Inc.

You need to design an exercise intervention for a female adult who has high social physique anxiety. What type of intervention would you design and why? Justify your answer based on current research on this topic.

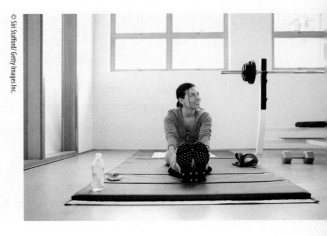
© Siri Stafford/Getty Images Inc.

What are the effects of chronic exercise on social physique anxiety? Pearson, Hall, and Gammage (2013) found that an exercise intervention results in improved social physique anxiety in overweight and obese sedentary women. As well, Kathleen Martin Ginis and her colleagues (2014) found that an 8-week exercise program for women with body-image concerns resulted in significant reductions in social physique anxiety and other related body image measures. Of importance, women who were assigned to the aerobic training condition had greater improvements in social physique anxiety and appearance evaluation compared to women in the strength-training condition.

■ Summary

Self-esteem and body image are important constructs for physical activity. Researchers have continually demonstrated that physical activity is associated with improved self-esteem and body image. In other words, people who are physically active have higher self-esteem, are less preoccupied with body measurements, and have better body image than nonactive people (Korn et al., 2013). The emerging research is revealing that sedentary behavior is negatively related with self-esteem and body image. In summary, physical activity can be used to enhance self-esteem and body image. It has a positive impact on males and females of all ages, but the greatest effects of physical activity are shown in people with low levels of self-esteem, body image, and physical activity.

KEY TERMS

body image
fitspiration
Physical Self-Perception Profile
self-concept

self-esteem
self-presentation
social physique anxiety

REVIEW QUESTIONS

1. What is the difference between self-esteem and self-concept?

2. Describe the Physical Self-Perception Profile.

3. Describe the study conducted by Justin Moore and his colleagues (2011). What was the main conclusion from this study?

4. Define *body image*. How does body image differ from self-esteem?

5. Describe the "ideal" physique for men versus women.

6. What is the relationship between body image and physical activity?

7. What is social physique anxiety? What is the relationship between social physique anxiety and physical activity behavior?

8. How does body image affect physical activity motivation?

9. Define the term *fitspiration*. Do you think that fitspirations are effective in increasing people's motivation to engage in physical activity?

APPLYING THE CONCEPTS

1. What concepts help explain how and why Divya's preoccupation with the way others perceived her impacted her exercise habits?

2. Why was Divya able to exercise in the woman's fitness facility more readily than at her school's gym?

3. Describe the shift in Divya's attitude toward exercise and her

self-awareness while engaging in it. How might this help explain the benefits she derived from her active lifestyle?

4. What changes did becoming active introduce into Divya's self-concept? How did these changes impact her self-esteem and body image?

REFERENCES

Arbour, K. P., & Martin Ginis, K. A. (2008). Improving body image one step at a time: Greater pedometer step counts produce greater body image improvements. *Body Image, 5*, 331–336.

Bellomy Research. (2014). TODAY/AOL "Ideal to Real" body image survey results. Retrieved March 12, 2014, from http://www.aol.com/article/2014/02/24/loveyourselfie/20836450/

Brudzynski, L., & Ebben, W. P. (2010). Body image as a motivator and barrier to exercise participation. *International Journal of Exercise Science, 1*, 14–24.

Campbell, A., & Hausenblas, H. A. (2009). Effects of exercise interventions on body image: A meta-analysis. *Journal of Health Psychology, 14*, 780–793.

Cash, T. F., & Fleming, E. C. (2002). Body image and social relations. In T. F. Cash & T. Pruzinsky (Eds.), *Body image: A handbook of theory, research, and clinical practice* (pp. 277–286). New York, NY: Guilford Press.

Cochane, G. H., & Pope, H. G. (2001). Body image in boys: A review of the literature. *International Journal of Eating Disorders, 29*, 373–379.

Crawford, S., & Eklund, R. C. (1994). Social physique anxiety, reasons for exercise, and attitudes toward exercise settings. *Journal of Sport and Exercise Psychology, 16*, 70–82.

Croghan, I. T., Bronars, C., Patten, C. A., Schroeder, D. R., Nirelli, L. M., Thomas, J. L., . . . Hurt, R. D. (2006). Is smoking related to body image satisfaction, stress, and self-esteem in young adults? *American Journal of Health Behavior, 30*, 322–333.

Ekeland, E., Heian, F., & Hagen, K. B. (2005). Can exercise improve self-esteem in children and young people? A systematic review of randomized controlled trials. *British Journal of Sports Medicine, 39*, 792–798.

Elavsky, S. (2010). Longitudinal examination of the exercise and self-esteem model in middle-aged women. *Journal of Sport and Exercise Psychology, 32*, 862–880.

Focht, B. C., & Hausenblas, H. A. (2003). State anxiety responses to acute exercise in women with high social physique anxiety. *Journal of Sport & Exercise Psychology, 25,* 123–144.

Focht, B. C., & Hausenblas, H. A. (2004). Perceived evaluative threat and state anxiety during exercise in women with high social physique anxiety. *Journal of Applied Sport Psychology, 16,* 361–368.

Focht B. C., & Hausenblas, H. A. (2006). Exercising in public and private environments: Effects on feeling states in women with social physique anxiety. *Journal of Applied Behavioral Research, 11,* 147–165.

Fox, K. R. (2000). Self-esteem, self-perceptions, and exercise. *International Journal of Sport Psychology, 31,* 228–240.

Fox, K. R., & Corbin, C. B. (1989). The physical self-perception profile: Development and preliminary validation. *Journal of Sport and Exercise Psychology, 11,* 408–430.

Frederick, D., A. Buchman, G. M., Sadehgi-Azar, L., Peplau, L. A., Haselton, M. G., & Berezovskaya, A. (2007). Desiring the muscular ideal: Men's body satisfaction in the United States, Ukraine, and Ghana. *Psychology of Men and Masculinity, 8,* 103–117.

Frederick, D. A., Fesler, D. M., & Haselton, M. G. (2005). Do representations of male muscularity differ in men's and women's magazines? *Body Image, 2,* 81–86.

Frederick, D. A., Peplau, L. A., & Lever, J. (2006). The swimsuit issue: Correlates of body image in a sample of 52,677 heterosexual adults. *Body Image: An International Journal of Research, 4,* 413–419.

Gollings, E. K., & Paxton, S. J. (2006). Comparison of Internet and face-to-face delivery of a group body image and disordered eating intervention for women: A pilot study. *Eating Disorders, 14,* 1–15.

Gruber, J. J. (1986). Physical activity and self-esteem development in children: A meta-analysis. In G. A. Stull & H. M. Eckert (Eds.), *Effects of physical activity on children: A special tribute to Mabel Lee* (pp. 30–48). Champaign, IL: Human Kinetics.

Hart, E. A., Leary, M. R., & Rejeski, W. J. (1989). The measurement of social physique anxiety. *Journal of Sport and Exercise Psychology, 11,* 94–104.

Haugen, T., Safvenborn, R., & Ommundsen, Y. (2011). Physical activity and global self-worth: The role of physical self-esteem indices and gender. *Mental Health and Physical Activity, 4,* 49–56.

Hausenblas, H. A., Brewer, B. W., & Van Raalte, J. L. (2004). Self-presentation and exercise. *Journal of Applied Sport Psychology, 16,* 3–18.

Hausenblas, H. A., & Fallon, E. A. (2006). Exercise and body image: A meta-analysis. *Psychology and Health, 21,* 33–47.

Hausenblas, H. A., & Martin, K. A. (2000). Bodies on display. Predictors of social physique anxiety in female aerobic instructors. *Women in Sport and Physical Activity Journal, 9,* 1–14.

Homan, K. J., & Tylka, T. L. (2014). Appearance-based exercise motivation moderates the relationship between exercise frequency and positive body image. *Body Image, 11,* 101–108.

Johnson, F., & Wardle, J. (2005). Dietary restraint, body dissatisfaction, and psychological distress: A prospective analysis. *Journal of Abnormal Psychology, 114,* 119–125.

Korn, L., Gonen, E., Shaked, Y., & Golan, M. (2013). Health perceptions, self and body image, physical activity, and nutrition among undergraduate students in Israel. *PLos One, 8:*e58543. doi:10.1371/ journal.pone.0058543

Leary, M. J. (1992). Self-presentation in exercise and sport. *Journal of Sport and Exercise Psychology, 14,* 339–351.

Lepage, M. L., & Crowther, J. H. (2010). The effects of exercise on body satisfaction and affect. *Body Image, 7,* 124–130.

Lindwall, M., Asci, F. H., Palmeira, A., Fox, K. R., & Hagger, M. S. (2011). The importance of importance in the physical self: Support for the theoretically appealing but empirically elusive model of James. *Journal of Personality, 79,* 303–334.

Martin, K. A., Rejeski, W. J., Leary, M. R., McAuley, E., & Bain, S. (1997). Is the Social Physique Anxiety Scale really multidimensional? Conceptual and statistical arguments for a unidimensional model. *Journal of Sport and Exercise Psychology*, *19*, 359–367.

Martin Ginis, K. A., Strong, H. A., Arent, S. M., Bray, S. R., & Bassett-Gunter, R. L. (2014). The effects of aerobic- versus strength-training on body image among young women with pre-existing body image concerns. *Body Image*, *11*, 219–227.

McAuley, E., Bane, S. M., & Mihalko, S. L. (1995). Exercise in middle-aged adults: Self-efficacy and self-perception outcomes. *Preventive Medicine*, *24*, 319–328.

McAuley, E., Elavsky, S., Motl, R. W., Konopack, J. F., Hu, L., & Marquez, D. X. (2005). Physical activity, self-efficacy, and self-esteem: Longitudinal relationships in older adults. *The Journals of Gerontology. Series B, Psychological Sciences and Social Sciences*, *60*, 268–275.

McDonald, D. G., & Hodgdon, J. A. (1991). The psychological effects of aerobic fitness training: Research and theory. New York, NY: Springer-Verlag.

McDonald, K., & Thompson, J. K. (1992). Eating disturbance, body image dissatisfaction, and reasons for exercising: Gender differences and correlational findings. *International Journal of Eating Disorders*, *11*, 289–292.

Moore, J. B., Mitchell, N. G., Bibeau, W. S., & Bartholomew, J. B. (2011). Effects of a 12-week resistance exercise program on physical self-perceptions in college students. *Research Quarterly for Exercise and Sport*, *82*, 291–301.

Niven, A., Rendell, E., & Chisholm, L. (2008). Effects of 72-h of exercise abstinence on affect and body dissatisfaction in healthy female regular exercisers. *Journal of Sports Science*, *26*, 1235–1242.

Pearson, E. S., Hall, C. R., & Gammage, K. L. (2013). Self-presentation in exercise: Changes over a 12-week cardiovascular programme for overweight and obese sedentary females. *European Journal of Sport Sciences*, *13*, 407–413.

Raevuori, A., Keski-Rahkonen, A., Bulick, C. M., Rose, R. J., Rissanen, A., & Kaprio, J. (2006). Muscle dissatisfaction in young adult men. *Clinical Practice and Epidemiology in Mental Health*, *2*, 1–8.

Rote, A. E., Swartz, A. M., & Klos, L. A. (2013). Associations between lifestyle activity and body image attitudes among women. *Women and Health*, *53*, 282–297.

Schmalz, D. L., Deane, G. D., Birch, L. L., & Krahnstoever Davison, K. (2007). A longitudinal assessment of the links between physical and self-esteem in early adolescent non-Hispanic females. *Journal of Adolescent Health*, *41*, 559–565.

Shavelson, R. J., Hubner, J. J., & Stanton, G. C. (1976). Self-concept: Validation of construct interpretations. *Review of Educational Research*, *46*, 407–441.

Slevec, J. H., & Tiggemann, M. (2011). Predictors of body dissatisfaction and disordered eating in middle-aged women. *Clinical Psychology Review*, *31*, 515–524.

Smith, J. J., Eather, N., Morgan, P. J., Plotnikoff, R. C., Faigenbaum, A. D., & Lubans, D. R. (2014). The health benefits of muscular fitness for children and adolescents: A systematic review and meta-analysis. *Sports Medicine*, *44*, 1209–1223.

Sonstroem, R. J., Harlow, L. L., & Josephs, L. (1994). Exercise and self-esteem: Validity of model expansion and exercise associations. *Journal of Sport and Exercise Psychology*, *16*, 29–42.

Sonstroem, R. J., & Morgan, W. P. (1989). Exercise and self-esteem: Rationale and model. *Medicine and Science in Sports and Exercise*, *21*, 329–337.

Speck, R. M., Courneya, K. S., Mâsse, L. C., Duval, S., & Schmitz K. H. (2010). An update of controlled physical activity trials in cancer survivors: A systematic review and meta-analysis. *Journal of Cancer Survivors*, *4*, 87–100.

Spence, J. C., McGannon, K. R., & Poon, P. (2005). The effect of exercise on global self-esteem: A quantitative review. *Journal of Sport and Exercise Psychology*, *27*, 311–334.

Stice, E., & Bearman, S. K. (2001). Body-image and eating disturbances prospectively predict increases in depressive symptoms in adolescent girls: A growth curve analysis. *Developmental Psychology, 37,* 597–607.

Stice, E., Presnell, K., & Spangler, D. (2002). Risk factors for binge eating onset: A prospective investigation. *Health Psychology, 21,* 131–138.

Thompson, J. K., Heinberg, L. J., Altabe, M., & Tantleff-Dunn, S. (1999). *Exacting beauty: Theory, assessment, and treatment of body image disturbance.* Washington, DC: American Psychological Association.

Tremblay, M. S., LeBlanc, A. G., Kho, M. E., Saunders, T. J., Larouche, R., Colley, R. C., . . . Gorber, S. C. (2011). Systematic review of sedentary behaviour and health indicators in school-age children and youth. *International Journal of Behavioral Nutrition and Physical Activity.* Sep 21;*8*:98. doi:10.1186/1479-5868-8-98

Trzesniewski, K. H., Donnellan, M. B., & Robins, R. W. (2003). Stability of self-esteem across the life span. *Journal of Personality and Social Psychology, 84,* 205–220.

Wiederman, M. W. (2002). Body image and sexual functioning. In T. F. Cash & T. Pruzinsky (Eds.), *Body image: A handbook of theory, research, and clinical practice* (pp. 287–294). New York, NY: Guildford Press.

CHAPTER 11

Stress and Pain

Vignette: Carla

When I'm feeling overwhelmed, my body gets stiff. My shoulders hunch up. I purse my lips. I clench my jaw. I tend to remain in whatever position I happen to be in. Because I work as the office manager of a small consulting firm, that position is usually seated. And because my boss and his underlings are never short on demands, criticisms, and tension-filled directives to bark in my direction, I'm usually stressed on most days.

I don't have the most intellectually rigorous job in the world but that doesn't mean I don't arrive at and leave my office exhausted and more than occasionally overwhelmed. We're a high-pressure environment, and there's a lot of people crammed into the open-plan setup all 52 employees currently occupy. But who am I to complain?

I've worked this job for going on 3 years now, and I've watched the firm grow. My bosses have been open to the idea of incorporating employee wellness into their ever-expanding business model. And as someone who resolves to "get in shape" every January 1st, I figured getting the whole office to go in with me on some type of fitness push would keep me from backtracking on my commitments—like I typically do, come March.

I've long known that exercise is a great means of ridding myself of anxiety and stress. In high school, I played volleyball and tennis, swam, and took frequent advantage of the

LEARNING OBJECTIVES

After completing this chapter, you will be able to

- Understand the relationship between exercise and pain.
- Understand the relationship between being physically active and responding to life stressors.
- Differentiate between the various types of pain and stress.
- Understand the relationship between pain and improvements in physiological function via involvement in exercise and sedentary behavior.

257

stationary bike my dad kept in our basement. Throughout my undergraduate years I was also relatively active. I stuck with the volleyball team for my freshman and sophomore years until I spent a year abroad. My senior year I was too busy interning to make practices, so instead of regular sports meetups I made use of my campus's fitness facilities.

I had a really difficult time finding a job right out of college. I moved back in with my parents in San Francisco and bounced between a few administrative assistant gigs until I found the firm where I currently work. The pay was enough that I could afford my own place. (As an only child, I was never one for roommates. I prefer to live alone, and I figured I'd stay with mom and dad until I could actually finance a room of my own.)

But since day one on the job, I've felt like my outlets to relax have diminished. Sure, I go out for happy hour with my girlfriends. I enjoy dating in my spare time. But I miss that general calm I used to feel back in college. (One could argue, however, that my mental ease then was more a function of having all my bills paid for at the time—not to mention being comfortably enveloped in my campus's friendly social environment.)

In fact, my blood pressure appears to have gone up slowly but consistently since I began this job, or so my primary care physician tells me. The one time it dipped back down to a level that elicited my doctor's nod of approval was when I'd gone through a phase of attending spin class. (That lasted about 3 months. Once I strained my knee on a bike, I stopped going.)

Hence why I volunteered to help coordinate this employee wellness program my bosses finally decided to move ahead with last summer. I'll admit, I was motivated selfishly. I wanted to do all these activities but I needed gym buddies. (Most of my friends were about as reliable as I was when it came to regularly going to classes, meaning that they were not reliable at all.)

First and foremost, I wanted to make sure we all had access to a gym and to fitness classes. Elliptical trainers, weights, treadmills . . . yoga, Pilates, Zumba—you name it! I figured if we were all granted access to these options most of us would take advantage of them. I managed, with the help of my bosses, to secure a pretty decent corporate rate at a gym that's a quick drive from our offices. (Technically, you could walk, but it takes about 30 minutes by foot, give or take traversing some busy roads.)

I also knew a few fellow employees with prior experience on team sports. In fact, several other men and women who work in this office have also, like me, played on volleyball teams. So I'm in the process of scheduling a small group of us to play one another at a beach volleyball court at the end of this month.

We're off to a good start. I'm impressed by how many people are actually making use of their fancy new gym memberships. (In part, I like it because it makes *me* more likely to join them. I call this positive peer pressure!) But what's even better about the new access our employees have to a fitness facility is that the general tone around the office seems to have gotten a bit, well, nicer.

I still get orders barked at me. I still overhear griping and sniping. My bosses are still overworked, testy, and occasionally cruel. But ever since we really got this employee wellness program up and running I'm noticing more smiles around the office and I swear I'm hearing a bit more laughter.

The tension in my own body also seems to be going down. (Not completely, of course.) But now that I'm back to taking regular yoga classes and meeting two of my officemates for an after-work gym session on Tuesdays and Thursdays, I'm getting closer to that college-calmness I had going on a decade ago.

Fitness may not be the solution to all my woes. But being able to get up from my desk, leave the office behind, and sweat out to some great music, good company, and a different environment really does wonders when it comes to maintaining my own mental sanity. Though in my greatest times of stress my initial response is still to freeze up and remain seated, I've been trying to use a lunch break here and there to head to the gym my company now belongs to.

Here's to hoping that this time the resolution lasts year round!

◼ Introduction

Everyone experiences stress and pain. How and why we experience stress and pain may change throughout our lives, but none of us can escape them. What does vary is how each of us responds to stress and pain and how these two psychobiological constructs affect us. In this chapter, we will examine the health significance of pain and stress and the role that exercise and sedentary behavior plays for both of these constructs. More specifically, the research examining the relationship between both experimentally induced and endogenous (i.e., naturally occurring) pain and physical activity is reviewed. As well, research pertaining to how our involvement in physical activity affects our reactivity to stressors is discussed.

◼ Stress

Exposure to stressful situations is one of the most common things people experience. Just think about how many times you have said "I am stressed" or "I feel stressed." Stressful situations can range from daily annoyances, such as forgetting your phone or wallet at your house, to the consequences of overstretched,

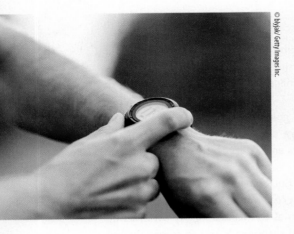

© blyjak/ Getty Images Inc.

time-pressured lifestyles, to events such as illness, loss, and natural disasters. So, what exactly is stress?

Despite the pervasiveness of stress, psychologists have not had an easy time coming up with an acceptable definition. To better understand stress, it is necessary to recognize the following critical distinction: the difference between stressors and stress. **Stress** is often defined as the process by which we perceive and respond to events called **stressors** that we appraise as either threatening or challenging. We must judge a challenging event to be either threatening or even beyond our ability to cope before we will be stressed by it.

CRITICAL THINKING ACTIVITY 11-1

© ecco/Shutterstock, Inc.

What is the difference between a stress and a stressor? Provide examples of each from your everyday life.

In other words, stress is the failure of a person to respond to mental, emotional, or physical demands, whether actual or imagined (Selye, 1956). More specifically, stress is a normal physical response to events that make you feel threatened or that upset your balance in some way. Stress usually happens in real time, such as when you are forced to manage many different things during the day, including work, school, family, friends, and sports.

Stressors are the outside forces that people must deal with. Stress is the individual's response to these stressors, such as increased anxiety. It is not so important what happens to a person (stressors), but rather how he or she relates and copes with it. It is our response to these stressors that largely determines the severity of stress in our lives.

We can experience both active and passive stressors, which can be further divided into laboratory and real-life stressors. **TABLE 11-1** provides examples of active and passive stressors. *Active stressors* are tasks or situations in which the person's response leads to a particular outcome. In other words, the response is under the individual's control. An example of a common laboratory active stressor is the Stroop color-word task in which colored words are presented with a conflict. The name of the color (e.g., blue, red, green) is printed in a color not denoted by the name (e.g., the word "red" printed in blue ink instead of red ink). In this reaction time stress test, the person is supposed to ignore the word and state the color of

TABLE 11-1 Types of Stressors

Type of Stressor	Laboratory Examples	Real-Life Examples
Passive	Films that elicit emotional reactions Exposure to unpleasant sounds	Dental procedures An in-flight emergency
Active	Stroop color-word task Reaction time tests Mental arithmetic	Public speaking Exams Parachuting Defending a dissertation

the letters of the word. In contrast, *passive stressors* are tasks or situations in which the individual's response has no bearing on the outcome. For example, most people have no control over situations such as pain or noise.

CRITICAL THINKING ACTIVITY 11-2

© ecco/Shutterstock, Inc.

Complete the Stroop color-word test. Several versions of this test are available online. How long did it take you to complete the task? Did you find this task to be stressful? What type of stressor is this?

When you sense danger—whether real or imagined—your body's defenses kick into high gear in a rapid, automatic process known as the **fight-or-flight response**, or the stress response. When you perceive a threat, your sympathetic nervous system responds to the stressful event by releasing a flood of stress hormones, including adrenaline and cortisol. These hormones rouse the body for emergency action, increasing the body's heart rate, sending more blood to the brain and muscles, raising blood sugar levels, causing sweaty palms and soles, dilating the pupils, and prompting the hair on your skin to stand erect.

Stroop color-word test

BLUE	RED	YELLOW	ORANGE
GREEN	BLUE	PURPLE	RED
PURPLE	YELLOW	RED	BLUE
ORANGE	BLUE	YELLOW	RED
RED	GREEN	ORANGE	BLUE
PURPLE	YELLOW	BLUE	ORANGE

In other words, when you are under stress your heart pounds faster, your muscles tighten, your blood pressure rises, your breath quickens, and your senses become sharper. These physical changes increase your strength and stamina, speed your reaction time, and enhance your focus—preparing you to either fight or flee from the stressor at hand.

The stress response is the body's way of protecting you. When working properly, it helps you stay focused, energetic, and alert. In emergency situations, stress can save your life by giving you the extra strength to defend yourself or spurring you to slam on the brakes to avoid an accident. The stress response also helps you rise to meet challenges. Stress is what keeps you on your toes during a presentation at work, sharpens your concentration when you are attempting a free throw, or drives you to complete an assignment or exam when you would rather be watching television or socializing. But beyond a certain point, stress stops being helpful and starts causing damage to your physical, psychological, and social health.

Types of Stress

Understanding stress can be a challenge because of its complexity. That is, stress may be either short-lived or long lasting, and it may be either positive or negative in nature. Let's take a closer look at the different types of stress we may encounter in our lives.

Acute Versus Chronic Stress

Acute stress is short-lived, and it is the reaction to an immediate threat. Acute stress can be beneficial and create motivation. For example, when a deadline is approaching, stress may help you to focus and complete your task before the deadline. College students may use this type of stress to complete projects and cram for exams. Other situations where people may experience acute stress are during a car accident, before competing in a race, and when giving a speech. Once the situation is resolved, the stress diminishes.

In comparison, chronic or long-term stress comes about as the result of a situation that has either not been resolved or that continues for many years prior to being resolved. This might be a traumatic event that happened during childhood. Although resolved, the feelings surrounding the situation may not have been dealt with, and chronic stress remains. Or, a person may be in an ongoing situation, such as an abusive relationship, a dysfunctional home, a high-pressure work environment, persistent financial worries, or an ongoing illness in the family. Chronic stress has the ability to create additional cognitive (e.g., memory problems), emotional (e.g., moodiness), physical (e.g., aches and pains), and behavioral health issues (e.g., eating too much or too little). See **TABLE 11-2** for examples of the effects of chronic stress.

Positive Versus Negative Stress

Hans Selye (1975) developed a model that divided stress into the two major categories: eustress and distress. **Eustress** is stress that is healthy or that gives one positive feelings, such as hope or vigor. It is usually related to a desired event in a person's life. In other words, it is good stress. Eustress tends to be short term, and

TABLE 11-2 Cognitive, Emotional, Physical, and Behavioral Symptoms of Chronic Stress

Cognitive	Emotional	Physical	Behavioral
Memory problems	Moodiness	Aches, pains	Eating more or less
Decreased concentration	Irritability	Nausea	Sleeping too much or too little
Constant worrying	Agitation	Frequent colds	Nervous habits (nail biting, pacing)
Seeing only the negative	Depression	Chest pain	Using alcohol, cigarettes, or drugs to relax
Poor judgment	Sense of loneliness	Diarrhea or constipation	Isolating yourself from others

it is perceived to be within our coping abilities. It tends to motivate and focus our energy, resulting in improved performance. Examples of eustress include coming in first place in a race, getting a job promotion, getting married, riding a roller coaster, and engaging in exercise. Thus, stress that enhances a person's physical or mental function is considered eustress.

In contrast, **distress**, the most commonly referred to type of stress, has negative implications. Distress can be either short or long term, and it is perceived as being outside of our coping abilities. Distress may lead to anxiety and depressive behaviors such as social withdrawal, crying, and avoidance. Both positive and negative stress can be equally taxing on the body and are cumulative in nature, depending on a person's way of adapting to a change that has caused it. It is important to emphasize that our body cannot physically discern between distress or eustress (Kabat-Zinn, 1996). See **TABLE 11-3** for a summary of the differences between eustress and distress.

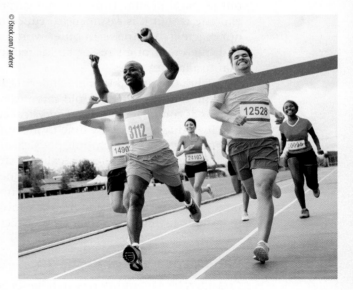

© iStock.com/ andrez

Stress, Exercise, and Sedentary Behavior

Stress is a subjective experience. Much of the stress we experience is based on our own perception of a situation; therefore, sources of stress can vary greatly

TABLE 11-3	Differences Between Eustress and Distress	
Type of Stress	**Characteristic**	**Example**
Eustress	Short term	Job promotion
	Perceived as within one's coping abilities	Marriage
	Motivates and focuses energy	Starting a new job
	Improves performance	Having a child
Distress	Short or long term	Death of a family member
	Perceived as outside one's coping abilities	Divorce
	Demotivates and drains our energy	Bankruptcy
	Can lead to mental and physical health issues	Legal problems
	Decreases performance	Injury or illness

from one person to another. The following two factors largely determine how we respond to stressful situations: (1) the way we perceive the situation and (2) our general state of physical health. We know that exercise has a positive effect on our physical health. Thus, it is not surprising then that one benefit espoused for exercise is that it is assumed to reduce how we react to stressful situations (i.e., our reactivity to stress). In other words, physical fitness helps people better cope with the onset of a stressor and it reduces the immediate physiological changes that result from stress.

Debra Crews and Daniel Landers (1987) suggested that two general processes through which exercise could serve to reduce stress are coping and inoculation. Insofar as coping is concerned, physical activity could provide a more efficient system by reducing recovery time in the autonomic nervous system. Similarly, inoculation might occur if chronic physical activity enhances the individual's physical and psychological abilities to deal with stress. So, for example, when an individual is faced with a stressor, the autonomic nervous system responds with its flight-or-fight response. For those individuals who are physically active, the stress response might be of less magnitude (i.e., at a lower level) and/or less time might be spent in a state of stress because of a faster recovery from the stress response.

Laboratory Stress Research

Considerable laboratory research has been undertaken to examine the association between exercise and reactivity to stressors. Typically, participants are exposed to a stressor such as an electric shock, a loud noise, or a cognitive task to be performed under time pressure. The question of interest is whether greater physical fitness or involvement in acute or chronic exercise helps protect the individual from the effects of a stressor (i.e., by reducing his or her reactivity) and/or help the person recover more quickly than an unfit or nonexercising person (Landers & Petruzzello, 1994).

Crews and Landers (1987) performed the first meta-analysis on the effects of aerobic exercise on psychosocial stress in an attempt to empirically summarize the research pertaining to this issue. They combined the results of 34 studies that included a total of 1,449 subjects. When Crews and Landers combined the results from all studies, they found that aerobically fit individuals have reduced reactivity to stress compared to unfit individuals (ES = .48).

Reduced reactivity and/or enhanced recovery from a stressor can be manifested through a variety of indices, such as heart rate, systolic blood pressure, diastolic blood pressure, skin response, and hormonal changes. Also, not surprisingly, different researchers have used different indices to assess stress reactivity. Because of this, Crews and Landers (1987) also carried out subanalyses using the different indices. An overview of the results for each of these physiological indices, as well as participants' self-reports of their reactivity and recovery, are presented in **TABLE 11-4** . Note that the smallest differences between aerobically fit and unfit individuals in stress reactivity was for hormonal changes (ES = .15), whereas the largest was for muscle tension (ES = .87).

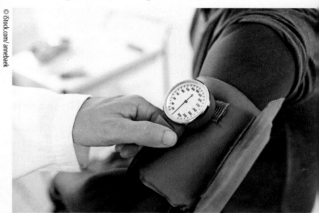

© iStock.com/ annebaek

TABLE 11-4 The Relationship Between Physical Activity and Reactivity to and Recovery from Stressors

Measure	Average Effect Size*
Overall reactivity/recovery to stressors	.48
Heart rate	.39
Systolic blood pressure	.42
Diastolic blood pressure	.40
Skin response	.67
Hormonal changes	.15
Muscle tension	.87
Psychological self-report	.57

*An effect size of .20 is small, .50 is medium, and .80 is large. The effect sizes are all positive, indicating reduced reactivity and enhanced recovery over control groups.

Adapted from Crews, D. J., & Landers, D. M. (1987). A meta-analytic review of aerobic fitness and reactivity to psychosocial stressors. *Medicine and Science in Sports and Exercise, 19*(Suppl. 5), S114–S120.

More recently, Mark Hamer and his colleagues (Hamer, Taylor, & Steptoe, 2006) conducted a review of randomized controlled trials that examined the effects of acute aerobic exercise on blood pressure responses to psychosocial laboratory tasks. The stressor tasks used in the studies reviewed included the Stroop color-word task, mental arithmetic, public speech, and cold pressor. The cold pressor task typically requires a person to submerse his or her hand or forearm in ice cold water for as long as can be tolerated. Of the 15 studies reviewed, 10 had significant reductions in postexercise stress-related blood pressure responses compared with the control. The mean effect sizes for systolic and diastolic blood pressure of .38 and .40, respectively, were similar to the earlier findings by Crews and Landers (1987). Of importance, Hamer et al. found that the exercise dose moderated the size of the effect, with greater exercise doses showing larger effects. In other words, more exercise resulted in better responses to the stressor. The researchers concluded that an acute bout of aerobic exercise has a beneficial impact on the blood pressure response to a psychosocial stressor.

Real-Life Stress Research

Stressful life events can contribute to both physical and psychological illness. Do stressful life events also affect our physical activity levels? Yes! Stressful life events tend to negatively affect our physical activity levels. In a systematic review of the literature, Matthew Stults-Kolehmainen and Rajita Sinha (2014) found that most of the research they reviewed revealed a negative association between stress and exercise. In fact, almost 73% of the studies reviewed supported the hypotheses that higher stress is related to lower levels of exercise. In other words, stress tends to lead to less exercise.

Researchers from Finland examined which stressful life-events are related to exercise behavior (Engberg et al., 2012). They conducted a systematic review of the literature examining the effects of life events on changes in exercise behavior. More specifically, they examined how the following positive and negative major life-changing events affect physical activity: transition to university; change in employment status; marital transitions and changes in relationships; pregnancy/having a child; experiencing harassment at work, violence, or disaster; and moving into an institution. The researchers found that for both men and women, transition to university, having a child,

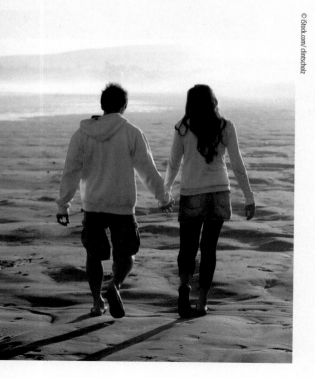

© iStock.com/ clintscholz

remarriage, and mass urban disaster resulted in decreased physical activity levels. In comparison, retirement resulted in increased physical activity levels.

They also found that in young women beginning work, changing work conditions, shifting from being single to cohabiting, getting married, becoming pregnant, experiencing a divorce/separation, and having a reduced income resulted in decreased exercise behavior. In contrast, starting a new personal relationship, returning to study, and harassment at work increased exercise behavior for young women.

In middle-aged women, changing work conditions, reduced income, personal achievement and death of a spouse/partner increased exercise, while experiencing violence and a family member being arrested or jailed decreased exercise. In older women, moving into an institution and interpersonal loss decreased exercise, while longer-term widowhood increased exercise. In addition, experiencing multiple simultaneous life events decreased exercise in both men and women. The researchers concluded that people experiencing life events could be an important target group for exercise promotion.

CRITICAL THINKING ACTIVITY 11-3

© ecco/Shutterstock, Inc.

What stressful life events have you experienced? How did this stress affect your exercise behavior?

Mechanisms of Effect

A potential reason for the positive effects of exercise on stress reactivity may be related to stress hormones. Heaney and colleagues (2014) examined the relationship between regular physical activity, life event–related stress, and the **cortisol** and **dehydroepiandrosterone (DHEA)** ratios in older adults. Cortisol and DHEA are **stress hormones**. Constant release of these stress hormones in response to continuous stressors can result in hormonal imbalances and adrenal dysfunction. The ultimate result of the release of these stress hormones over time is negative effects on overall health, such as sleep and mood disturbances and a suppressed immune system.

In their study, Heaney et al. (2014) had 36 older adults (aged 65 years or older) self-report on their physical activity and stress levels. Regarding stress levels, the older adults indicated if a particular event had happened to them in the past year (i.e., stress incidence) and how stressful they perceived the event to be (i.e., stress severity). Saliva samples were also obtained to determine the adults' salivary cortisol and DHEA secretion.

The researchers found that the older adults with higher stress severity for life events had higher cortisol:DHEA ratio. The observed association between stress severity and the cortisol:DHEA was driven by lower DHEA values in those reporting more severe stress, rather than higher levels of cortisol. Interestingly, the older adults' level of physical activity had an effect on their cortisol:DHEA levels. More specifically, older adults with higher stress incidence scores who did not participate in aerobic exercise had higher cortisol to DHEA ratios than those who regularly participated in aerobic exercise. This study suggests that life event stress may have a negative impact on the cortisol:DHEA ratio in older adults, and exercise may buffer against the effects of stress on the cortisol:DHEA ratio.

Stress Disorders and Exercise

When we are in danger, our natural response is to feel afraid. This fear triggers many split-second changes in the body as it prepares to defend against the danger or to avoid it. This fight-or-flight response is a healthy reaction meant to protect a person from harm. However, in **posttraumatic stress disorder (PTSD)** this reaction is either changed or damaged.

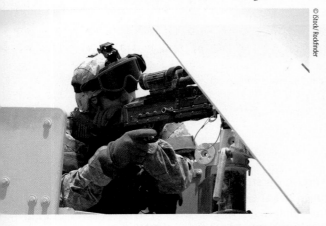
© iStock/Rockfinder

People who suffer from PTSD may feel stressed or frightened even when they are no longer in danger. PTSD is a traumatic stress disorder that develops after a distressing event, such as sexual assault, serious injury, or the threat of death. PTSD can also develop in those who have witnessed a harmful event that happened to loved ones or strangers. The disturbance, regardless of its trigger, causes clinically significant distress or impairment in the individual's social interactions, capacity to work, and other important areas of quality of life, such as sleep. See **TABLE 11-5** for a list of common PTSD symptoms.

TABLE 11-5   Symptoms of Posttraumatic Stress Disorder

Symptom Category	Specific Symptoms
Mood	Emotional distress, hopelessness, anger, fear, depression, inability to feel pleasure, guilt, and nervousness
Behavioral	Loss of interest in usual activities, self-harm, hypervigilance, irritability, aggression, agitation, self-destructive behavior (e.g., self-harm), and hostility
Psychological	Hallucination, severe anxiety, panic attack, mistrust, sleep disturbances, and flashbacks
Cognitive	Thoughts of suicide or unwanted thoughts
Social	Loneliness, social isolation, withdrawal from friends and family

People who suffer from PTSD tend to have lower rates of vigorous, moderate, and light physical activity compared to those who do not have PTSD (Rosenbaum et al., 2011; Zen, Whooley, Zhao, & Cohen, 2012). Pilot research has also revealed that aerobic exercise and moderate-intensity walking has positive effects on the severity of PTSD symptoms (Diaz & Motta, 2008; Newman & Motta, 2007). For example, Diaz and Motta (2008) conducted a nonrandomized study involving 12 female adolescents diagnosed with PTSD. Their results showed that 91% of adolescents had reductions in PTSD symptoms following participation in a walking program.

Using a prospective study design, Lisa Talbot and her colleagues (2014) examined the relationship between physical activity and sleep in 258 patients with PTSD. At baseline the participants rated their sleep quality. One year later they rated their sleep quality again and reported how physically active they were.

The researchers found that people suffering from PTSD had lower physical activity levels 1 year later. They also found that sleep quality mediated the relationship between baseline PTSD status and physical activity at the 1-year follow up, providing preliminary evidence that the association of reduced sleep quality with reduced physical activity could comprise a behavioral link to negative health outcomes such as obesity. In other words, sleep quality was more strongly associated with physical activity 1 year later than was having a diagnosis of PTSD.

Researchers from Australia examined the effects of a 12-week exercise program in addition to usual care for 81 patients with PTSD (Rosenbaum, Sherrington, & Tiedemann, 2015). The patients were randomized to receive either usual care or exercise in addition to usual care. The exercise intervention involved three, 30-minute resistance-training sessions a week and a walking program. The usual care consisted of psychotherapy, pharmaceutical interventions, and group therapy.

The researchers found that patients in the exercise in addition to usual care group had significantly reduced PTSD symptoms, compared with the usual care group. As well, the exercise in addition to usual care group showed significant improvements in depressive symptoms, waist circumference, sleep quality, and sedentary time compared to the usual care group. The researchers concluded that exercise may be a viable therapy to reduced PTSD symptoms.

■ Pain

Pain is frequently associated with physical activity, as evidenced by the common saying of "no pain, no gain." This exercise motto promises greater rewards for the price of a hard or even painful workout. This mentality, however, may serve as a deterrent for many people to not engage in exercise, because they may feel that exercise is always related to pain and discomfort. Luckily, researchers have found that exercise does not need to be painful to be beneficial, and exercise may even help us tolerate pain. Let's take a closer look at what pain is, the health significance of pain, and the relationship among exercise, sedentary behavior, and pain.

Pain is defined as "an unpleasant sensory and emotional experience associated with actual or potential tissue damage, or described in terms of such damage" (Merskey & Bogduk, 1994, p. 210). Implied in this definition of pain are three specific ideas. First, pain is always a subjective experience. One person who experiences a first-degree burn may report being in excruciating pain, whereas another person may report that it only hurts a little. Second, emotions are always an element of pain. For example, after a person is burned, he or she might have some emotional distress. Third, the perception of pain is not always related to the amount of tissue damage (O'Connor & Cook, 1999).

Pain is often divided into the following three general categories: acute, recurrent, and chronic. **Acute pain** is sharp, stinging pain that is usually localized in an injured area of the body. This type of pain is short-lived and usually related to tissue damage. Examples of acute pain include burns and factures. **Recurrent pain** involves episodes of discomfort interspersed with periods in which the person is relatively pain free for more than 3 months. Examples of recurrent pain include migraines and recurrent back pain. Finally, **chronic pain** is pain that lasts 6 month or longer. Chronic pain can be mild or excruciating, episodic or continuous, merely inconvenient, or totally incapacitating. The most common sources of chronic pain stem are headaches, joint pain, pain from injury, and backaches.

Millions of people suffer from either acute pain, recurrent pain, and/or chronic pain every year, and the effects of pain exact tremendous healthcare costs, as well as place an emotional and financial burden on patients and their families, friends, and coworkers. In fact, more than half of Americans live with chronic or recurrent pain (ABC News/USA Today/Stanford Medical Center Poll, 2005). Leading causes of recurrent or persistent pain affecting Americans are headache pain, back pain, and neck pain. About 40% of Americans say that pain interferes with their mood, activities, sleep, ability to do work, or enjoyment of life.

The costs of unrelieved pain can result in longer hospital stays, increased rates of rehospitalization, increased outpatient visits, and decreased ability to function fully. As such, a person's unrelieved chronic pain can often result in an inability to work and maintain health insurance. It is estimated that pain costs American society at least $560 to $635 billion annually, an amount equal to about $2,000 for everyone living in the United States (Institute of Medicine of the National Academies Report, 2011). Pain is also the most common reason for healthcare use, accounting for more than 50% of emergency room visits (Cordell et al., 2002), and pain is present in 30% of family practice visits (Hasselström, Liu-Palmgren, & Rasjö-Wrååk, 2002). As well, pain becomes more common as people approach death. A study of 4,703 patients found that 26% had pain in the last 2 years of life, increasing to 46% in the last month of life (Abu-Saad Huijer, 2010).

Not only is pain a costly and common problem, it causes functional and activity impairment in 3% to 13% of the population (Andersson, 1994). Functional impairments such as restricted mobility can significantly impact a person's daily activities. In addition, pain is associated with drug abuse and psychological disorders (Kouyanou, Pither, & Wessely, 1997). Furthermore, poor pain management can lengthen hospital stays and increase morbidity and mortality (Rauck, 1996).

In short, pain is common, disabling, and difficult to manage. The combination of these factors makes pain very costly to society.

The prevalence of pain also has a tremendous impact on business, with a recent report by the Institute of Medicine indicating that the annual value of lost productivity in 2010 dollars ranged between $297.4 and $335.5 billion. The value of lost productivity is based on the following three estimates: (1) days of work missed ($11.6 to $12.7 billion), (2) hours of work lost ($95.2 to $96.5 billion), and (3) lower wages ($190.6 to $226.3 billion) (Institute of Medicine of the National Academies Report, 2011).

An inability to effectively manage pain and the economic pressures to decrease its impact on healthcare costs have resulted in increased interest in non-surgical and nonpharmacological treatments for pain. One adjunct to traditional pain treatment is physical activity (O'Connor & Cook, 1999). Clinical practice guidelines that recommend physical activity as a modality for pain are based on research that can be categorized into two general categories: (1) investigations into the effects of regular exercise on endogenous (i.e., naturally occurring) pain and (2) research examining the effects of an acute bout of exercise on experimentally induced pain. Research in each of these areas, as well as the components of pain, are discussed below.

CRITICAL THINKING ACTIVITY 11-4

© ecco/Shutterstock, Inc.

Do you think the "no pain, no gain" slogan for exercise behavior is a motivator or rather a deterrent for sedentary behavior?

Components of Pain

Pain is a multidimensional construct that is composed of four components: nociception, perception of pain, emotion, and behavior . The first component, **nociception**, is the detection of tissue damage by sensory receptors known as *nociceptors*. A nociceptor is a sensory receptor that responds to potentially damaging stimuli by sending nerve signals to the spinal cord and brain. This process (i.e., nociception) usually causes the perception of pain. For example, when a person burns a finger on a hot plate, nociceptive signals of tissue damage travel quickly to the central nervous system. Common categories of nocioceptive pain include thermal (i.e., heat or cold), mechanical (i.e., crushing, tearing), and chemical (e.g., iodine in a cut, pepper spray in eyes).

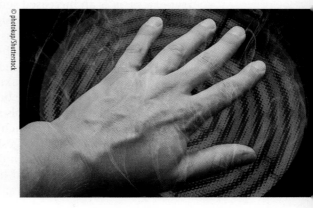

© photokup/Shutterstock

The second component is the perception of pain, and it can be experienced with or without actual tissue damage. An example of the latter event is phantom limb pain, which is pain from a part of the body that has been lost or from which the brain no longer receives signals. Phantom limb pain is a common experience of amputees, with the prevalence of phantom pain in upper limb amputees being nearly 82% (Kooijman, Dijkstra, Geertzen, Elzinga, & van der Schans, 2000). It is also possible for nocioception to occur without the perception of pain. For instance, **myocardial ischemia**, a disorder that causes reduced blood flow to the heart, occurs without pain in 4 to 5 million people in the United States each year.

The third component of pain is emotion. According to Price and Harkins (1992), pain-related emotion consists of two stages. The first stage is characterized by unpleasantness, distress, or annoyance. The level of the emotion in this stage corresponds to the intensity of the pain stimulus and amount of arousal. The second stage is characterized by an emotional reaction to the cognitive appraisal of

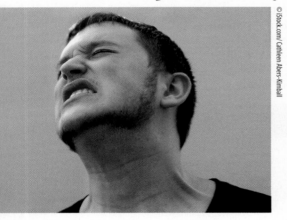

© iStock.com/Cathleen Abers-Kimball

how the pain influences one's life and activities of daily living. Cognitive appraisal is dependent on the context of pain, which includes such issues as the perceived origin of the pain and the perceived ability to control the pain.

Behavior, the fourth component of pain, refers to activities that are either performed or avoided as a result of the perception of pain. Healthcare-seeking, medication consumption, moaning, crying, complaining, pain-related body postures, facial expressions, and activity avoidance are all pain behaviors. These behaviors communicate the perception of pain to others (Keefe & Williams, 1992).

Pain, Exercise, and Sedentary Behavior

Hyperalgesia is an increased sensitivity to pain that may be caused by damage to nociceptors. In contrast, **hypoalgesia** occurs when nociceptive (painful) stimuli are either interrupted or decreased somewhere along the path between the input (nociceptors) and the places where they are processed and recognized as pain in our conscious mind. Hypoalgesic effects can be mild, such as massaging a stubbed toe to make it hurt less or taking aspirin to decrease a headache. Hypoalgesic effects can also be severe, like being under strong anesthesia. Hypoalgesia can be caused by exogenous chemicals such as opioids, as well as by chemicals produced by the body in phenomena such as exercise-induced hypoalgesia.

Exercise-induced hypoalgesia is the phenomena whereby during and following exercise people have a diminished sensitivity to pain (Kolytn, 2002). In other words, exercise-induced hypoalgesia is characterized by elevations in pain thresholds and pain tolerances, as well as reductions in pain ratings during and following both aerobic and resistance exercise (Umeda, Newcomb, Ellingson, & Kolytn, 2010; Umeda, Newcomb, & Koltyn, 2009). Many studies have shown the direct link between exercise and decreased pain perception by having participants exercise and then having them rate their pain responses.

However, despite a great deal of research, the mechanism of action responsible for the exercise-induced hypoalgesia is poorly understood. It has been shown that the triggering mechanism for the hypoalgesic effects is the increase in blood pressure that accompanies a good workout. We will now examine the research that has examined the effects of exercise and sedentary behavior for both endogenous (i.e., naturally occurring) and experimentally induced pain.

Effects of Exercise and Sedentary Behavior on Endogenous Pain

Endogenous pain is naturally occurring pain. Researchers examining endogenous pain typically access either patients or population-based samples. This type of survey research assesses large numbers of individuals for their pain, including those who may not be under the supervision of a healthcare professional. However, such survey research is limited by the inability to control the amount of nociception. Anecdotes from athletes who continue strenuous exercise in the face of severe injuries and later report that they felt no pain have contributed to the notion that physical activity can alter people's pain perception (Koltyn, 2000).

Much of the research on regular physical activity and naturally occurring pain has concentrated on musculoskeletal pain (Fuentes, Armijo-Olivo, Magee, & Gross, 2011). Musculoskeletal pain is pain that affects the muscles, ligaments, and tendons, as well as the bones. Research has revealed that aerobic and strengthening exercises may have beneficial effects on reducing musculoskeletal pain associated with osteoarthritis, rheumatoid arthritis (Minor & Brown, 1993), low back problems (Lahad, Malter, Berg, & Deyo, 1994), fibromyalgia (Newcomb, Koltyn, Morgan, & Cook, 2011), **peripheral artery disease** (Gardner & Poehlman, 1995), neck pain (Andersen et al., 2010), menstruation pain (Hightower; 1997), and labor pain (Artal, 1992). The mechanisms for why exercise may be helpful in reducing endogenous pain remain unknown (O'Connor & Cook, 1999).

Fibromyalgia is a chronic musculoskeletal disorder that is characterized by widespread pain with distinct tender points that are often referred to as *trigger points* (Wolfe et al., 1990). The defining symptoms of fibromyalgia are chronic and widespread pain, fatigue, and heightened pain in response to tactile pressure. Other symptoms may include sleep disturbance, weakness in the limbs, and joint stiffness. This disorder is often accompanied by fatigue, memory problems, and depression. Fibromyalgia is estimated to affect 2% to 4% of the American population, with a female-to-male incidence ratio of about 9 to 1 (Buskila & Cohen, 2007).

The pathophysiology of this disorder is poorly understood, and its cause remains unknown. Thus, some medical experts challenge its very existence. To diagnose fibromyalgia, healthcare professionals often check for tender points or

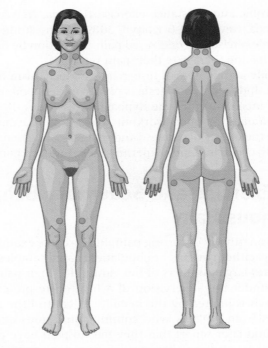

 FIGURE 11-1   Tender Points

trigger points on the body. These trigger points tend to be painful when pressed and may spread pain to other parts of the body (see **FIGURE 11-1**). There is no cure for fibromyalgia, and treatment usually requires a multidisciplinary perspective using both pharmacological and nonpharmacological approaches. The treatments for fibromyalgia are often symptom based and generally unsatisfactory. Preliminary research, however, is revealing that exercise may be a viable treatment for fibromyalgia (Clauw, 2014).

But just how physically active are people who suffer with fibromyalgia? A cross-sectional study by Jonatan Ruiz and his colleagues (2013) examined levels of objectively measured sedentary time and physical activity in women with fibromyalgia. They found that over 60% of the women met the physical activity guidelines, which were defined as 30 minutes per day of moderate to vigorous physical activity on 5 or more days of the week. They also found that these women spent about 71% (about 10 hours a day) of their waking time in sedentary activities (see **FIGURE 11-2**). In other words, although most women met the physical activity guidelines, they spent the majority of their waking hours being sedentary.

Lauren Newcomb and her colleagues (2011) examined the influence of a preferred-versus a prescribed-intensity exercise session on pain in 21 women

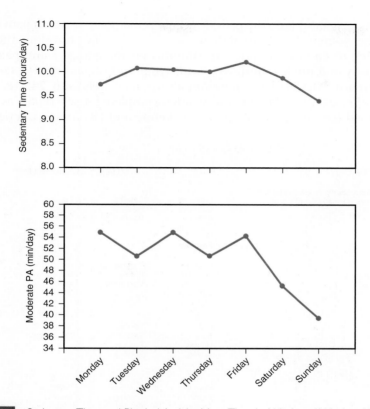

FIGURE 11-2   Sedentary Time and Physical Activity Mean Time by Week and Weekend Days

Reproduced from BMJ Open, Ruiz, J. R., Segura-Jimenez, V., Ortega, F. B., Alvarez-Gallardo, I. C., Camiletti-Moiron, D., et al. (2013). With permission from BMJ Publishing Group Ltd.

(mean age = 44 years) with fibromyalgia. In their study, the women with fibromyalgia completed two randomly assigned exercise sessions on separate days consisting of 20 minutes of cycle ergometry at a self-selected intensity level or a prescribed moderate-intensity level.

Multiple aspects of pain were assessed. First, muscle pain was assessed every 5 minutes during exercise using a muscle pain intensity scale, whereby participants verbally rated the intensity of pain, with 1 being no pain and 10 being extremely intense pain (almost unbearable). Second, experimental pain perception was assessed before and after each exercise session using a pressure stimulator. Force was applied to the right forefinger for a maximum of 2 minutes. This force creates a painful sensation but does not cause short- or long-term tissue damage. The women then reported their **pain thresholds**, which is the elapsed time from the initial application of the pressure stimulus until the participant perceives the stimulus to be painful (i.e., the pain threshold is the point at which pain begins to be felt). The women also reported their **pain tolerance** (i.e., how long the women were willing to endure the pressure stimulus on their finger) and pain ratings (i.e., intensity and unpleasantness). Third, symptoms of pain were assessed with the Short-Form McGill Pain Questionnaire immediately and 24, 48, 72, and 96 hours after exercise. Finally, the women completed a self-report assessment of their mood (i.e., Profile of Mood States) before and 15 minutes after exercise.

McGill Pain Questionnaire

Part 1 **Where Is Your Pain?**

Please mark on the drawing below the areas where you feel pain.Put E if external, or I if internal near the areas you mark. Put EI if both external and internal.

Part 2 **What Does Your Pain Feel Like?**

1 Flickering Quivering Pulsing Throbbing Beating Pounding	2 Jumping Flashing Shooting	3 Pricking Boring Drilling Stabbing Lancinating	4 Sharp Cutting Lacerating
5 Pinching Pressing Gnawing Camping Crushing	6 Tugging Pulling Wrenching	7 Hot Burning Scalding Searing	8 Tingling Itchy Smarting Stinging
9 Dull Sore Hurting Aching Heavy	10 Tender Taut Rasping Splitting	11 Tiring Exhausting	12 Sickening Suffocating
13 Fearful Frightful Terrifying	14 Punishing Grueling Cruel Vicious Killing	15 Wretched Blinding	16 Annoying Troublesome Miserable Intense Unbearable
17 Spreading Radiating Penetrating Piercing	18 Tight Numb Drawing Squeezing Tearing	19 Cool Cold Freezing	20 Nagging Nauseating Agonizing Dreadful Torturing

Part 3 **How Does Your Pain Change With Time?**

1. Which word or words would you use to describe the <u>pattern</u> of your pain?

1	2	3
Continuous Steady Constant	Rhythmic Periodic Intermittent	Brief Momentary Transient

2. What kind of things <u>relieve</u> your pain?

3. What kind of things <u>increase</u> your pain?

Part 4 **How Strong Is Your Pain?**

People agree that the following 5 words represent pain of increasing intensity. They are:

1	2	3	4	5
Mild	Discomforting	Distressing	Horrible	Excruciating

To answer each question below, write the number of the most appropriate word in the space beside the question.

1. Which word describes your pain right now? ____
2. Which word describes it at its worst? ____
3. Which word describes it when it is least? ____
4. Which word describes the worst toothache you ever had? ____
5. Which word describes the worst headache you ever had? ____
6. Which word describes the worst stomachache you ever had? ____

The researchers found that the women preferred a lower intensity of exercise than what was prescribed. Muscle pain in the legs, however, was similar in the two conditions, and it was significantly increased during exercise. Pain thresholds increased significantly after exercise, with larger effects being evidenced after the preferred exercise. This meant that the effect for the preferred intensity was large compared to small for the prescribed intensity. Also, pain tolerances increased significantly after exercise, indicating that the women were able to endure the noxious stimulation for a longer duration. The peak pain ratings of pain intensity and pain unpleasantness decreased after exercise. Furthermore, self-reported pain in the follow-up period was found to be lower than baseline. Finally, the women reported significant improvements in levels of depression, anger, fatigue, confusion, and overall mood following exercise. The authors concluded that women with fibromyalgia who participated in this study experienced significant improvements in pain after exercise. The researchers concluded that recommendations for exercise prescription for individuals with fibromyalia should consider the preferred-intensity exercise model as a strategy to reduce pain.

Reviews of the literature have revealed that many types of physical activity (e.g., resistance training, yoga, lifestyle physical activity) are effective treatments for adults with fibromyalgia (Busch et al., 2013; Nelson, 2015). Exercise results in reductions of pain and depression and improvement in total health and physical function. A gradual intensity progression for deconditioned individuals with fibromyalgia toward moderate intensity is recommended (Busch et al., 2011).

Effects of Exercise on Experimentally Induced Pain

In contrast to endogenous pain, experimentally induced pain provides an opportunity to control the amount of nociception. Pain stimuli can be used to induce nociception, and such stimuli can be applied to either healthy participants or pain patients. These stimuli can also be applied in either laboratory or clinical settings.

How is pain experimentally induced? Common experimental pain stimuli include pressure pain, electrical pain, thermal pain, ischemic pain, and cold-pressor pain (see **TABLE 11-6**). Typically, the noxious stimulus is applied before and following exercise to see if relief occurs following physical activity (Koltyn, 2000). Reviews of the research on the effects of a single episode of exercise on pain have concluded that exercise can be an analgesic depending on the types of experimentally induced pain and characteristics of the exercise bout (Koltyn, 2000; O'Connor & Cook, 1999).

Kelli Koltyn and her colleagues (Koltyn, Garvin, Gariner, & Nelson, 1996) examined pain threshold following exercise and quiet rest in 16 adults (mean age = 29 years). As discussed earlier, pain thresholds are measured by gradually increasing the intensity of a stimulus such as an electric current or heat applied to the body. The pain perception threshold is the point at which the stimulus begins

TABLE 11-6	Common Experimental Pain Stimuli
Type of Pain	**Example**
Pressure pain	A weighted edge applied to a finger or a football cleat applied against the tibia
Electrical pain	Electric current sent to electrodes attached to the skin or dental pulp
Thermal pain	Cutaneous application of heat to the forearm
Ischemic pain	Use of a blood pressure cuff to restrict blood flow to the hands
Cold-pressor pain	Immersion of a hand in a container of cold water

to hurt, and the pain tolerance threshold is reached when the subject acts to stop the pain.

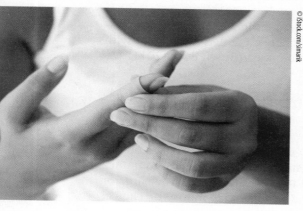

© iStock.com/simarik

In their study, participants were assigned to an exercise condition or a no-exercise control group. The exercise session was 30 minutes of cycle ergometer exercise at 75% of VO$_2$ max. The control condition consisted of resting quietly for 30 minutes. Pressure was applied to each participant's finger for 2 minutes before, immediately following, and 15 minutes after the exercise and control conditions. Pain threshold and pain ratings were assessed during the 2-minute pain exposure. Pain threshold was defined as the elapsed time from the initial application of the pain stimulus until the subject perceived the stimulus to be painful. Pain ratings were provided by the participants every 15 seconds during the 2-minute pain exposure.

The researchers found that pain threshold was significantly elevated immediately and 15 minutes following exercise. In contrast, pain threshold did not change following the quiet rest condition (see **FIGURE 11-3**). Also, pain ratings were significantly lower following exercise in comparison to the control condition. The researchers concluded that an acute bout of exercise results in increased pain threshold and significantly lower pain ratings. The mechanisms responsible for exercise-induced analgesia, however, are not fully understood (Koltyn, 2000).

In a more recent study, Umeda and colleagues (2010) examined exercise-induced hypoalgesia in 50 young healthy men and women to determine whether different magnitudes of blood pressure elevations induced by isometric exercise influenced pain perception. Isometric exercise is a type of strength training in which the joint angle and muscle length do not change during contraction. The adults performed four laboratory sessions consisting of a baseline session and three

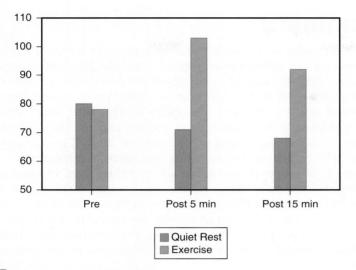

| **FIGURE 11-3** | Experimental Pain and Exercise |

Note: Values on *y*-axis on pain threshold in seconds. Mean scores for pain threshold responses in the exercise and quiet rest condition.

Koltyn, K. F., Garvin, A. W., Gardiner, G. R., & Nelson, T. F. (1996). Perception of pain following aerobic exercise. *Medicine and Science in Sports and Exercise, 28*, 1418–1421.

isometric exercise sessions of varying duration (i.e., 1, 3, and 5 minutes) while blood pressure and pain perception were assessed. Pain perception was assessed before and after isometric exercise using a pressure pain stimulator applied to the forefinger of the dominant hand for a maximum of 2 minutes. During the pain pressure task, the participants' pain threshold, pain intensity, and pain unpleasantness were assessed.

The researchers found that blood pressure was significantly elevated while pain intensity and pain unpleasantness were lower immediately following isometric exercise. As well, pain thresholds were found to be elevated following exercise. Of importance, the results did not follow a dose–response relationship. The researchers concluded that isometric exercise produced exercise-induced hypoalgesia in healthy men and women, but that there was not a dose–response relationship between blood pressure and exercise-induced hypoalgesia.

CRITICAL THINKING ACTIVITY 11-5

What are some possible mechanisms for why exercise results in an analgesic effect?

■ Summary

Feelings of stress arise when we perceive an imbalance between the demands of the situation and our ability to meet those demands. The body responds with a flight-or-fight response caused by changes in the autonomic nervous system that result in increased heart rate, blood pressure, and so on. The good news, however, is that physical activity enhances our ability to deal with stress. With repeated exposures to physical activity, our overall reaction improves in terms of elevations in heart rate, blood pressure, and muscle tension, as well as changes in various skin conductivity responses (i.e., sweating, temperature increases).

Everyone experiences pain at some point in their lives. Physical activity can help to alleviate that pain. Research has shown that involvement in physical activity can have beneficial effects on both experimentally induced and endogenous pain, such as the pain associated with osteoarthritis, rheumatoid arthritis, low back problems, peripheral artery disease, menstruation, and childbirth. Further research is needed to determine the mechanisms of this exercise-induced analgesic effect.

KEY TERMS

acute pain
chronic pain
cortisol
dehydroepiandrosterone (DHEA)
distress
eustress
fibromyalgia
fight-or-flight response
hyperalgesia
hypoalgesia
myocardial ischemia

nocioception
pain
pain threshold
pain tolerance
peripheral artery disease
posttraumatic stress disorder (PTSD)
recurrent pain
stress
stress hormones
stressor

REVIEW QUESTIONS

1. What is fibromyalgia? Is exercise an effective treatment for this disease? Justify your answer with research support.

2. Define *posttraumatic stress disorder* (PTSD). Can physical activity be used as an effective treatment for PTSD? Explain why or why not.

3. Describe what is meant by exercise-induced hypoalgesia.

4. What is the difference between endogenous versus experimentally

induced pain? Provide examples of each category of pain.

5. What is the relationship between acute stress and exercise?

APPLYING THE CONCEPTS

1. How might participating in regular yoga sessions and meeting her colleagues for after-work gym sessions have enabled Carla to better handle the stress of her job?

2. What non-work-related events would make Carla less likely to take advantage of her company's new gym membership?

REFERENCES

ABC News/USA Today/Stanford Medical Center Poll. (2005). Poll: Americans searching for pain relief. New poll shows nearly 4 in 10 American adults suffer from pain on a regular basis. Retrieved December 14, 2011, from http://abcnews.go.com/images/Politics/979a1TheFightAgainstPain.pdf

Abu-Saad Huijer, H. (2010). Chronic pain: A review. *The Lebanese Medical Journal, 58*, 21–27.

Andersen, L. L., Christensen, K. B., Holtermann, A., Poulsen, O. M., Sjøgaard, G., Pedersen, M. T., & Hansen, E. A. (2010). Effect of physical exercise interventions on musculoskeletal pain in all body regions among office workers: A one-year randomized controlled trial. *Manual Therapy, 15*, 100–104.

Andersson, H. I. (1994). The epidemiology of chronic pain in a Swedish rural sample. *Quality of Life Research, 3*, S19–S26.

Artal, R. (1992). Exercise and pregnancy. *Clinics in Sports Medicine, 11*, 363–377.

Busch, A. J., Webber, S. C., Brachaniec, M., Bidonde, J., Dal Bello-Haas, V., Danyliw, A. D., . . . Schachter, C. L. (2011). Exercise therapy for fibromyalgia. *Current Pain and Headache Reports, 15*, 358–367.

Busch, A. J., Webber, S. C., Richards, R. S., Bidonde, J., Schachter, C. L., Schafer, L. A., . . . Overend, T. J. (2013). Resistance exercise training for fibromyalgia. *Cochrane Database of Systematic Reviews*. doi:10.1002/14651858.CD010884

Buskila, D., & Cohen, H. (2007). Comorbidity of fibromyalgia and psychiatric disorders. *Current Pain and Headache Reports, 11*, 333–338.

Clauw, D. J. (2014). Fibromyalgia: A clinical review. *JAMA, 311*, 1547–1555.

Cordell, W. H., Keene, K. K., Giles, B. K., Jones, J. B., Jones, J. H., & Brizendine, E. J. (2002). The high prevalence of pain in emergency medical care. *American Journal of Emergency Medicine, 20*, 165–169.

Crews, D. J., & Landers, D. M. (1987). A meta-analytic review of aerobic fitness and reactivity to psychosocial stressors. *Medicine and Science in Sports and Exercise, 19* (Suppl. 5), S114–S120.

Diaz, A. B., & Motta, R. (2008). The effects of an aerobic exercise program on posttraumatic stress disorder symptom severity in adolescents. *International Journal of Emergency Mental Health, 10*, 49–59.

Engberg, E., Alen, M., Kukkonen-Harjula, K., Peltonen, J. E., Tikkanen, H. O., & Pekkarinen, H. (2012). Life events and change in leisure time physical activity: A systematic review. *Sports Medicine, 42*, 433–447.

Fuentes, C. J. P., Armijo-Olivo, S., Magee, D. J., & Gross, D. P. (2011). Effects of exercise therapy on endogenous pain-relieving peptides in musculoskeletal pain: A systematic review. *The Clinical Journal of Pain, 27*, 365–374.

Gardner, A. W., & Poehlman, E. T. (1995). Exercise rehabilitation programs for the treatment of claudication pain: A meta-analysis. *JAMA, 274*, 975–980.

Hamer, M., Taylor, A., & Steptoe, A. (2006). The effect of acute aerobic exercise on stress-related blood pressure responses: A systematic review and meta-analysis. *Biological Psychology, 71*, 183–190.

Hasselström, J., Liu-Palmgren, J., & Rasjö-Wrååk, G. (2002). Prevalence of pain in general practice. *European Journal of Pain, 6*, 375–385.

Heaney, J. L. J., Carroll, D., & Phillips, A. C. (2014). Physical activity, life events stress, cortisol, and DHEA in older adults: Preliminary findings that physical activity may buffer against the negative effects of stress. *Journal of Aging and Physical Activity, 22*, 465–473.

Hightower, M. (1997). Effects of exercise participation on menstrual pain and symptoms. *Women and Health, 26*, 15–27.

Institute of Medicine of the National Academies Report. (2011). *Relieving pain in America: A blueprint for transforming prevention, care, education, and research.* Washington, DC: The National Academies Press.

Kabat-Zinn, J. (1996). *Full catastrophe living—how to cope with stress, pain, and illness using mindfulness meditation.* Piatkus Books.

Keefe, F. J., & Williams, D. A. (Eds.). (1992). *Assessment of pain behaviors.* New York, NY: Guilford Press.

Koltyn, K. F. (2000). Analgesia following exercise: A review. *Sports Medicine and Physical Fitness, 29*, 85–98.

Koltyn, K. F. (2002). Exercise-induced hypoalgesia and intensity of exercise. *Sports Medicine, 32*, 477–487.

Koltyn, K. F., Garvin, A. W., Gardiner, G. R., & Nelson, T. F. (1996). Perception of pain following aerobic exercise. *Medicine and Science in Sports and Exercise, 28*, 1418–1421.

Kooijman, C. M., Dijkstra, P. U., Geertzen, J. H., Elzinga, A., & van der Schans, C. P. (2000). Phantom pain and phantom sensations in upper limb amputees: An epidemiological study. *Pain, 87*, 33–41.

Lahad, A., Malter, A. D., Berg, A. O., & Deoy, R. A. (1994). The effectiveness of four interventions for the prevention of low back pain. *JAMA, 272*, 1286–1291.

Landers, D. M., & Petruzzello, S. J. (1994). The effectiveness of exercise and physical activity in reducing anxiety and reactivity to psychosocial stressors. In H. A., Quinney, L. Gauvin, & A. E. Wall (Eds.). *Toward active living* (pp. 77–82). Champaign, IL: Human Kinetics.

Loeser, J. D., & Melzack, R. (1999). Pain: An overview. *Lancet, 353*, 1607–1609.

Merskey H., & Bogduk N. (1994). *Classification of chronic pain.* Seattle: IASP Press.

Minor, M. A., & Brown, J. D. (1993). Exercise maintenance of persons with arthritis after participation in a class experience. *Health Education Quarterly, 20*, 83–95.

Nelson, N. L. (2015). Muscle strengthening activities and fibromyalgia: A review of pain and strength outcomes. *Journal of Bodywork and Movement Therapy, 19*, 370–376.

Newcomb, L. W., Koltyn, K. F., Morgan, W. P., & Cook, D. B. (2011). Influence of preferred versus prescribed exercise on pain in fibromyalgia. *Medicine and Science in Sports and Exercise, 43*, 1106–1113.

Newman, C. L., & Motta, R. W. (2007). The effects of aerobic exercise on childhood PTSD, anxiety, and depression. *International Journal of Emergency Mental Health, 9*, 133–158.

O'Connor, P. J., & Cook, D. B. (1999). Exercise and pain: The neurobiology, measurement, and laboratory study of pain in relation to exercise in humans. *Exercise and Sports Sciences Reviews, 27*, 119–166.

Price, D. D., & Harkins, S. W. (Eds.). (1992). *Psychophysical approaches to pain measurement and assessment.* New York, NY: Guilford Press.

Rauck, R. L. (1996). Cost-effectiveness and cost/benefit ratio of acute pain management. *Regional Anesthesia, 21*, 139–143.

Rosenbaum, S., Nguyen, D., Lenehan, T., Tiedemann, A., van der Ploeg, H., & Sherrington, C. (2011). Exercise augmentation compared to usual care for posttraumatic stress disorder: A randomized controlled trial (The REAP study: Randomised exercise augmentation for PTSD). *BMC Psychiatry.* doi:10.1186/1471-244X-11-115

Rosenbaum, S., Sherrington, C., & Tiedemann, A. (2015). Exercise augmentation compared with usual care for posttraumatic stress disorder: A randomized controlled trial. *Acta Psychiatrica Scandinavia, 131*, 350–359.

Ruiz, J. R., Segura-Jimenez, V., Ortega, F. B., Alvarez-Gallardo, I. C., Camiletti-Moiron, D., Femia, P., . . . Delgado-Fernandez, M. (2013). Objectively measured sedentary time and physical activity in women with fibromyalgia: A cross-sectional study. *BMJ Open, 3*, pii: e002722. doi: 10.1136/bmjopen-2013-002722

Selye, H. (1956). *The stress of life.* New York, NY: McGraw-Hill.

Selye, H. (1975). Confusion and controversy in the stress field. *Journal of Human Stress, 1*, 37–44.

Stults-Kolehmainen, M. A., & Sinha, R. (2014). The effects of stress on physical activity and exercise. *Sports Medicine, 44*, 81–121.

Talbot, L. S., Neylan, T. C., Metzler, T. J., & Cohen, B. E. (2014). The mediating effect of sleep quality on the relationship between PTSD and physical activity. *Journal of Clinical Sleep Medicine, 10*, 795–801.

Umeda, M., Newcomb, L. W., Ellingson, L. D., & Koltyn, K. F. (2010). Examination of the dose–response relationship between pain perception and blood pressure elevations induced by isometric exercise in men and women. *Biological Psychology, 85*, 90–96.

Umeda, M., Newcomb, L. W., & Koltyn, K. F. (2009). Influence of blood pressure elevations by isometric exercise on pain perception in women. *International Journal of Psychophysiology, 74*, 45–52.

Wolfe, F., Smythe, H. A., Yunus, M. B., Bennett, R. M., Bombardier, C., Goldenberg, D. L., . . . Clark, P. (1990). The American College of Rheumatology 1990 criteria for the classification of fibromyalgia. Report of the multicenter criteria committee. *Arthritis and Rheumatism, 33*, 160–172.

Zen, A. L., Whooley, M. A., Zhao, S., & Cohen, B. E. (2012). Posttraumatic stress disorder is associated with poor health behaviors: Findings from the heart and soul study. *Health Psychology, 31*, 194–201.

Vignette: Omar

I'm not sure when, exactly, I became such a terrible sleeper. It might have been when my family moved from a small town in Connecticut when I was 10 to Chicago, where my mother had been relocated for business and my father was able to start a new job. We downsized our living arrangements, so I ended up splitting a bedroom with my younger brother, who was a snorer. I would frequently wake up and shake the top of the bunk bed we shared in an effort to wake him so he'd be quieter.

I started to worry I had insomnia after I began technical college in Wisconsin. I worked at a restaurant during some evenings and weekend mornings to help pay for the apartment I rented with a fellow student roommate. And on days I was on my feet a lot, running back and forth between the kitchen and tables, I'd have an easier time falling asleep. But when I spent most of my day sitting in the library, in class, or watching sports on TV during the weekend, I found myself wide awake at odd hours of the night.

My doctor at the time offered to write me a prescription for sleeping pills. He said sleeplessness could be more common among folks like myself who didn't get a lot of sunlight and kept odd hours, due to my work and school schedule. I was hesitant to take them, though, having heard horror stories of friends of friends sleepwalking on Ambien. So the bottle of pills pretty much remained tucked inside a bathroom cabinet.

LEARNING OBJECTIVES

After completing this chapter, you will be able to

- Understand the relationship between being physically active and sleeping behavior.
- Define the stages of sleep.
- Describe the health effects of sleep deprivation.
- Understand the relationship between exercise and various sleep disorders.
- Describe the potential mechanisms for why exercise results in improved sleep.

285

One night at work, just before I was about to end my shift and head back to my apartment, I slipped on the staircase leading to the downstairs employee locker room. I landed hard on my tailbone and wrenched my spine, resulting in what I'd find out weeks later was a severely herniated disc.

The pain just kept getting worse in the days after my fall. I iced my back and took over-the-counter painkillers, but to no avail. Needless to say, my sleep schedule got even more interrupted, as it was barely possible to find a position to lie in that wasn't excruciating for my spine.

I was angry and frustrated at having to take time off work after I literally could no longer hold up a tray without wincing. I knew something was seriously wrong, and I was terrified that I'd have to get surgery—as a couple of different doctors I consulted with suggested. With the worker's compensation I received for the fall—turns out my employer had a series of violations that resulted in them swiftly footing my medical bills—I enrolled in physical therapy. It took almost 6 months before I was able to resume my normal life without wincing in agony with every move.

I put on a fair bit of weight during this time. And once I was okayed by the physical therapist to start an exercise program, I desperately sought her advice. The woman who treated me strongly suggested I take up swimming. So, in part to shed some pounds, but also to help keep my back in good shape to keep my recovery going, I started doing laps a few times a week at a local YMCA.

I felt rather ridiculous stepping into a pool in my swimming trunks, what with the gut I'd grown during my time off from work. But I tried to swallow my pride and self-consciousness, dive in, and see what I could make happen.

The relief of feeling weightless in the water was helpful in keeping me motivated to come back. I was breathless within seconds of starting a forward crawl. And for the first few weeks I started swimming I could only last in the pool about 15 minutes max. Boy, was I also sore. From head to toe the days after I got out of the pool I was made aware of muscles in my body I didn't even know were there simply by their achiness following exertion.

But a surprisingly pleasant thing happened beginning no later than the first night after I tried my arms and legs at swimming. I came home, had dinner, and passed out on the couch. I woke up about 5 hours later, groggy and slightly disoriented. I picked myself up and crawled back into bed for another 2 or so hours of sleep, and then woke up feeling—though incredibly sore—surprisingly refreshed.

It took me a while to get in shape. But the longer I was able to swim, the better I became at going to bed. It was almost like I didn't have a choice. My body would just be ready for bed after dinnertime and I'd have to give in. In a few months' time, I'd nearly forgotten I'd ever struggled to fall and remain asleep. My roommate even asked me if I was finally taking those sleeping pills I'd told him about. I was so proud to say that I didn't even have to.

By the time I got my associate's degree in accounting I'd been swimming regularly for almost a year. I'd mastered that crawl like you wouldn't believe! Then I got offered a job as a payroll clerk at a small accounting firm in Milwaukee after a month or so of searching, which got in the way of my workout schedule.

I had to cut back on the number of days a week I went swimming. I moved to an apartment that wasn't close to any fitness centers with pools. And as I've gotten accustomed to my new work hours, I've found little time to get to and from the nearest YMCA. Not surprisingly, my sleep started getting lighter again, and I found myself desperately considering taking those pills.

I've since been searching for alternative exercise programs, like treadmill walks or investing in some fitness equipment for my home. But I'm not well versed in how to go about all this. And whatever I've tried hasn't compared to the freedom I feel when propelling myself through water.

I make a point to get to the pool on weekends and I force myself to wake up early at least once during the work week to swim. I'm hoping within the next year to find a more convenient place to live—one that puts me nearer to a pool than to work. I'm not sure I realized how crucial swimming was to my health, happiness, and ability to get a good night's rest until I couldn't do it as often as I wanted.

■ Introduction

Mark Twain is an American icon who wrote with insight and humor. Not surprisingly then, he has often been quoted for his perspectives on a variety of topics. One of the topics on which he advanced an opinion was exercise: "I have never taken any exercise except sleeping and resting and I never intend to take any" (Twain, 1905). As this quote indicates, Mark Twain was not a strong proponent of being physically active. Ironically, if he were alive today and consulted with healthcare professionals, he likely would be advised to exercise more frequently to improve his sleep! As Shawn Youngstedt, Patrick O'Connor, and Rod Dishman (1997) stated, "few behaviors are as closely linked with enhanced sleep as exercise" (p. 203). In this chapter, the suspected link between physical activity and sleep is explored. Before we examine this growing body of research, let's first determine what sleep is and why it is so important to our health.

■ What Is Sleep?

Sleep is a naturally recurring state of rest for the mind and body in which the eyes usually close and consciousness is either completely or partially lost. When we

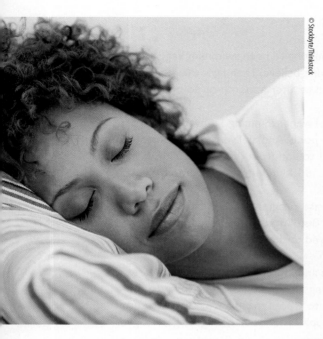

© Stockbyte/Thinkstock

sleep there is a decrease in bodily movement and responsiveness to the things around us (American Heritage Medical Dictionary, 2007). Sleep affects how we look, feel, and perform on a daily basis, and it can have a major impact on our overall quality of life. Sleep helps us thrive by contributing to a healthy immune system, and it can balance our appetites by helping regulate levels of hormones that play a role in our feelings of hunger and fullness. So when we are sleep deprived, we may feel the need to eat more, which can lead to weight gain. So the third of our lives that we spend sleeping is far from unproductive. Let's take a closer look at what happens to us when we sleep.

When we sleep we follow a pattern of alternating between REM (rapid eye movement) and NREM (nonrapid eye movement) sleep in a cycle that repeats itself about every 90 minutes. We spend about 75% of our sleep time in NREM sleep. As we begin to fall asleep, we enter NREM sleep, which is composed of four stages (see **TABLE 12-1** for a description of each stage). Stage 1 is the period of transition between wakefulness and the onset of sleep, and it occupies about 5% (1 to 7 minutes) of our night's sleep. Stage 2 signals the onset of sleep where we become disengaged from our surroundings and our body temperature drops. We are in Stage 2 of NREM approximately 45% of the time. Stages 3 and 4 of NREM are the deepest and most restorative sleep and represent about 25% of our sleep time. REM sleep, as the name suggests, is characterized by rapid eye movements. REM represents 25% of our nightly sleep.

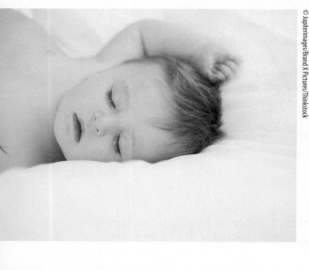

© Jupiterimages/Brand X Pictures/Thinkstock

■ How Much Sleep Do We Need?

The first thing sleep experts will tell you is that there is no "magic number" for how much sleep we need each night. The reason there is no magic number is complex, but it can be partly explained by the following three reasons. First, different age groups need different amounts of sleep. Although researchers cannot pinpoint an exact amount of sleep

TABLE 12-1 Stages of Sleep

Stage	Percent of Total Sleep Time	Characteristics
NREM	75%	
Stage 1	5%	Being awake and falling asleep Light sleep
Stage 2	45%	Onset of sleep Becoming disengaged from surroundings Breathing and heart rate are regular Body temperature drops
Stages 3 and 4	25%	Deepest and most restorative sleep Blood pressure drops Breathing becomes slower Muscles relax Blood supply to muscle increases Tissue growth and repair occurs Energy is restored Hormones are released (e.g., growth hormone)
REM	25%	Provides energy to brain and body Supports daytime performance Brain is active and dreams occur Eyes dart back and forth

Data from the National Sleep Foundation website. Retrieved September 12, 2015, from http://sleepfoundation.org/how-sleep-works/what-happens-when-you-sleep.

TABLE 12-2 Rule of Thumb for Amount of Sleep Needed at Night by Age

Age Group	Nightly Hours of Sleep
Newborns (0–2 months)	12–18
Infants (3–11 months)	14–15
Toddlers (1–3 years)	12–14
Preschoolers (3–5 years)	11–13
School-age children (5–10 years)	10–11
Teens (10–17 years)	8.5–9.25
Adults	7–9

people need at different ages, [TABLE 12-2] shows the rule-of-thumb amounts of sleep different age groups need (Hirschkowitz, 2015).

CRITICAL THINKING ACTIVITY 12-1

© ecco/Shutterstock, Inc.

How many hours a night do you typically sleep? Are you getting enough sleep to maintain your overall health?

Second, not only do different age groups need different amounts of sleep, but sleep needs also vary by individual. Just like any other characteristic you are born with, the amount of sleep you need to perform at your best may be different for you than for another person of the same age. While you may be at your best sleeping 8 hours a night, someone else may need only 6 hours to function optimally.

The third reason is related to a person's basal sleep and sleep debt. **Basal sleep** is defined as the amount of sleep we need on a regular basis for optimal performance. **Sleep debt** is the accumulated sleep that is lost each night. For example, we can lose sleep due to poor sleep habits, sickness, staying up too late to watch TV, and awakening due to environmental factors (e.g., loud noises). Researchers have found that healthy adults have a basal sleep need of 7 to 8 hours a night, but

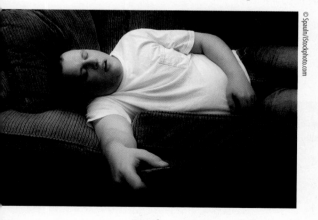

© Spauln/iStockphoto.com

where things get complicated is the interaction between basal sleep and sleep debt (Van Dongen, Rogers, & Dinges, 2003). Our basal sleep is in competition with our sleep debt; that is, we constantly need our basal sleep to pay down our sleep debt. For example, if your basal sleep is 8 hours a night and you only get 7 hours of sleep, you have a sleep debt of 1 hour that you need to try to make up. And this could accumulate over a week, for example, and your sleep debt would then be 7 hours. Luckily, a short nap of 20 minutes or less can equate to 1 hour of "extra" night-time sleep (Home, 2011).

So the question of the magic number of hours of sleep a night is difficult to answer. Another way to look at this question is how much sleep each night is needed for optimal health. Francesco Cappuccio and his colleagues (2010) conducted a meta-analysis that included over 1.3 million participants to determine the relationship between the number of hours of sleep a night and mortality. They found that short sleepers (commonly defined as people who sleep less than 7 hours per night) have a 12% greater risk of dying than people who sleep 7 to 8 hours per night. As well, long sleepers (commonly defined as people who sleep

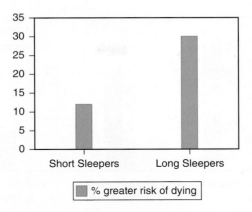

FIGURE 12-1   Percent Greater Risk of Dying for Short and Long Sleepers Compared to People Who Sleep 7 to 8 Hours per Night

Data from Cappuccio, F. P., D'Elia, L., Strazzullo, P., & Miller, M. A. (2010). Sleep duration and all-cause mortality: A systematic review and meta-analysis of prospective studies. *Sleep, 33,* 585–592.

greater than 8 or 9 hours per night) have a 30% greater risk of dying than people who sleep 7 to 8 hours per night. Researchers describe this relationship as the U-shaped curve, where both sleeping too little and sleeping too much may put a person at risk for increased mortality (Cappuccio, D'Elia, Stazzullo, & Miller, 2010; Grandner & Drummond, 2007; Youngstedt & Kript, 2004; see **FIGURE 12-1**). Unfortunately, about 37% of U.S. adults aged 20 years or older put their health at risk by sleeping 6 hours or less a night (Frenk & Chong, 2013).

Sleep, Exercise, and Sedentary Behavior

Most of us hold the common belief that exercise promotes sleep. Indeed, survey studies have consistently shown a link between exercise and better sleep (Youngstedt & Kline, 2006). One noteworthy survey on this topic was an epidemiological study undertaken in Tampere, Finland, with a large random sample of 1,190 men and women between the ages of 36 and 50 (Vuori, Urponen, Hasan, & Partinen, 1988). **Epidemiology** is the science that studies the patterns, causes, and effects of health and disease conditions in defined populations. Rather than asking potentially suggestive questions about whether exercise improved their sleep, the participants were provided with the following open-ended statement: "Please state, in their order of importance, three habits, practices, or actions that you have observed to best promote your falling asleep immediately or perceived quality of sleep." Interestingly, exercise was ranked number one. Exercise was most frequently listed as the "most important habit" for improved sleep by 33%

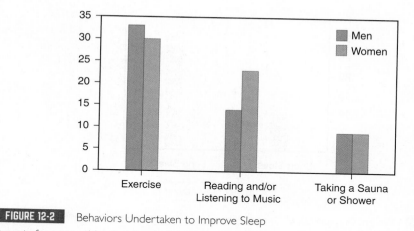

FIGURE 12-2 Behaviors Undertaken to Improve Sleep

Percent of survey participants stating the importance various practices have on promoting their sleep.

Reproduced from Vuori, I., Urponen, H., Hasan, J., & Partinen, M. (1988). Epidemiology of exercise effects on sleep. *Acta Physiologica Scandinavica, 133*(S574), 3–7.

of the men and 30% of the women, followed by reading and/or listening to music (14% of men and 23% of women), and taking a sauna/shower (9% of men and 9% of women) (see **FIGURE 12-2**).

So, at first glance, it might seem that we should exercise to improve our sleep quality. However, self-reports on both sleep and exercise have been questioned from both reliability and validity perspectives. For example, most of us hold the common belief that physical activity promotes sleep. So, if asked, we would likely report that being physically active causes us to have longer and deeper sleep. Is this really the case? Most of us also hold the common belief that alcohol promotes sleep when, in fact, it disrupts sleep. So, our self-reporting on physical activity and sleep could be as invalid as our self-reporting on alcohol and sleep.

To overcome this research limitation, Paul Loprinzi and Brad Cardinal (2011) examined the association between objectively measured physical activity (i.e.,

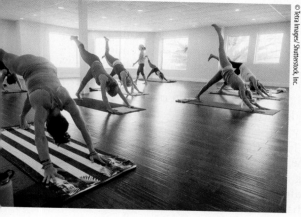

accelerometry) and a variety of self-reported sleeping parameters. Accelerometry provides an objective measure of physical activity and allows the frequency, intensity, and duration of exercise to be assessed over many days.

In their study, Loprinzi and Cardinal (2011) studied a nationally representative sample of over 3,000 men and women between the ages of 18 and 85 years. The participants wore an accelerometer on their right hip for a week and then answered questions examining their sleepiness and quality of sleep. The researchers found that people who engaged in at least 150 minutes of moderate intensity or 75 minutes of vigorous intensity exercise per week, or a combination of the two, had 65% better sleep quality than people who exercised less. The exercisers also felt less tired throughout the day, had less difficulty concentrating when tired, and had fewer leg cramps while sleeping compared to the nonexercisers.

The National Sleep Foundation has conducted the Sleep in America® poll since 1991. This poll is representative of the U.S. population between the ages of 23 and 60 years. The 2013 poll, which sampled 1,000 American adults, focused on the relationship between sleep and physical activity (Hirschkowitz et al., 2013). The results of the poll revealed that exercisers reported better sleep than nonexercisers, even though both exercisers and nonexercisers said they sleep the same amount each night. With regard to exercise intensity, vigorous exercise appeared to produce the best sleep results. People who engaged in vigorous exercise were about twice as likely as nonexercisers to report "I had a good night's sleep" every night or almost every night during the week. As well, people who exercised, regardless of the intensity, had better overall quality of sleep compared to nonexercisers (see █ FIGURE 12-3 █).

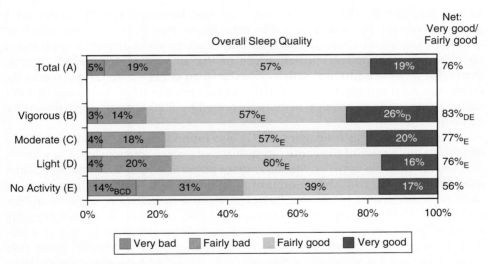

Net: Very good/ Fairly good

Overall Sleep Quality

		Net: Very good/ Fairly good
Total (A)	5% 19% 57% 19%	76%
Vigorous (B)	3% 14% 57%$_E$ 26%$_D$	83%$_{DE}$
Moderate (C)	4% 18% 57%$_E$ 20%	77%$_E$
Light (D)	4% 20% 60%$_E$ 16%	76%$_E$
No Activity (E)	14%$_{BCD}$ 31% 39% 17%	56%

0%   20%   40%   60%   80%   100%

■ Very bad   ■ Fairly bad   ■ Fairly good   ■ Very good

Base = Total sample (Total n = 1,000; Vigorous n = 183; Moderate n = 250; Light n = 477; No activity n = 88)
Letters indicate significant differences at the 95% confidence level.

FIGURE 12-3 Exercise Is Good for Sleep

Data from the 2013 Sleep in America® poll overwhelmingly support the proposition that "Exercise is good for sleep." Although those who exercise and do not exercise report very similar sleep needs and sleep patterns, those who exercise are more likely to say, "I had a good night's sleep" on both worknights and nonworknights. The proportion of those who categorize themselves as vigorous exercisers, moderate exercisers, and light exercisers and report very good or fairly good overall sleep quality (83%, 77%, and 76%, respectively) is significantly higher than those who categorize themselves as no activity or nonexercisers (56%).

Reproduced from 2013 Sleep in America Poll: Exercise and Sleep. National Sleep Foundation. 2013.

CRITICAL THINKING ACTIVITY 12-2

© ecco/Shutterstock, Inc.

Do you think that exercise intensity (i.e., mild, moderate, or strenuous) has an effect on the quality and quantity of sleep?

Emerging research is revealing that sedentary behavior is negatively related to sleep quality in a variety of populations. For example, screen-based sedentary behavior is related to sleep problems in adolescent girls (Costigan, Barnett, Plotnikoff, & Lubans, 2013). As well, there is a strong relationship between low physical activity, not getting enough sleep, and high television time for adolescents (Laurson, Lee, & Eisenmann, 2014). For adults, excess sitting is associated with poor sleep quality; and sitting while watching television is associated with relatively poor sleep quality and obstructive sleep apnea risk (Buman et al., 2015).

Affects of Acute and Chronic Exercise on Sleep

Shawn Youngstedt, Patrick O'Connor, and Rod Dishman (1997) conducted a meta-analysis on 38 studies with 401 participants that examined the influence of acute exercise on sleep. They found that acute physical activity has no effect on either the time it takes to fall asleep or the amount of wakefulness during the night. However, physical activity does have an effect—a significant moderate effect—on total duration of sleep. They found that the total sleep time of individuals after bouts of physical activity increased by 9.90 minutes over nonactive controls.

Youngstedt and his colleagues (1997) also found that exercise duration was a consistent moderator of the acute physical activity–sleep relationship. They found that the relationship between the duration of physical activity and total sleep time is linear in nature, with the amount of time spent in physical activity increasing sleep duration. A note of caution, however, was interjected by Youngstedt and his colleagues. They pointed out that because reliable increases in sleep were only obtained in their meta-analysis for activity periods greater than 1 hour in duration, most of the population is unlikely to experience these benefits given that most people are not physically active generally, let alone for periods greater than 1 hour.

It is important to point out that Youngstedt et al. (1997) did attach a strong qualifier to the findings from their meta-analysis. Research on the impact of acute exercise on sleep has been undertaken with people who are good sleepers. In short, a ceiling effect was present in the research they reviewed. People who already sleep well are unlikely to show large increases in the amount and/or type of sleep they experience.

A more recent meta-analysis of 66 studies by Kredlow and colleagues (Kredlow, Capozzoli, Hearon, Calkins, & Otto, 2015) found that acute exercise has small beneficial effects on total sleep time, sleep onset latency, sleep efficiency, stage 1 sleep, rapid eye movement, and slow-wave sleep. The researchers also found that acute exercise had a moderate beneficial effect on wake time after sleep onset. They also found that regular exercise has small beneficial effects on total sleep time and sleep efficiency, small-to-medium beneficial effects on sleep onset latency, and a moderate beneficial effect on sleep quality.

Researchers have also examined the effects of exercise with people who report impaired sleep quality. For example, in a longitudinal study of adults with impaired sleep quality, Matt Buman and his colleagues (Buman, Hekler, Bliwise, & King, 2011a, 2011b) examined the effects of a 12-month moderate-intensity exercise program on adults' sleep quality. Underactive male and female adults aged 55 years and older with mild to moderate sleep complaints were randomized to either 12 months of a moderate-intensity endurance exercise group (*n* = 36) or a health education control group (*n* = 30). Daily sleep logs, sleep quality, and in-home polysomnographic sleep recordings were collected at baseline, 6 months, and 12 months. **Polysomnography** is a comprehensive recording on the biophysiological changes that occur during sleep.

They found that 12 months of moderate-intensity exercise reduced night-to-night fluctuations in self-rated time to fall asleep, and this relationship was independent of mean-level time to fall asleep. They also found that less active individuals with higher initial physical function and poorer sleep quality had the best improvements in their sleep.

Evening Exercise and Sleep

A common assumption is that engaging in vigorous bouts of exercise just prior to bedtime will disrupt a person's sleep. However, research has consistently found that engaging in either moderate or vigorous exercise in the evening does *not* impair sleep quality (Myllymaki, Kyrolainen, et al., 2011). In fact, increasing either exercise intensity or duration in the evening does not seem to disrupt sleep quality. For example, results for the 2013 National Sleep Foundation Sleep in America Poll revealed that evening exercise was not associated with worse sleep. In fact, most people who did vigorous evening exercise believed that their sleep was of either equal or better quality (97%) and duration (98%) on days they exercised compared to when they did not exercise (Buman, Phillips, Youngstedt, Kline, & Hirschkowitz, 2014). In other words, people who exercise close to bedtime compared to earlier in the day do not have a difference in their self-reported sleep

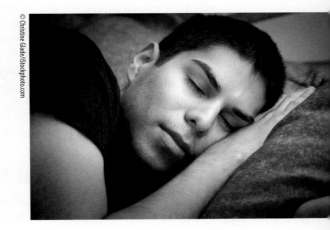
© Christine Glade/iStockphoto.com

quality. In fact, for most people, exercise at any time during the day seems to be better for sleep than no exercise at all (Hirschkowitz et al., 2013).

CRITICAL THINKING ACTIVITY 12-3

© ecco/Shutterstock, Inc.

What would you tell people who say they do not exercise because the only time they would be able to fit exercise in is at night, and evening exercise would make it difficult for them to fall asleep? Is this really a valid reason to not exercise?

Using an experimental design, a group of Finnish researchers (Myllymaki, Rusko, et al., 2011) examined the effects of various exercise intensities and durations on actigraphic and subjective sleep quality of 14 moderately physically active healthy men (mean age = 36 years). The actigraphs were watch shaped and determined the amount of movement and time spent sleeping. The participants also completed a subjective visual analogue sleep quality assessment in the morning after awakening using the question, "How did you sleep last night?" with verbal instructions to answer on a scale of 0 to 100, where 0 was "extremely badly" and 100 was "extremely well."

The men performed five different exercises on separate nights starting at 6:00 p.m. The effect of duration was studied with 30, 60, and 90 minutes of moderate exercise. The effect of intensity was studied with 30 minutes of exercise at mild, moderate, and vigorous intensities. Thus, on separate nights the men performed 30 minutes of mild, moderate, or strenuous exercise and 60 or 90 minutes of moderate exercise. The researchers found that neither exercise intensity nor duration had any impact on actigraphic or subjective sleep quality.

This finding has important implications for exercise adherence. As Youngstedt (2000) observed, evening is a practical time for many people to exercise. However, many people indicate that they do not exercise in the evenings because it may negatively affect their sleep quality. Thus, an unsubstantiated assumption that sleep might be negatively affected by evening activity represents an unnecessary barrier to a physically active lifestyle.

Also, many recommendations about exercise and sleep almost invariably added the caveat that late-night exercise (usually defined as within 4 to 6 hours of sleep) will impair sleep, especially if it is vigorous exercise. The aforementioned research clearly contradicts the long-standing sleep hygiene tip not to exercise close to bedtime. The National Sleep Foundation has recently amended its sleep recommendations for "normal" sleepers to encourage exercise without any caveat to time of day as long as it is not at the expense of sleep. See **TABLE 12-3** for other good **sleep hygiene** tips (Institute of Medicine, 2011).

Exercise and Clinical Sleep Disorders

For most people, sleep is an inevitable, natural daily experience. However, it is estimated that 1 in 6 people in the United States have a **sleep disorder**. A sleep

TABLE 12-3	Good Sleep Hygiene Practices
Recommendation	**Examples**
Sleep schedule	Establish a consistent sleep and wake schedule, even on weekends.
	Create a regular, relaxing bedtime routine, such as soaking in a hot bath or listening to soothing music.
	Don't go to bed unless you are sleepy.
Sleep environment	Sleep in a dark, quiet, comfortable, and cool room.
	Use bedroom only for sleep and sex (keep "sleep stealers" like watching TV or using your computer in bed out of the bedroom).
Activities	Vigorous exercise is best, but even light exercise is better than no activity. Exercise at any time of day, but not at the expense of your sleep.
Food and substances	Finish eating at least 2 to 3 hours before your regular bedtime.
	Avoid caffeine and alcohol close to bedtime.
	Quit smoking.
	Reduce your fluid intake before bedtime.

disorder, or somnipathy, is a medical disorder of the sleep patterns. The International Classification of Sleep Disorders currently lists more than 80 distinct sleep disorders (American Academy of Sleep Medicine, 2014). Common sleep disorders are sleep apnea, insomnia, restless leg syndrome, narcolepsy, and night terrors. See **TABLE 12-4** for a description of these common sleep disorders.

Some sleep disorders are serious enough to interfere with normal physical, mental, and social functioning. According to the National Commission on Sleep Disorders Research (1993), a lack of sleep can result in psychiatric disturbances, reduced productivity, and increased incidence of accidents. In fact, it has been suggested that major world catastrophes such as, for example, the Chernobyl nuclear plant accident, can be traced to employee sleepiness (U.S.D.H.H.S., 1993–1995).

As a consequence, there is an interest—particularly on the part of people suffering from sleep disorders—in determining how

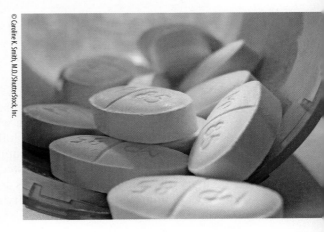

© Caroline K. Smith, M.D./ShutterStock, Inc.

TABLE 12-4	Description of Common Sleep Disorders
Sleep Disorder	**Description**
Sleep apnea	Characterized by pauses in breathing or instances of shallow or infrequent breathing during sleep.
Insomnia	Characterized by difficulty falling and/or staying asleep.
Restless legs syndrome	Characterized by an irresistible urge to move one's body to stop uncomfortable or odd sensations.
Narcolepsy	A neurological disorder that affects the control of sleep and wakefulness. People with narcolepsy experience excessive daytime sleepiness and intermittent, uncontrollable episodes of falling asleep during the daytime.
Night terrors	Episodes of screaming, intense fear, and flailing while still asleep.

sleep can be facilitated. One common approach taken to improve the quality and quantity of sleep has been medication in the form of sleeping pills. However, sleeping pills do not seem to be the answer. In their recent review of the exercise and sleep literature, Matt Buman and Abby King (2010) noted that people can become dependent on sleeping pills and develop tolerance to prescribed dosages. Also, sleeping pills are often associated with profound rebound insomnia. Even more important, however, is the fact that regular use of sleeping pills is the mortality equivalent of smoking one to two packs of cigarettes a day. So, sleeping pills do not work well over the long term, and their chronic use represents a health risk.

CRITICAL THINKING ACTIVITY 12-4

© ecco/Shutterstock, Inc.

How would you convince someone who is taking sleep medication that exercise is a better option to treat their sleep disorder?

Although historically research on the relationship between exercise and sleep has focused on good sleepers, more recently researchers have begun to examine the effects of exercise on people with sleep problems and sleep disorders (Yang, Ho, Chen, & Chiene, 2012), including restless legs syndrome (Aukerman et al., 2006; Giannaki et al., 2013), insomnia (Passos et al., 2011), and obstructive sleep apnea (Iftikhar, Kline, & Youngstedt, 2013; Kline et al., 2011). Although preliminary, the results of these studies are promising, illustrating that exercise is effective in improving the sleep quality of people suffering with these sleep disorders.

Obstructive sleep apnea is the most common type of sleep apnea, and it is caused by obstruction of the upper airway during sleep. This leads to a lack of sufficient deep sleep and is often accompanied by snoring. It is characterized by repetitive pauses in breathing during sleep, despite the effort to breathe, and it is often related to a reduction in blood oxygen saturation. These pauses in breathing, called **apneas**, usually last 20 to 40 seconds. People with obstructive sleep apnea are rarely aware of having difficulty breathing, even upon awakening. Common signs of obstructive sleep apnea include unexplained daytime sleepiness, restless sleep, and loud snoring that is often followed by periods of silence followed by gasps. Emerging research is revealing that exercise is an effective nonsurgical and nonpharmacological treatment for obstructive sleep apnea (Dobrosielski, Patil, Schwartz, Bandeen-Roche, & Stewart, 2015).

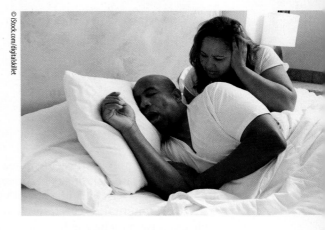

Restless legs syndrome is a neurological disorder characterized by an irresistible urge to move one's body to stop uncomfortable or odd sensations (Earley, 2003). It most commonly affects the legs, but can affect the arms, torso, head, and even phantom limbs. The odd sensations range from pain or an aching in the muscles to "an itch you can't scratch," an unpleasant "tickle that won't stop," or even a "crawling" feeling (Skidmore et al., 2009). The sensations typically begin or intensify during quiet wakefulness, such as when relaxing, reading, studying, or trying to sleep (Allen et al., 2003). Symptoms occur primarily at night when a person is relaxing or at rest and can increase in severity during the night. Moving the legs relieves the discomfort.

Insomnia, or sleeplessness, is one of the most common sleep disorders. The prevalence of chronic insomnia is between 10% and 15% worldwide (Ohayon, 2002). Insomnia is characterized by long-term difficulties with initiating or maintaining sleep. People with insomnia have one or more of the following symptoms: (1) difficulty falling asleep, (2) waking up often during the night and having trouble going back to sleep, (3) waking up too early in the morning, and (4) feeling tired upon waking. Thus, an individual with insomnia may have an inability to either fall asleep or stay asleep as long as desired. Insomnia is often defined as a positive response to either of the following two questions (Roth, 2007):

1. Do you experience difficulty sleeping?
2. Do you have difficulty falling or staying asleep?

About 50% of middle-age and older adults complain of symptoms of chronic insomnia, such as having a hard time falling asleep and/or staying asleep and having impaired daytime functioning. The results of insomnia include fatigue,

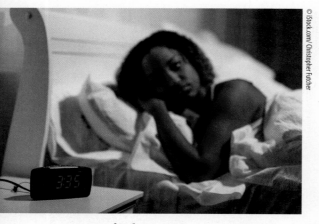

© iStock.com/ Christopher Futcher

increased accidents while driving a vehicle, poor mood, decreased concentration, and poor quality of life (American Academy of Sleep Medicine, 2005; Ohayon, 2002).

Using poll data from 1,000 American adults, Max Hirschkowitz and his colleagues (2013) found that more than two-thirds of vigorous exercisers say they rarely or never (in the past 2 weeks) had symptoms commonly associated with insomnia. In contrast, 50% of nonexercisers say they woke up during the night, and 24% had difficulty falling asleep every night or almost every night. The researchers also found that nonexercisers had more symptoms of sleep apnea. They found that 44% of nonexercisers exhibited a moderate risk of sleep apnea, compared to 26% of light exercisers, 22% of moderate exercisers, and 19% of vigorous exercisers.

Experimental research by Reid and colleagues (2010) has revealed that aerobic exercise may be the best prescription to battle chronic insomnia. They studied 17 middle-age sedentary adults (mean age = 61.6 years) with insomnia. Participants were randomly assigned for 16 weeks to either an exercise and sleep hygiene education group or a nonexercise and sleep hygiene control group. The exercise program included at least two of the following aerobic activities: walking, stationary biking, or using a treadmill. In the control group, participants took part in either recreational or educational activities such as attending a cooking class or listening to a museum lecture. The control group met for about 45 minutes three to five times a week for 16 weeks.

All participants received sleep hygiene education, which consisted of an appointment with a board-certified sleep specialist who provided verbal and written sleep hygiene instructions and counseling. The researchers found that the exercise group improved in sleep quality, **sleep latency** (i.e., amount of time to fall asleep), sleep duration, daytime function, and sleep efficiency compared to the control group. The exercise group also had reductions in depressive symptoms, daytime sleepiness, and improvements in vitality. The researchers concluded that aerobic exercise with sleep hygiene education is an effective treatment approach to improve sleep quality, mood, and quality of life in older adults with chronic insomnia.

Researchers from Iran found that aerobic exercise results in improved signs of restless legs syndrome in patients with **end-stage renal disease** who must undergo chronic **hemodialysis** (Mortazavi et al., 2013). The researchers randomly assigned 26 patients to either an exercise ($n = 13$) or a control condition ($n = 13$). The exercise group performed aerobic exercise (i.e., biking for 30 minutes three times a week) during their hemodialysis for 16 weeks. The patients' quality of life and severity of restless legs syndrome were assessed at weeks 1 and 16 of the study.

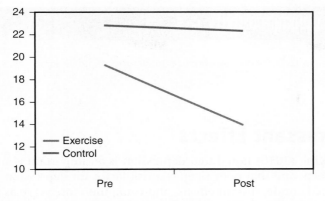

FIGURE 12-4   Restless Legs Syndrome Scoring in Exercise and Control Groups

Note: Difference of means between the first week of experiment and the final week was −5.5 ± 4.96 in the exercise group and −0.53 ± 2.3 in the control group.

Data from Mortazavi, M., Vadhatpour, B., Ghasempour, A., Taheri, D., Shahidi, S., et al. (2013). Aerobic exercise improves signs of restless legs syndrome in end-stage renal disease patients suffering chronic hemodialysis. *The Scientific World Journal*, Nov 6;628142. doi: 10.1155/2013/628142.

Results revealed that aerobic exercise resulted in improvements in symptoms of restless legs syndrome compared to the control group (see **FIGURE 12-4**). No significant difference was evidenced for quality of life between the two groups. Thus, the researchers concluded that aerobic exercise improves the symptoms of restless legs syndrome. However, exercise did not result in improved quality of life.

Mechanisms of How Exercise Affects Sleep

Several mechanisms have been proposed for how exercise helps people sleep better (Buman & King, 2010; Youngstedt & Kline, 2006). Some of the commonly accepted mechanisms are briefly reviewed below.

Anxiety Reduction

Perhaps the most plausible mechanism through which exercise could promote sleep is anxiety reduction (Youngstedt & Kline, 2006). Disturbed sleep is a hallmark of anxiety, and chronic insomnia has been associated with increased physiological arousal. Therefore, stimuli that reduce anxiety may promote sleep. It is well established that acute exercise reduces state anxiety and that chronic exercise results in stable reductions in trait anxiety.

CRITICAL THINKING ACTIVITY 12-5

How can the anxiolytic effect of exercise help those with sleep disorders?

Antidepressant Effects

Buman and King (2010) noted that depression is an important contributing factor to poor sleep, and that poor sleep is a risk factor for depression. Exercise has well-established antidepressant effects, and could therefore serve as an important mediator of the depression–sleep relationship.

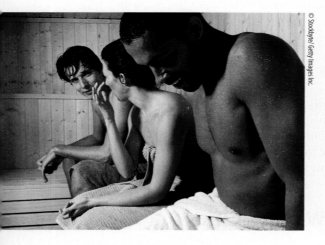

Thermoregulation

Our body temperature drops as we fall asleep (Driver & Taylor, 2000). Temperature elevation (e.g., due to warm baths, saunas, or exercise prior to bedtime) can activate temperature downregulation, which is associated with deeper forms of sleep (Bauman & King, 2010). Thus, increasing body temperature before bed can improve sleep quality. Youngstedt (2005) has suggested that chronic exercise could support a more efficient temperature regulation process during the sleep–wake cycle, resulting in better sleep.

Circadian Rhythms

Circadian rhythms (commonly referred to as our body clock) are the physical, mental, and behavioral changes that follow a roughly 24-hour cycle. For example, our body temperature tends to be lowest at 4:30 a.m., we have our sharpest rise in blood pressure at 6:45 a.m., and we have greater cardiovascular and muscle strength at 5:00 p.m. Our circadian system is affected by both endogenous (e.g., body temperature, melatonin) and exogenous (e.g., bright light, exercise, meal timing) cues that regulate the sleep–wake cycle. Disturbed sleep may occur when endogenous and exogenous cues are not synchronized, such as during jet-lagged travel and shift work. Common circadian rhythm sleep disorders include jet lag, shift work sleep disorder, and delayed sleep phase syndrome.

Jet lag consists of symptoms such as excessive sleepiness and a lack of daytime alertness in people who travel across time zones. Shift-work sleep disorder affects people who frequently rotate shifts or work at night. Delayed sleep phase syndrome is a disorder of sleep timing where people tend to fall asleep at very late times and have difficulty waking up in time for work, school, or social engagements.

The strongest synchronizer of our circadian rhythms is light, particularly artificial bright light, natural light, and domestic lighting conditions. Exercise has also been implicated in such synchronization effects. While research has been hampered because of a lack of control of light and exercise characteristics, a review by Edwards, Reilly, and Waterhouse (2009) suggests that exercise bouts of various intensities and durations can mediate phase shifts, independent of the effects produced by light alone.

Summary

Research has proven that exercise improves sleep. In fact, people often list that exercise is the most important thing they can do to improve their sleep (Vuori et al., 1988). Clinical trials have supported this self-reported finding, illustrating that exercise improves both the quality and quantity of sleep in both "normal sleepers" and people suffering with a clinical sleep disorder such as restless legs syndrome or insomnia. Because researchers continually find that exercise improves sleep, physical activity is included as a good sleep hygiene recommendation. It is recommended to exercise at any time of day, but not at the expense of sleep.

KEY TERMS

apnea
basal sleep
end-stage renal disease
epidemiology
hemodialysis
insomnia
obstructive sleep apnea

polysomnography
restless legs syndrome
sleep
sleep debt
sleep disorder
sleep hygiene
sleep latency

REVIEW QUESTIONS

1. Describe the stages of sleep.

2. What is the difference between basal sleep and sleep debt?

3. Loprinzi and Cardinal (2011) conducted a sleep study on a nationally representative sample of over 3,000 men and women. The participants wore an accelerometer on their right hip for a week and then they completed questions examining their

sleepiness and quality of sleep. What did the researchers find?

4. How does acute physical activity impact sleep?

5. What is insomnia?

6. Define *obstructive sleep apnea*. Can physical activity be used as an effective treatment for sleep apnea?

7. Describe the various proposed mechanisms of how exercise affects sleep.

APPLYING THE CONCEPTS

1. What mechanisms might explain how regular swimming improved Omar's ability to fall and stay asleep?

2. Without easy and regular access to swimming due to his new job, Omar's sleep may likely be impaired once again. What might this put him at risk for?

REFERENCES

Allen, R., Picchietti, D., Hening, W. A., Trenkwalder, C., Walters, A. S., & Montplaisi, J. (2003). Restless legs syndrome: Diagnostic criteria, special considerations, and epidemiology: A report from the restless legs syndrome diagnosis and epidemiology workshop at the National Institutes of Health. *Sleep Medicine, 4*, 101–119.

American Academy of Sleep Medicine. (2005). *International classification of sleep disorders, revised: Diagnostic and coding manual.* Westchester, IL: Author.

American Academy of Sleep Medicine. (2014). *International classification of sleep disorders—third edition (ICSD-3).* Darien, IL.

American Heritage Medical Dictionary. (2007). Sleep definition. New York, NY: Houghton Mifflin Company.

Aukerman, M. M., Aukerman, D., Bayard, M., Tudiver, F., Thorp, L., & Bailey, B. (2006). Exercise and restless legs syndrome: A randomized controlled trial. *Journal of the American Board of Family Medicine, 19,* 487–493.

Buman, M. P., Hekler, E. B., Bliwise, D. L., & King, A. C. (2011a). Exercise effects on night-to-night fluctuations in self-rated sleep among older adults with sleep complaints. *Sleep Research, 20,* 28–37.

Buman, M. P., Hekler, E. B., Bliwise, D. L., & King, A. C. (2011b). Moderators and mediators of exercise-induced objective sleep improvements in midlife and older adults with sleep complaints. *Health Psychology, 30,* 579–587.

Buman, M. P., & King, A. C. (2010). Exercise as a treatment to enhance sleep. *American Journal of Lifestyle Medicine, 6,* 500–513.

Buman, M. P., Kline, C. E., Youngstedt, S. D., Phillips, B., Tulio de Mello, M., & Hirschkowitz, M. (2015). Sitting and television viewing: Novel risk factors for sleep disturbance and apnea risk? Results for the 2013 National Sleep Foundation Sleep in America Poll. *Chest, 147,* 728–734.

Buman, M. P., Phillips, B. A., Youngstedt, S. D., Kline, C. E., & Hirschkowitz, M. (2014). Does night-time exercise really disturb sleep? Results for the 2013 National Sleep Foundation Sleep in America Poll. *Sleep Medicine, 15,* 755–761.

Cappuccio, F. P., D'Elia, L., Strazzullo, P., & Miller, M. A. (2010). Sleep duration and all-cause mortality: A systematic review and meta-analysis of prospective studies. *Sleep, 33,* 585–592.

Costigan, S. A., Barnett, L., Plotnikoff, R. C., & Lubans, D. R. (2013). The health indicators associated with screen-based sedentary behavior among adolescent girls: A systematic review. *Journal of Adolescent Health, 52,* 382–392.

Dobrosielski, D. A., Patil, S., Schwartz, A. R., Bandeen-Roche, K., & Stewart, K. J. (2015). Effects of exercise and weight loss in older adults with obstructive sleep apnea. *Medicine and Science in Sports and Exercise, 47,* 20–26.

Driver, H. S., & Taylor, S. R. (2000). Exercise and sleep. *Sleep Medicine Reviews, 4,* 387–402.

Earley, C. J. (2003). Restless legs syndrome. *New England Journal of Medicine, 348,* 2103–2109.

Edwards, B. J., Reilly, T., & Waterhouse, J. (2009). Zeitgeber-effects of exercise on human circadian rhythms: What are alternative approaches to investigating the existence of a phase-response curve to exercise? *Biological Rhythm Research, 40,* 53–69.

Frenk, S. M., & Chong, Y. (2013). QuickStats: Sleep duration among adults aged ≥20 years, by race/ethnicity—National Health and Nutrition Examination Survey, United States, 2007–2010. *MMWR, 62,* 755.

Giannaki, C. D., Sakkas, G. K., Karatzaferi, C., Hadjigeorgiou, G. M., Laydas, E., Koutedakis, Y., & Stefanidis, I. (2013). Effect of exercise training and dopamine agonists in patients with uremic restless legs syndrome: A six-month randomized, partially double-blind, placebo-controlled comparative study. *BMC Nephrology, 14,* 194.

Grandner, M. A., & Drummond, S. P. (2007). Who are the long sleepers? Towards an understanding of the mortality relationship. *Sleep Medicine Reviews, 11,* 341–360.

Hirschkowitz, M. (2015). The National Sleep Foundation's sleep time duration recommendations: Methodology and results summary. *Sleep Health.* Retrieved September 12, 2015, from http://sleepfoundation.org/sites/default/files/STREPchanges_1.png

Hirshkowitz, M., Buman, M., Kline, C., Tulio de Mello, M., & Youngstdet, S. D. (2013). 2013 Sleep in America® poll. Exercise and Sleep. Summary of findings. *National Sleep Foundation.* Retrieved December 5, 2013, from http://www.sleepfoundation.org/sites/default/files/RPT336%20Summary%20of%20Findings%2002%2020%202013.pdf

Home, J. (2011). The end of sleep: 'Sleep debt' versus biological adaptation of human sleep to waking needs. *Biological Psychology, 87,* 1–14.

Iftikhar, I. H., Kline, C. E., & Youngstedt, S. D. (2013). Effects of exercise training on sleep apnea: A meta-analysis. *Lung, 29,* epub.

Institute of Medicine, Committee on Sleep Medicine and Research. (2006). *Sleep disorders and sleep deprivation: An unmet public health problem.* Washington, DC: National Academies Press.

Kline, C. E., Crowley, E. P., Ewing, G. B., Burch, J. B., Blair, S. N., Durstine, J. L.,… Youngstedt, S. D. (2011). The effect of exercise training on obstructive sleep apnea and sleep quality: A randomized controlled trial. *Sleep, 34,* 1631–1640.

Kredlow, M. A., Capozzoli, M. C., Hearon, B. A., Calkins, A. W., & Otto, M. W. (2015). The effects of physical activity on sleep: A meta-analytic review. *Journal of Behavioral Medicine, 38,* 427–449.

Laurson, K. R., Lee, J. A., & Eisenmann, J. C. (2014). The cumulative impact of physical activity, sleep duration, and television time on adolescent obesity: 2011 Youth Risk Behavior Survey. *Journal of Physical Activity and Healthy, 12,* 355–360.

Loprinzi, P. D., & Cardinal, B. J. (2011). Association between objectively-measured physical activity and sleep, NHANES 2005–2006. *Mental Health and Physical Activity, 4,* 65–69.

Mortazavi, M., Vadhatpour, B., Ghasempour, A., Taheri, D., Shahidi, S., Moeinzadeh, F.,… Dolat-khah, S. (2013). Aerobic exercise improves signs of restless legs syndrome in end-stage renal disease patients suffering chronic hemodialysis. *The Scientific World Journal,* Nov 6;628142. doi:10.1155/2013/628142

Myllymaki, T., Kyrolainen, H., Savolainen, K., Hokka, L., Jakonen, R., Juuti, T.,… Rusko, H. (2011). Effects of vigorous late-night exercise on sleep quality and cardiac autonomic activity. *Journal of Sleep Research, 20,* 146–153.

Myllynaki, T., Rusko, H., Syvaoja, H., Juuti, T., Kinnunen, M. L., & Kyrolainen, H. (2011). Effects of exercise intensity and duration on nocturnal heart rate variability and sleep quality. *European Journal of Applied Physiology, 112,* 801–809.

Ohayon, M. M. (2002). Epidemiology of insomnia: What we know and what we still need to learn. *Sleep Medicine Reviews, 6,* 97–111.

Passos, G. S., Poyares, D., Santana, M. G., D'Aurea, C. V. R., Youngstedt, S. D. Tufik, S., & de Mello, M. T. (2011). Effects of moderate aerobic exercise training on chronic primary insomnia. *Sleep Medicine, 12,* 1018–1027.

Reid, K. J., Baron, K. G., Lu, B., Naylor, E., Wolfe, L., & Zee, P. C. (2010). Aerobic exercise improves self-reported sleep and quality of life in older adults with insomnia. *Sleep Medicine, 11,* 934–940.

Roth, T. (2007). Insomnia: Definition, prevalence, etiology, and consequences. *Journal of Clinical Sleep Medicine, 3*(5 Suppl), S7–S10.

Skidmore, F. M., Drago, V., Foster, P. S., & Heilman, K. M. (2009). Bilateral restless legs affecting a phantom limb, treated with dopamine agonists. *Journal of Neurology, Neurosurgery, and Psychiatry, 80,* 569–570.

Twain, M. (1905). Seventieth birthday speech. Retrieved December 5, 2013, from http://www.pbs.org/marktwain/learnmore/writings_seventieth.html

U.S.D.H.H.S. (1993–1995). *Wake up America: A national sleep alert: Report of the National Commission on Sleep Disorder Research.* Washington: DC.

Van Dongen, H. P., Rogers, N., L., & Dinges, D. (2003). Sleep debt: Theoretical and empirical issues. *Sleep and Biological Rhythms, 1,* 5–13.

Vuori, I., Urponen, H., Hasan, J., & Partinen, M. (1988). Epidemiology of exercise effects on sleep. *Acta Physiologica Scandinavica, 133*(S574), 3–7.

Yang, P. Y., Ho, K. H., Chen, H. C., & Chiene, M. Y. (2012). Exercise training improves sleep quality in middle-age and older adults with sleep problems: A systematic review. *Journal of Physiotherapy, 58,* 157–163.

Youngstedt, S. D. (2000). The exercise-sleep mystery. *International Journal of Sport Psychology, 31,* 241–255.

Youngstedt, S. D. (2005). Effects of exercise on sleep. *Clinics in Sports Medicine, 24,* 355–365.

Youngstedt, S. D., & Kline, C. E. (2006). Epidemiology of exercise and sleep. *Sleep and Biological Rhythms, 4,* 215–221.

Youngstedt, S. D., & Kript, D. F. (2004). Long sleep and mortality: Rationale for sleep restriction. *Sleep Medicine Reviews, 8,* 159–174.

Youngstedt, S. D., O'Connor, R. K., & Dishman, R. K. (1997). The effects of acute exercise on sleep: A quantitative synthesis. *Sleep, 20,* 203–214.

Health-Related Quality of Life and Positive Psychology

Runner © Izf/Shutterstock

Vignette: Beverly

I received a devastating diagnosis of cancer shortly after my 34th birthday. My husband and I had begun putting aside money for a second child, and our first was about to turn 6. My husband was the first person who noticed a lump in my left breast. And because my paternal grandmother died of cancer before I was born, I didn't waste any time seeking medical attention.

An ultrasound by the end of the week produced inconclusive but concerning results. So I immediately underwent a biopsy. The 4 days I had to wait for the results were agonizing. I barely slept, ate, or remained emotionally present at the elementary school I then worked at as an English teacher. About 30 days after hearing the confirmation that I had stage 2A breast cancer, I began treatment.

In my case, this meant a mastectomy in order to forgo radiation and an immediate reconstruction. It took me about 3 weeks to fully recover my strength and feel comfortable enough to come off the pain killers I'd been put on. And about the only exercise I could do was to walk slowly around our house while performing the basic arm movements a physical therapist showed me the morning after my surgery.

LEARNING OBJECTIVES

After completing this chapter, you will be able to

- Distinguish among quality of life, standard of living, and health-related quality of life.
- Measure your own health-related quality of life using assessment tools.
- Understand how physical activity and sedentary behavior affect health-related quality of life in a variety of populations.
- Define positive psychology and happiness.
- Explain how exercise and sedentary behavior are related to our levels of happiness.
- Describe how an acute bout of exercise affects feeling states.

I continued to work with a physical therapist for months after I was able to return to work. After I was cleared for exercise by my doctor, I went on to work with a personal trainer who helped me rebuild my upper body strength with a simple weight training regimen and elastic band routine I could do at home. The trainer also helped me find a cardiovascular program appropriate for my energy levels, schedule, and preferred pace of movement. Eventually, she introduced me to cycling.

My husband, a former football player in college, had outfitted our home with a weight rack and treadmill. And once I expressed to him my desire to take charge of my health by making physical activity a regular part of my life, he agreed to join me at a cycling studio that offered daily classes.

It was important to me to impart to my son how important mommy's new routine was, now that she was out of the hospital. At first, he was sad that I'd go to the gym after work on most days of the week rather than bring him to baseball or soccer practice. But once I convinced him that my going to the gym was a way for me to stay home for good—and be around to be his mommy for longer—he eventually got the message. In fact, he even started asking me, over dinners, "Mommy, did you do your exercise today?"

Cancer, to me, was a horrifying experience. I've been in remission for 2 years now, but I'm still worried I might not be in the clear. I was diagnosed relatively young, which increases my odds that I could have a reoccurrence. Hence why it's so crucial to me to have not just a means of keeping my body in its healthiest form ever, but also finding activities that keep me feeling empowered and in control of my life.

I derive immense joy from being a mother and a wife and from teaching English at the magnet school I now work at, but few things compare to the feeling I get when I reach that 15-mile mark on my bike or when I round the final bend of a 3-mile jog around my neighborhood, make it through 10 pushups without touching my knees on the floor, or reach the peak of the mountain my husband and son hike up with me on some weekends without feeling winded.

I would never in a million years have asked to be diagnosed with cancer. It's a traumatic experience for anyone, and its imprint will always linger on my life, as well as on the lives of everyone who has known and loved me. But that it galvanized me to take charge of my health and be more aware of my body—not to mention the time I have here on earth and its meaning—has indeed been a blessing (albeit a very unexpected, hidden, and conflicting one).

I can honestly say that at 36 I feel healthier than I've ever felt in my life. I have more energy. I enjoy my days more. And I come home from my workouts with more of me to share with the family I deeply and truly love. I will, of course, have to adjust my workout schedule slightly over the next year, because my husband and I are, at long last, finally expecting that second child.

■ Introduction

Historically, researchers focused on how physical activity could reduce negative mood states and psychological disorders such as anxiety and depression. This line of research has found that exercise is a viable intervention to reduce these negative mood states in both healthy and diseased populations. The flip side to this line of inquiry is the following question: Can exercise be used to improve positive mood states such as happiness, vigor, energy, and enthusiasm and overall quality of life?

Like many people, Martin Luther King Jr. believed that quality of life is very important, as evidenced in his following quote: "The quality, not the longevity, of one's life is what is important." (n.d.). In other words, it is the quality of one's life, not the quantity of life, that needs to be fostered. In fact, research has revealed that if you increase people's quality of life, their quantity of life will also increase (Brown, Thompson, Zack, Arnold, & Barile, 2013).

The purpose of this chapter is to examine how exercise and sedentary behavior affect people's health-related quality of life (HRQoL) in healthy as well as special populations (e.g., cancer patients, diabetics, and older adults). First, we will define and determine how HRQoL is measured, and then we will examine the effects of exercise and sedentary behavior on HRQoL in a variety of special populations. Finally, we will define positive psychology and examine its relationship to our quality of life, in particular the relationship between happiness and positive mood states and physical activity and sedentary behavior.

■ Health–Related Quality of Life

Quality of life is a broad multidimensional term that assesses a person's perceived quality of his or her daily life. In other words, quality of life is a subjective evaluation of both positive and negative aspects of people's general well-being and their ability to function in daily tasks. This includes, for example, emotional (e.g., joy, stress, sadness, anger), social (e.g., family, friends, church groups), and physical (e.g., healthy, overweight, chronic disease) aspects of the individual's life. Quality of life research began in the 1970s to describe and measure the impact of different conditions on people's daily lives, taking into account emotional, social, and physical functions.

Although many different conceptualizations of quality of life exist, the World Health Organization (WHO) envisions quality of life as a broad concept consisting of the following six domains: physical health, psychological health, independence, social relationships, spirituality, and the environment (WHO, 1997; see **FIGURE 13-1**). **TABLE 13-1** provides a description of each of these domains. **FIGURE 13-2** presents another multidimensional quality of life model (Gill et al., 2011). This model

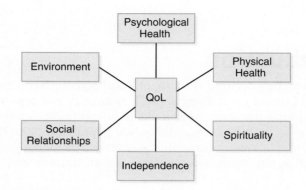

FIGURE 13-1 WHO Quality of Life

Data from World Health Organization. (1997). WHOQOL. Measuring quality of life. Retrieved from http://www.who.int/mental_health/media/68.pdf.

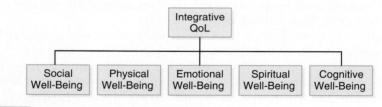

FIGURE 13-2 Integrative Quality of Life

Modified from Gill, D. L., Chang, Y. K., Murphy, K. M., Speed, K. M., Hammond, C. C., Rodriguez, E. A.,... Shang, Y.-T. (2011). Quality of life assessment for physical activity and health promotion. *Applied Research in Quality of Life, 6,* 181–200. With kind permission from Springer Science and Business Media.

TABLE 13-1	World Health Organization Multidimensional Quality of Life Model
Domain	**Quality of Life Example**
1. Physical health	Energy and fatigue, pain and discomfort, sleep and rest
2. Psychological health	Body image and appearance, negative feelings, positive feelings, self-esteem, thinking, learning, memory, and concentration
3. Independence	Mobility, activities of daily living, dependence on medicinal substances and medical aids, work capacity
4. Social relationships	Personal relationships, social support, sexual activity
5. Environment	Financial resources, freedom, physical safety and security, health and social care, home environment, recreation opportunities
6. Spirituality	Religion, personal beliefs

Reproduced from World Health Organization. (1997). WHOQOL. Measuring quality of life. Retrieved from http://www.who.int/mental_health/media/68.pdf.

similarly envisions the domains of social, physical, cognitive, emotional, and spiritual well-being all contributing to an integrative quality of life.

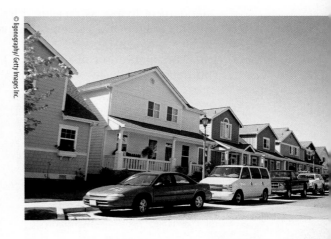

Factors that play a role in people's quality of life vary according to personal preferences, but they often include financial security, job satisfaction, family life, health, and safety. For example, financial decisions usually involve a tradeoff whereby quality of life is either decreased by saving money or increased by spending money. A person may buy that new car she has been eyeing, or she may decide to not buy the car and save her money in order to purchase a house in the near future instead of continuing to rent a small apartment.

Commuting to work provides another good example of something that can affect people's quality of life. Many people save money on housing by living further away from work. However, living farther from work requires a longer commute (usually both in distance and time) to the office. The extra time spent traveling reduces the available time that the commuter will have with family, friends, and doing leisure activities, but it offers more affordable housing and suburban amenities. In popular job centers, such as major urban areas like New York City, it is not uncommon for people to spend 2 hours commuting one way in order to live in more affordable and larger housing in the suburbs. Some people consider this tradeoff worthwhile for their quality of life, whereas others choose to maximize their quality of life by spending more money on housing to live closer to work. In short, perceptions of quality of life vary greatly from person to person.

CRITICAL THINKING ACTIVITY 13-1

© ecco/Shutterstock, Inc.

What is more important to your quality of life? To live close to work or to live in the suburbs?

The terms *quality of life* and *standard of living* are often incorrectly used interchangeably. **Standard of living** refers to levels of wealth, comfort, and material goods. Although standard of living is often measured by a person's income, it can include many other factors, such as quality and availability of employment, class disparity, poverty rate, quality and affordability of housing, inflation rate, number of holiday days per year, affordable (or free) access to quality health care, quality and availability of education, life expectancy, incidence of disease, cost of goods and services, economic and political stability, political and religious freedom, environmental quality, climate, and safety. In comparison, quality of life is related to how people feel about their lives and themselves. A person can have a very high standard of living, as measured by having a high income level, yet have a low quality of life. Or a person can have a low standard of living and a high quality of life.

The application of quality of life to the impact of diseases and treatments on people's daily lives and their ability to function has given rise to a field of 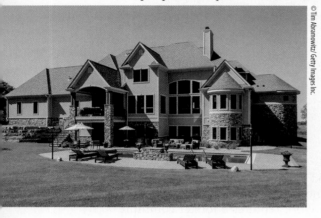 research called **health-related quality of life (HRQoL)**. The field of HRQoL assesses how people's quality of life affects their physical, social, and mental health. **Health** is defined as a state of complete physical, mental, and social well-being, not merely the absence of disease (WHO, 1948). Most people would agree that either increasing or maintaining your health improves your overall quality of life. Not surprisingly, people with chronic diseases (e.g., diabetes, cancer, stroke, arthritis, and hypertension) tend to have lower HRQoL than healthy people.

Measurement of Health–Related Quality of Life

HRQOL-14 Measure

A number of assessment tools have been developed to measure HRQoL. One of the more popular HRQoL assessment tools is the Centers for Disease Control and Prevention's (CDC) HRQOL-14 Measure. The HRQOL-14 Measure has been used since 1993 in epidemiological studies to assess behavioral risk factors for health in the United States. This measure has three modules. The Healthy Days Core Module includes four core questions (see **TABLE 13-2**). These questions are useful at the national level to identify health disparities and track population trends. For example, almost 16% of Americans report that they have either fair or poor health (question 1 of the Healthy Days Core Module; Zack, 2013). Certain groups are more at risk for poor HRQoL. For example, groups with higher percentages of fair or poor health and who report more physically and mentally unhealthy days include women, older adults, obese individuals, minority racial/ethnic groups, those with less education, those who speak another language besides English at home, and those with a disability (Zack, 2013; Zack, Moriarty, Stroup, Ford, & Mokdad, 2004).

CRITICAL THINKING ACTIVITY 13-2

© ecco/Shutterstock, Inc.

Complete the Healthy Days Core Module. What does this tell you about your HRQoL? What can you do to improve your HRQoL?

TABLE 13-2	CDC HRQOL-14: Healthy Days Core Module

1. Would you say that in general your health is (circle one):

   Excellent   Very Good   Good   Fair   Poor

2. Now thinking about your PHYSICAL HEALTH, which includes physical illness and injury, how many days during the past 30 days was your physical health NOT good?

   _____ Number of Days

3. Now thinking about your MENTAL HEALTH, which includes stress, depression, and problems with emotions, how many days during the past 30 days was your mental health NOT good?

   _____ Number of Days

4. During the past 30 days, how many days did POOR PHYSICAL OR MENTAL HEALTH keep you from doing your usual activities, such as self-care, work, or recreation?

   _____ Number of Days

Reproduced from National Center for Chronic Disease Prevention and Health Promotion | Division of Population Health.

With regard to age, a negative linear relationship with HRQoL is evidenced, with 9% of adults ages 18 to 24 years reporting either fair or poor health, compared to 30.1% of adults aged 75 or older. As well, a positive relationship exists between education level and overall health, with 37% of people with less than a high school education reporting either fair or poor health, compared to 7.1% of people who have graduated college. For weight status, 37.5% of people who are overweight or obese report either fair or poor health, compared to 10.9% of normal weight individuals (National Center for Chronic Disease Prevention and Health Promotion, 2011). In short, demographic variables (such as age, weight status, and education) are directly related to people's HRQoL.

The Activity Limitations Module contains five questions that assess physical, mental, or emotional problems or limitations a person may have in his or her daily life (see **TABLE 13-3**). Finally, the Healthy Days Symptoms Module contains five questions that assess a person's recent pain, depression, anxiety, sleeplessness, and vitality and the cause, duration, and severity of a current activity limitation an individual may have had in his or her life during the past 30 days (see **TABLE 13-4**).

SF-36 Scale

Another widely used quality of life measure is the Short-Form (SF)-36 scale (Ware & Sherbourne, 1992). The SF-36 assesses the following eight physical and/or mental health concepts: (1) limitations in quality of life physical activities because of health problems; (2) limitations in social activities because of physical or emotional problems; (3) limitations in usual role activities because of physical health problems; (4) bodily pain; (5) general mental health (psychological distress

TABLE 13-3 CDC HRQOL–14: Activity Limitations Module
These next questions are about physical, mental, or emotional problems or limitations you may have in your daily life.
1. Are you LIMITED in any way in any activities because of any impairment or health problem? YES or NO
2. What is the MAJOR impairment or health problem that limits your activities? a. Arthritis/rheumatism b. Back or neck problem c. Fractures, bone/joint injury d. Walking problem e. Lung/breathing problem f. Hearing problem g. Eye/vision problem h. Heart problem i. Stroke problem j. Hypertension/high blood pressure k. Diabetes l. Cancer m. Depression/anxiety/emotional problem n. Other impairment/problem
3. For HOW LONG have your activities been limited because of your major impairment or health problem? a. Days b. Weeks c. Months d. Years
4. Because of any impairment or health problem, do you need the help of other persons with your PERSONAL CARE needs, such as eating, bathing, dressing, or getting around the house? a. Yes b. No
5. Because of any impairment or health problem, do you need the help of other persons in handling your ROUTINE needs, such as everyday household chores, doing necessary business, shopping, or getting around for other purposes? a. Yes b. No

Reproduced from National Center for Chronic Disease Prevention and Health Promotion | Division of Population Health.

and well-being); (6) limitations in usual role activities because of emotional problems; (7) vitality (energy and fatigue); and (8) general health perceptions (see TABLE 13-5 for the dimensions and sample items). The SF-36 has been widely used and has excellent psychometric properties. Research that has used both of these HRQoL scales will be discussed below.

TABLE 13-4 CDC HRQOL-14: Healthy Days Core Module

Please indicate the number of days that represent your response to each item.	# of Days
During the past 30 days, how many days did PAIN make it hard for you to do your usual activities, such as self-care, work, or recreation?	
During the past 30 days, how many days have you felt SAD, BLUE, or DEPRESSED?	
During the past 30 days, how many days have you felt WORRIED, TENSE, or ANXIOUS?	
During the past 30 days, how many days have you felt you did NOT get ENOUGH REST or SLEEP?	
During the past 30 days, how many days have you felt VERY HEALTHY and FULL OF ENERGY?	

Reproduced from National Center for Chronic Disease Prevention and Health Promotion | Division of Population Health.

TABLE 13-5 SF-36 Sample Items

Health Dimension	Scale	Sample Item (paraphrased)
Physical	Physical functioning	Does your health limit you in the amount of vigorous activities you do, such as running, lifting heavy objects, or participating in strenuous sports?
Physical	Physical role functioning	Have you cut down the amount of time you spent on work or other activities because of your physical health?
Physical	Bodily pain	How much bodily pain have you experienced during the past 4 weeks?
Physical and mental	General health perceptions	I am as healthy as anyone I know.
Physical and mental	Vitality	Do you feel full of pep?
Mental	Social role functioning	Has your health interfered with your normal social activities (like visiting friends and relatives)?
Mental	Emotional role functioning	Have you accomplished less than you would like because of any emotional problems (such as feeling depressed or anxious)?
Mental	Mental health	Have you felt downhearted and blue?

Data from Ware, J. E. & Sherbourne, C. D. (1992). The MOS 36-Item Short-Form Health Survey (SF-36): I. Conceptual framework and item selection. *Medical Care*, 30, 473–483.

■ Health–Related Quality of Life, Exercise, and Sedentary Behavior

General Population

Exercise is positively associated with higher HRQoL across the lifespan (Blacklock, Rhodes, & Brown, 2007; Gopinath, Hardy, Baur, Burlutsky, & Mitchell, 2012; Luncheon & Zack, 2011; Penedo & Dahn, 2005). In other words, physical activity enhances people's HRQoL (Bize, Johnson, & Plotnikoff, 2007; Gillison, Skevington, Sato, Standage, & Evangelidou, 2009). For example, data obtained from the Healthy Days Core Module of the CDC HRQOL-14 reveals that physical activity is positively related to HRQoL. With regard to exercise, 11.3% of active people report to be in either fair or poor health, compared to 30.2% of inactive people (National Center for Chronic Disease Prevention and Health Promotion, 2011).

Nonactive people also report poorer physical and mental health than active individuals. For example, nonactive people report that of the past 30 days their physical health was not good for an average of 6.6 days, compared to 2.6 days for active people. Similarly, nonactive people report of the past 30 days that their mental health was not good for 5.1 days, compared to 3.0 for active people. Finally, nonactive people report that of the past 30 days their poor physical or mental health kept them from doing their usual activities (e.g., self-care, work, or recreation activities) for an average of 4.6 days, compared to 1.5 days for active individuals (see FIGURE 13-3).

Whereas physical activity positively influences HRQoL, obesity negatively influences HRQoL. But which has more of an impact on HRQoL, physical activity or weight status? Herman, Hopman, Vanderkerhof, and Rosenberg (2012) attempted to answer this question using a cross-sectional sample of 110,986 adults who completed measures of their HRQoL and activity levels. The researchers found that inactive individuals had a greater likelihood of worse health and activity limitation due to either illness or injury at all body mass index (BMI) levels. Conversely, in active individuals, being underweight, overweight, or obese had little effect on health and activity limitation due to illness or injury. They thus concluded that when examining BMI and physical activity in combination, exercise is the more important correlate of HRQoL, regardless of weight status. This reinforces the importance of physical activity to health outcomes over and above the benefits related to either weight loss or maintenance.

How does sedentary behavior affect HRQoL? The limited research has revealed that people who spend more time engaged in sedentary behaviors such as television viewing, computer and video game use, and reading have lower HRQoL than their less sedentary counterparts (Gopinath et al., 2012).

In addition, it appears that quality of life is a main motivator of physical activity; that is, people start exercising because it contributes to their HRQoL (Bagoien, Halvari, & Nesheim, 2010; Standage, Gillison, Ntoumanis, & Treasure, 2012).

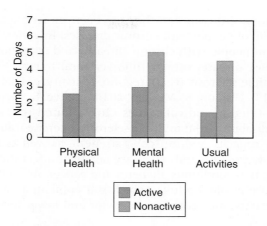

Leisure-Time Physical Activity and Health-Related Quality of Life Responses to the Healthy Days Core Module

Note: Healthy Days Core Module (Questions 2–4)

2. Now thinking about your physical health, which includes physical illness and injury, for how many days during the past 30 days was your physical health not good?
3. Now thinking about your mental health, which includes stress, depression, and problems with emotions, for how many days during the past 30 days was your mental health not good?
4. During the past 30 days, for about how many days did poor physical or mental health keep you from doing your usual activities, such as self-care, work, or recreation?

Data from National Center for Chronic Disease Prevention and Health Promotion. (2011). HRQOL tables and maps. Retrieved March 7, 2014, from http://www.cdc.gov/hrqol/data.htm.

Future research is needed to understand how HRQoL serves as a motivator for both increasing physical activity and for decreasing sedentary behavior.

Health–Related Quality of Life and Exercise in Special Populations

People suffering with chronic diseases such as diabetes, hypertension, asthma, heart disease, and stroke have lower HRQoL than people without these chronic diseases (Jia, Zack, & Thompson, 2013). Thus, it is important to examine ways to increase the HRQoL of these special populations. Common types of interventions to increase HRQoL include behavioral interventions, medication, education, pharmacotherapy, and surgery (Zhang, Norris, Chowdhury, Gregg, & Zhang, 2007).

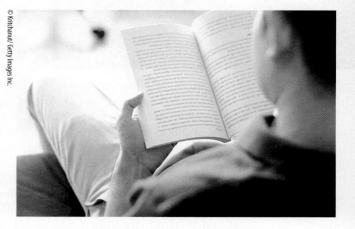

Exercise is also an intervention that has been undertaken in an attempt to improve the HRQoL of people with chronic diseases. In general, physical activity improves HRQoL in people with chronic diseases and conditions such as cancer, chronic pain, kidney disease, osteoporotic vertebral fracture, intermittent claudication, and multiple sclerosis (Giangregorio, Macintyre, Thabane, Skidmore, & Papaioannou, 2013; Guidon & McGee, 2010; Heiwe & Jacobson, 2011). For example, Latimer-Cheung and colleagues (2013) found that among those with mild to moderate disability from multiple sclerosis, exercise training is effective for improving aerobic capacity and muscular strength, as well as HRQoL. Let's take a closer look at how exercise and sedentary behavior affect the HRQoL of people with the following two conditions: diabetes and cancer. As well, we will examine HRQoL and exercise in older adults, which is a population at increased risk for both physical inactivity and sedentary behavior and lower levels of HRQoL than younger populations.

Cancer Populations

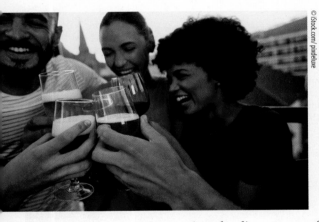

Cancer is a broad group of diseases involving unregulated cell growth. Cancer can affect any part of the body, and its defining feature is the rapid creation of abnormal cells that grow beyond their usual boundaries. These unregulated cells can then invade adjoining parts of the body and spread to other organs. The causes of cancer are diverse, complex, and only partially understood. About 30% of cancer deaths are directly related to the following five risk factors: (1) high BMI, (2) low fruit and vegetable intake, (3) lack of physical activity, (4) tobacco use, and (5) alcohol use.

Cancer is a leading cause of death worldwide, accounting for 8.2 million deaths in 2012 (WHO, 2012). The most common forms of this disease are lung cancer, stomach cancer, liver cancer, colorectal cancer, and breast cancer. Prevalence and incidence rates of cancer are rising largely due to the fact that people are living longer and lifestyle changes resulting in increased obesity and inactivity (Jemal et al., 2011).

A **cancer survivor** is a person with cancer of any type who is still living. The number of cancer survivors in the United States increased from 3 million in 1971 to 9.8 million in 2001 and to 11.7 million in 2007. This represents an increase in cancer survivors from 1.5% to 4% of the U.S. population. Cancer survivors largely consist of people who are 65 years of age or older and women (CDC, 2011). Many people with cancer live a long time after diagnosis.

Cancer survivors face many physical and emotional challenges throughout their treatment and recovery, including persistent and profound adverse effects on their HRQoL. Because HRQoL is an important determinant of cancer survivorship, it is important to examine methods to increase HRQoL in this special population both during and after the end of active treatment. Research reveals that exercise interventions are an advantageous intervention that can improve HRQoL in cancer survivors during active treatment. For example, in a large-scale review, Shiraz Mishra and her colleagues (2012a) found that exercise improves HRQoL in cancer patients undergoing active treatment.

What are the effects of physical activity on cancer survivors who have finished cancer treatment? Shiraz Mishra and her colleagues (2012b) also reviewed this area of research, and they found that exercise had a positive impact on certain HRQoL domains. More specifically, exercise resulted in improvements in body image, self-esteem, emotional well-being, anxiety, social functioning, sleep, and levels of fatigue and pain. No effect of exercise, however, was found on the HRQoL domains of cognitive function, physical functioning, general health perspective, role function, and spirituality.

These meta-analytic findings echo the recent roundtable by the American College of Sports Medicine that exercise is safe during and after cancer treatment and that physical activity results in improved HRQoL for this special population (Schmitz et al., 2010). In fact, the benefits to HRQoL are sufficient for the recommendation that cancer survivors follow the current physical activity guidelines, with specific exercise program adaptations based on disease and treatment-related adverse events.

While exercise is beneficial in improving HRQoL among cancer survivors, evidence is limited on the independent role of sedentary behavior in doing so. Stephanie George and her colleagues (2014) attempted to examine this important research gap. Using a cross-sectional design, they studied the relationship between sedentary behavior and HRQoL among 54 cancer survivors who were, on average, 3.4 years post-diagnosis. At baseline, the researchers objectively measured sedentary time (i.e., amount of waking time spent sitting and lying), moderate- to vigorous-intensity physical activity, and self-reported HRQoL with the SF-36. They found that survivors with higher sedentary time had poorer physical functioning, general health, and physical health. No association was found between sedentary time and role-physical, bodily pain, vitality, social functioning, role-emotional, or mental health. Based on these findings, it appears that sedentary time is associated with aspects of physical HRQoL in cancer survivors.

Diabetic Populations

The term **diabetes** refers to a group of diseases that affect how the body uses blood glucose (also known as blood sugar). People with diabetes have high blood sugar, meaning that they have too much glucose in their blood, which can lead to serious health issues. Worldwide, diabetes is estimated to affect 382 million people, and it is the eighth leading cause of death. The number of people with diabetes is expected to rise to 592 million by 2035 (International Diabetes Foundation, 2014). Understanding how to prevent and treat diabetes is a major public health concern because of its high prevalence and serious negative side effects.

Low levels of HRQoL are associated with increased mortality in people with diabetes (McEwen et al., 2009). Chia-Lin Li and colleagues (Li, Chang, Hsu, Lu, & Fang, 2013) found that increased mortality risk was associated with reduced HRQoL in diabetic patients who reported no exercise, indicating that engaging in exercise may improve survival in diabetic patients who have poor quality of life. As well, Ron Plotnikoff and his colleagues (Imayama, Plotnikoff, Courneya, & Johnson, 2011) found a positive relationship between physical activity levels and HRQoL in diabetic patients.

Older Adults

Older adults are typically defined as persons 60 years of age and older. The world population is rapidly aging. Between 2000 and 2050, the proportion of the world's

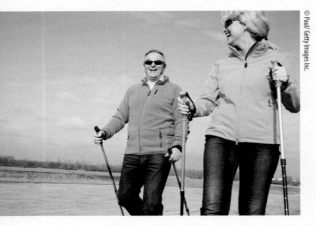

population aged 60 years and older will double from about 11% to 22%. The absolute number of people aged 60 years and older is expected to increase from 605 million to 2 billion over the same period (WHO, 2014). As we become more of an aged society, understanding how HRQoL later in life can be maintained or improved by exercising is an important public health question. A review of the literature examining the relationship between physical activity and quality of life in older adults has found strong evidence for the beneficial effects of physical activity for HRQoL among older adults (Motl & McAuley, 2010).

What about sedentary behavior and HRQoL in older adults? Using a prospective cohort design, Balboa-Castillo and his colleagues (Balboa-Castillo, Leon-Munoz, Rodriguez-Artalejo, & Guallar-Castillon, 2011) examined if both sedentary behavior and exercise were associated with HRQoL in older adults. Participants self-reported their exercise behavior, sedentary behavior (i.e., number of hours sitting per week), and HRQoL using the SF-36. The data were collected on a large representative sample of older adults living in Spain over a 9-year period. The researchers found a positive relationship between exercise behavior and the HRQoL dimensions of physical functioning, physical role, bodily pain, social functioning, vitality, emotional role, and mental health. They also found that the number of sitting hours showed a gradual and inverse relationship with most of the SF-36 scales. In short, the researchers found that more exercise and less sitting were independently associated with better long-term HRQoL in older adults.

In general, increased levels of physical activity and decreased levels of sedentary behavior are related to improving HRQoL in both healthy and diseased populations. As the number of people with chronic diseases increases, further understanding of the dose–response effects of both physical activity and sedentary behavior on HRQoL is needed.

CRITICAL THINKING ACTIVITY 13-3

© ecco/Shutterstock, Inc.

What effect do you think sedentary behavior has on adolescents' HRQoL? Provide research from other populations to justify your response.

Positive Psychology

Psychology traditionally has focused on people with mental illness (e.g., personality disorders, anxiety disorders, and depressive disorders) or other psychological problems and how to treat these issues. **Positive psychology**, by contrast, is a relatively new field that focuses on how to help people prosper and lead healthy, happy lives (Seligman & Csikszentmihalyi, 2000; Seligman, Steen, Park, & Peterson, 2005). Positive psychology was founded on three ideas: that people want to (1) lead meaningful and fulfilling lives, (2) foster what is best within themselves, and (3) enhance their experiences of love, work, and play. Positive psychology has three central concerns: positive emotions, positive individual traits, and positive institutions (see **TABLE 13-6** for a description of these concerns).

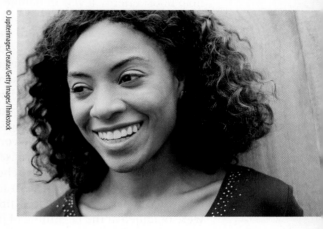

© Jupiterimages/Creatas/Getty Images/Thinkstock

TABLE 13-6 Central Concerns of Positive Psychology	
Concern	**Description of Research Focus**
Positive emotions	Study of contentment with the past, happiness in the present, and hope for the future
Positive individual	Study of strengths and virtues (e.g., capacity for love and work, courage, compassion, resilience, creativity, curiosity, integrity, self-knowledge, moderation, self-control, and wisdom)
Positive institutions	Study of the meaning and purpose as well as the strengths that foster better communities, such as justice, responsibility, civility, parenting, nurturance, work ethic, leadership, teamwork, purpose, and tolerance

Positive Psychology, Exercise, and Sedentary Behavior

Not surprisingly, most of the scientific research in the psychology of exercise and sedentary behavior has focused on the impact of these behaviors on negative psychological states such as depression and anxiety (Wipfli, Rethorst, & Landers, 2008). More recently, researchers have studied the effects of exercise and sedentary behavior on positive mood states such as happiness, vigor, energy, and tranquility (Reed & Ones, 2006). In this section, we will examine how various positive psychology concepts are related to both physical activity and sedentary behavior.

Can exercise give you more energy? It might seem counterintuitive that expending energy through exercise would increase feelings of energy and reduce feelings of fatigue. When a person is tired, the last thing he or she wants to do is exercise. However, research has shown that regular, low-intensity exercise may help boost energy levels in people suffering from fatigue.

Tim Puetz and his colleagues (Puetz, Flowers, & O'Connor, 2008) studied whether exercise can be used to treat fatigue in a laboratory-based exercise study. The participants were 36 young adults who were not regular exercisers and who also complained of persistent fatigue. People who reported fatigue due to serious medical conditions, such as those with chronic fatigue syndrome, were excluded from the study. One group of fatigued adults was randomized to a prescribed 20 minutes of moderate-intensity aerobic exercise three times a week for 6 weeks. The second group of adults engaged in low-intensity aerobic exercise for the same time period. A third group, the control group, did not exercise.

The participants in the exercise conditions exercised on bikes in the laboratory because this enabled the researchers to control their level of exertion. The low-intensity exercise was equivalent to a leisurely, easy walk. The more intense exercise was similar to a fast-paced uphill walk. Vigor and fatigue mood state scores were obtained at the beginning of the third exercise session each week for 6 weeks.

Both of the exercise groups had about a 20% increase in energy levels by the end of the study, compared to the control group. Interestingly, for fatigue, the low-intensity group reported a 65% drop in feelings of fatigue, compared to a 49% drop in the group doing moderate-intensity biking. The researchers concluded that for people with low activity levels, lower-intensity exercise may be the most effective way to reduce fatigue, because a moderate-intensity exercise regime may be too intense for their fitness level.

Meta-analyses provide further confirmation that exercise increases people's feelings of energy and reduces their feelings of fatigue in both healthy populations and populations enrolled in cardiac rehabilitation programs (Puetz, Beasman, & O'Connor, 2006; Puetz, O'Connor, & Dishman, 2006). Thus, lacing up your running shoes and doing some physical activity may provide that burst of energy that you are looking for. Let's take a closer look at these meta-analyses.

Puetz, Beasman, and O'Connor (2006) conducted a meta-analysis to examine the effects of chronic exercise on feelings of energy and fatigue in 70 randomized controlled trials that enrolled a total of 6,807 subjects. They found that chronic exercise increased feelings of energy and lessened feelings of fatigue compared with control conditions (mean ES = .37). In a second meta-analysis, Puetz, O'Connor, and Dishman (2006) found that this positive energy-enhancing effect of exercise was also evidenced in people enrolled in cardiac rehabilitation exercise programs. In their review of 36 studies consisting of a total of 4,765 subjects, they found that exercise improved feelings of energy and decreased fatigue for this special population.

In another meta-analysis, Justy Reed and Deniz Ones (2006) examined the effects of acute aerobic exercise on self-reported positive affect. They reviewed 158 studies with a total sample size of 13,101 participants. They found that people in the exercise groups reported higher positive affect levels compared with the inactive control groups. They also noted that the positive effects of exercise on affect lasted for at least 30 minutes after exercise before returning to baseline levels.

Most of the studies integrated into these meta-analyses refer to either specific exercise programs or to physical activity that is planned and structured. These studies generally do not refer to unstructured daily activities, such as going for a walk or gardening. More recently, researchers have attempted to measure the association between physical activity and mood in everyday life. Understanding this association and the manner in which exercise contributes to enhanced positive feelings in everyday life may help to answer whether people can manage their mood through their lifestyle physical activities.

An interesting research technique called **ecological momentary assessment** enables researchers to comprehensively examine the association between daily mood experience and physical activity because the data are assessed in real time when the assumed effect of exercise on mood happens. Ecological momentary assessment refers to a category of methods that involve the collection of real-time data about current states (e.g., mood, activity) in the natural environment repeatedly over time. This technique reduces recall bias because the data are recorded when events actually occur and enables researchers to obtain data that have higher ecological validity compared with data collected in the laboratory (Stone, Shiffman, Atienza, & Nebeling, 2007). In addition, multiple assessments of mood from each participant allow for higher-power analyses. In short, ecological momentary assessment provides a strong external validity of within-subject variations in physical activity and mood.

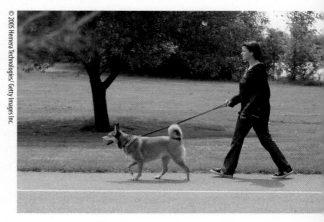

© 2005 Hemera Technologies/ Getty Images Inc.

To date, only a few ecological momentary assessment studies of physical activity and positive mood have been undertaken (Schwerdtfeger, Eberhardt, & Chmitorz, 2008). For example, Heather Hausenblas and her colleagues (Hausenblas, Gaurin, Symons Down, & Duley, 2008) analyzed the effects of abstinence from regular exercise on feeling states with ecological momentary assessment. Participants were deprived of their scheduled exercise on 3 days and maintained their regular exercise routine on 3 other days. After controlling for diurnal variations in mood, they found that feeling states were significantly better after exercise.

In a more recent study, Martina Kanning and Wolfgang Schlicht (2010) examined the relationship between daily activities and mood in healthy people during their everyday life. They had 13 participants complete a standardized diary and report their mood (i.e., valence, energetic arousal, and calmness) over a 10-week period, resulting in 1,860 measurement points. They found that the participants felt more content (valence), awake (energetic arousal), and calm (calmness) after being physically active (e.g., walking and gardening) compared to when they were inactive. They also found that the positive mood–exercise relationship was affected by the individual baseline mood level, with the greatest effect seen when the participants' mood was depressed.

CRITICAL THINKING ACTIVITY 13-4

© ecco/Shutterstock, Inc.

What would you tell someone who says they do not exercise because they are too tired? Is this a valid excuse for not engaging in exercise?

Happiness

A main area of inquiry in positive psychology is how to help people become happier. **Happiness** is a state of mind or a feeling characterized by contentment, love, satisfaction, pleasure, or joy; it is a fundamental human goal. Research in this rapidly growing field often studies what makes people happy and how they can lead fulfilling and satisfying lives. Emerging evidence indicates that happiness also influences health. Conversely, unhappiness (i.e., not being cheerful, joyful, or glad) is related to mental and physical problems such as depression, cardiovascular disease, lower immune response, and a shorter lifespan (Chida & Steptoe, 2008). Positive psychology interventions are designed to raise positive feelings, positive cognitions, and/or positive behaviors, as opposed to interventions aimed at reducing symptoms, problems, or disorders (Bolier et al., 2013).

Chida and Steptoe (2008) conducted a meta-analysis to examine the relationship between positive psychological well-being and physical health in both healthy and diseased populations ($N = 70$ studies). They found that both positive affect (e.g., emotional well-being, positive mood, joy, happiness, vigor, energy) and positive trait-like dispositions (e.g., life satisfaction, hopefulness, optimism, sense of humor) were associated with reduced mortality in healthy and diseased populations. Interestingly, the protective effects of positive psychological well-being were independent of negative affect. The authors concluded that positive psychological well-being has a favorable effect on survival in a variety of populations.

Are people who exercise and stand more often happier? It appears that people who exercise are happier than people who are inactive or sedentary in both the short and the long term (Matheson, 2014; Richards et al., 2015). Wang and colleagues (2012) conducted a longitudinal study to examine the association between changes in leisure-time physical activity and happiness. The participants were 17,276 randomly selected Canadians older than 12 years of age. People who reported clinical depression or the use of antidepressants at baseline or follow-up were excluded from the study. As well, people who reported preexisting unhappiness at baseline were also excluded from the study. To assess happiness, participants answered the following question: "Would you describe yourself as being usually _____" by selecting one of the following predefined responses of: "happy and interested in life," "somewhat happy," "somewhat unhappy," "unhappy with little interest in life," and "so unhappy that life is not worthwhile." The researchers combined "happy and interested in life" with "somewhat happy" responses into an overall "happy" category and combined the remaining responses as "unhappy."

Happy participants were classified as physically active or inactive at baseline and then followed up on to examine whether they became unhappy. The researchers found that people who exercised were less likely to be unhappy after 2 years and 4 years. In contrast, people who were inactive over time were more than twice as likely to be unhappy as those who remained active. Compared with those who became active, inactive participants who remained inactive were also more likely to become unhappy. As well, people who went from active to inactive were more likely to become unhappy. In short, exercise is associated with maintaining happiness and avoiding unhappiness in the long term.

Satisfaction with life is related to peoples' physical and mental health and is a key determinant of happiness throughout the lifespan. Participation in physical activity is related to enhanced satisfaction with life in a variety of populations, including college students, middle-age adults, and older adults (Elavsky & McAuley, 2005; Elavsky et al., 2005; Maher et al., 2013; McAuley et al., 2008). In other words, people report greater satisfaction with life on days when they are more active.

What is the relationship between satisfaction with life and sedentary behavior? Jaclyn Maher and her colleagues (Maher, Doerksen, Elavsky, & Conroy, 2014) examined whether physical activity and sedentary behavior were related to satisfaction of life in college students. They selected college students because satisfaction with life appears to worsen more during young adulthood (18 to 25 years) than any other time in the adult lifespan. Thus, college students represent a high-risk group for decreased satisfaction with life. Using an ecological momentary assessment design, they had 128 college students wear an accelerometer to objectively measure physical activity and sedentary behavior for 14 days.

The participants were also asked to complete self-report assessments of their physical activity, sedentary behavior, and satisfaction with life at the end of each day. To assess satisfaction with life, the study used the following single item: "I was satisfied with my life today." The students rated this item on a visual analogue scale ranging from 0 ("strongly disagree") to 100 ("strongly agree"). They found that the students' daily satisfaction with life was related to greater amounts of physical activity and lower amounts of sedentary behavior. In other words, increasing daily physical activity and reducing daily sedentary behavior can improve satisfaction with life in college students.

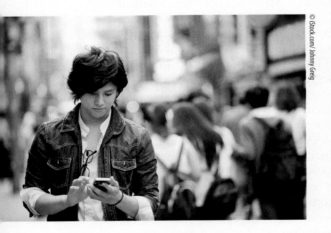

Smartphones are central to college students' lives, keeping them constantly connected with friends, family, and the Internet. Emerging research is revealing that high cell phone use has negative health outcomes. For example, cell phone use is related to lower cardiorespiratory fitness and more sedentary behavior in college students (Lepp, Jacob, Barkley, & Karpinski, 2014). In another study, Andrew Lepp and his colleagues (2013) found that cell phone use is negatively related to GPA and happiness and positively related to anxiety in college students. In other words, high-frequency cell phone users tended to have lower GPAs, higher anxiety, and lower satisfaction with life (happiness) relative to their peers who used their cell phones less often. These results suggest that students should reduce their cell phone use so that it does not negatively affect their academic performance, mental and physical health, and overall well-being or happiness.

CRITICAL THINKING ACTIVITY 13-5

© ecco/Shutterstock, Inc.

Does your cell phone use have a positive or negative affect on your exercise behavior?

Exercise-Induced Feelings

A commonly used measure to assess positive feeling states induced through exercise is the Exercise-Induced Feeling Inventory. This scale was developed by Lise Gauvin and Jack Rejeski (1993) to assess feeling states that people often feel following exercise, such as happy, refreshed, and upbeat. The **Exercise-Induced Feeling Inventory** is a 12-item multidimensional inventory consisting of four 3-item subscales: positive engagement, revitalization, tranquility, and physical exhaustion. Participants are asked to rate the extent to which they are

TABLE 13-7 Items from the Exercise–Induced Feeling Scale	
Subscale	**Items**
Positive engagement	Enthusiastic Happy Upbeat
Revitalization	Refreshed Energetic Revived
Tranquility	Calm Relaxed Peaceful
Physical exhaustion	Fatigued Tired Worn-out

Modified from Gauvin, L., & Rejeski, W. J. (1993). The Exercise-Induced Feeling Inventory: Development and initial validation. *Journal of Sport and Exercise Psychology*, *15*, 403–423.

currently experiencing each of the 12 items on a scale ranging from 0 ("do not feel") to 4 ("feel very strongly"). See **TABLE 13-7** for information on the items from the Exercise-Induced Feeling Inventory.

A common research design is to have participants complete the Exercise-Induced Feeling Inventory immediately before they exercise and then immediately after they finish. Researchers continually have found that people report improvements on all four measures of the Exercise-Induced Feeling Inventory immediately following exercise compared to their pre-exercise scores (Bryan, Pinto Zipp, & Parasher, 2012; Rendi, Szabo, Szabo, Velenczei, & Kovacs, 2008; Szabo & Abraham, 2013). This positive mood–inducing effect is seen for a variety of types of exercises (e.g., aerobic or weight training), exercise levels (regular exercisers, sedentary people), and age groups (young adults and older adults; Annesi, 2002; Annesi & Westcott, 2007). That is, immediately following exercise, people typically report increased positive engagement, revitalization, and tranquility, and decreased physical exhaustion.

Although most of the research reveals that exercise induces positive feelings, there are some exceptions to this "rule." The positive feeling state effect following exercise is not evidenced in all populations and exercise environments. For example, Brian Focht and his colleagues (Focht, Gauvin, & Rejeski, 2004) found that older, obese adults with knee osteoarthritis did not exhibit improvements in feeling states that are often observed following acute exercise in younger, more physically active populations. In another study, Brian Focht and Heather Hausenblas (2006) found that women with high social physique anxiety only had improvements in their Exercise-Induced Feeling State scores when they exercised alone in a private environment. When these women with high social physique anxiety exercised in a public environment (i.e., coed gym), they did not experience improvements in their mood. The researchers hypothesized that for women with high social physique anxiety, exercising in a public coed gym is anxiety provoking. This finding suggests that women with body image concerns may have better adherence to home-based or private exercise compared to gym-based exercise programs.

As another example, outdoor exercise tends to result in better improvements in mood and feeling states compared to indoor exercise. Researchers from Canada found that postmenopausal women reported better affective responses to exercise and exercise adherence during outdoor exercise compared to indoor exercise (Lacharite-Lemieux, Brunelle, & Dionne, 2014). In a 12-week trial, the researchers randomized 23 healthy postmenopausal women (age range = 52 to 69 years) to either an outdoor training or an indoor training exercise program. Each condition exercised three times a week for 1 hour durations of both aerobic and resistance training. After the 12 weeks of exercise, the researchers found that the outdoor exercise group had better improvements in exercise-induced feelings, affect, and depressive symptoms compared to the indoor exercise group. As well, adherence was significantly higher in the outdoor exercise program compared to those who participated in the indoor exercise program.

■ Summary

In this chapter, we examined how physical activity and sedentary behavior affects people's positive mood and health-related quality of life (HRQoL) in a variety of populations. In general, exercise improves people's HRQoL and sedentary behavior decreases people's HRQoL. As well, both acute and chronic bouts of exercise improve our positive mood states. In other words, people who exercise report that they are happier and have more energy than their sedentary counterparts. More research is needed in this emerging area of inquiry.

KEY TERMS

cancer
cancer survivor
diabetes
ecological momentary assessment
Exercise-Induced Feeling Inventory
happiness

health
health-related quality of life (HRQoL)
positive psychology
quality of life
standard of living

REVIEW QUESTIONS

1. Define the terms *quality of life* and *standard of living*. How do these two terms differ? Provide examples.

2. Describe the domains of World Health Organization conceptualization of quality of life.

3. Define *health-related quality of life*.

4. The CDC's Healthy Days Core Module items are useful at the national level to identify health disparities and track population trends. Based on the results of surveys using the module, which groups are more at risk for poor HRQoL?

5. What is ecological momentary assessment? Describe an ecological momentary assessment study and its main findings.

6. What is positive psychology? How is positive psychology related to physical activity and sedentary behavior?

APPLYING THE CONCEPTS

1. What HRQoL domains did Beverly's adoption of physical activity help her improve?

2. How did Beverly's standard of living contribute to her overall quality of life, despite having and being in remission from cancer?

REFERENCES

Annesi, J. J. (2002). Relation of rated fatigue and changes in energy after exercise and over 14 weeks in previously sedentary women exercisers. *Perceptual and Motor Skills, 95,* 719–729.

Annesi, J. J., & Westcott, W. L. (2007). Relations of physical self-concept and muscular strength with resistance Exercise-Induced Feeling State scores. *Perceptual and Motor Skills, 104,* 183–190.

Bagoien, T. E., Halvari, H., & Nesheim, H. (2010). Self-determined motivation in physical education and its links to motivation for leisure-time physical activity, physical activity, and well-being in general. *Perceptual and Motor Skills, 111,* 407–432.

Balboa-Castillo, T., Leon-Munoz, L. M., Rodriquez-Artalejo, F., & Guallar-Castillon, P. (2011). Longitudinal association of physical activity and sedentary behavior during leisure time with health-related quality of life in community-dwelling older adults. *Health and Quality of Life Outcomes, 9,* 1–14.

Bize, R., Johnson, J. A., & Plotnikoff, R. C. (2007). Physical activity level and health-related quality of life in the general adult population: A systematic review. *Preventive Medicine, 45*, 401–415.

Blacklock, R. E., Rhodes, R. E., & Brown, S. G. (2007). Relationship between regular walking, physical activity, and health-related quality of life. *Journal of Physical Activity and Health, 4*, 138–152.

Bolier, L., Haverman, M., Westerhof, G. J., Riper, H., Smit, F., & Bohlmeijer, E. (2013). Positive psychology interventions: A meta-analysis of randomized controlled studies. *BMC Public Health, 13*, 119.

Brown, D. S., Thompson, W. W., Zack, M. M., Arnold, S. E., & Barile, J. P. (2013). Associations between health-related quality of life and mortality in older adults. *Preventive Science*, epub.

Bryan, S., Pinto Zipp, G., & Parasher, R. (2012). The effects of yoga on psychosocial variables and exercise adherence: A randomized, controlled pilot study. *Alternative Therapies in Health and Medicine, 18*, 50–59.

Centers for Disease Control and Prevention (CDC). (2011). Cancer survivors—United States, 2007. *MMWR, 60*, 269–272.

Chida, Y., & Steptoe, A. (2008). Positive psychological well-being and mortality: A quantitative review of prospective observational studies. *Psychosomatic Medicine, 70*, 741–756.

Elavsky, S., & McAuley, E. (2005). Physical activity, symptoms, esteem, and life satisfaction during menopause. *Maturitas, 52*, 374–385.

Elavsky, S., McAuley, E., Motl, R. W., Konopack, J. F., Marquez, D. Z., Jerome, G. J., & Diener, E. (2005). Physical activity enhances long-term quality of life in older adults: Efficacy, esteem, and affective influences. *Annals of Behavioral Medicine, 30*, 138–145.

Focht, B. C., Gauvin, L., & Rejeski, W. J. (2004). The contribution of daily experiences and acute exercise to fluctuations in daily feeling states among older, obese adults with knee osteoarthritis. *Journal of Behavioral Medicine, 27*, 101–121.

Focht, B. C., & Hausenblas, H. A. (2006). Exercising in public and private environments: Effects on feeling states in women with social physique anxiety. *Journal of Applied Biobehavioral Research, 11*, 147–165.

Gauvin, L., & Rejeski, W. J. (1993). The Exercise-Induced Feeling Inventory: Development and initial validation. *Journal of Sport & Exercise Psychology, 15*, 403–423.

George, S. M., Alfano, C. M., Groves, J., Karabulut, Z., Haman, K. L., Murphy, B. A., & Matthews, C. E. (2014). Objectively measured sedentary time is related to quality of life among cancer survivors. *PLoS One, 5*, e87937. doi:10.1371/journal.pone.0087937

Giangregorio, L. M., Macintyre, N. J., Thabane, L., Skidmore, C. J., & Papaioannou, A. (2013). Exercise for improving outcomes after osteoporotic vertebral fracture. *Cochrane Database of Systematic Reviews*, Jan 31;1:CD008618. doi:10.1002/14651858.CD008618.pub2

Gill, D. L., Chang, Y. K., Murphy, K. M., Speed, K. M., Hammond, C. C., Rodriguez, E. A.,... Shang, Y.-T. (2011). Quality of life assessment for physical activity and health promotion. *Applied Research in Quality of Life, 6*, 181–200.

Gillison, F. B., Skevington, S. M., Sato, A., Standage, M., & Evangelidou, S. (2009). The effects of exercise interventions on quality of life in clinical and healthy populations: A meta-analysis. *Social Science and Medicine, 68*, 1700–1710.

Gopinath, B., Hardy, L. L., Baur, L. A., Burlutsky, G., & Mitchell, P. (2012). Physical activity and sedentary behaviors and health-related quality of life in adolescents. *Pediatrics, 130*, e167–e174.

Guidon, M., & McGee, H. (2010). Exercise-based interventions and health-related quality of life in intermittent claudication: A 20-year (1989–2008) review. *European Journal of Cardiovascular Prevention and Rehabilitation, 17*, 140–154.

Hausenblas, H. A., Gauvin, L., Symons Downs, D., & Duley, A. R. (2008). Effects of abstinence from habitual involvement in regular exercise on feeling states: An ecological momentary assessment study. *British Journal of Health Psychology, 13*, 237–255.

Heiwe, S., & Jacobson, S. H. (2011). Exercise training for adults with chronic kidney disease. *Cochrane Database Systematic Review,* Oct 5;(10):CD003236. doi:10.1002/14651858.CD003236.pub2

Herman, K. M., Hopman, W. M., Vanderkerhof, E. G., & Rosenberg, M. W. (2012). Physical activity, body mass index, and health-related quality of life in Canadian adults. *Medicine and Science in Sports and Exercise, 44,* 625–636.

Imayama, I., Plotnikoff, R. C., Courneya, K. S., & Johnson, J. A. (2011). Determinants of quality of life in adults with type 1 and type 2 diabetes. *Health and Quality of Life Outcomes, 9,* 115. doi:10.1186/1477-7525-9-115

International Diabetes Foundation. (2014). *Diabetes atlas.* Retrieved April 13, 2014, from https://www. idf.org/diabetesatlas

Jemal, A., Bray, F., Center, M. M., Ferlay, J., Ward, E., & Forman, D. (2011). Global cancer statistics. *CA: A Cancer Journal for Clinicians, 61,* 69 – 90.

Jia, H., Zack, M. M., & Thompson, W. W. (2013). The effects of diabetes, hypertension, asthma, heart disease, and stroke on quality-adjusted life expectancy. *Value Health, 16,* 140–147.

Kanning, M., & Schlicht, W. (2010). An ecological momentary assessment of physical activity and mood. *Journal of Sport and Exercise Psychology, 32,* 253–261.

Lacharite-Lemieux, M., Brunelle, J. P., & Dionne, I. J. (2014). Adherence to exercise and affective responses: Comparison between outdoor and indoor training. *Menopause, 22,* 731–740.

Latimer-Cheung, A. E., Pilutti, L. A., Hicks, A. L., Martin Ginis, K. A., Fenuta, A. M., MacKibbon, K. A., & Motl, R. W. (2013). Effects of exercise training on fitness, mobility, fatigue, and health-related quality of life among adults with multiple sclerosis: A systematic review to inform guideline development. *Archives of Physical Medicine and Rehabilitation, 94,* 1800–1823.

Lepp, A., Barkley, J. E., Sanders, G. J., Rebold, M., & Gates, P. (2013). The relationship between cell phone use, physical and sedentary activity, and cardiorespiratory fitness in a sample of U.S. college students. *International Journal of Behavioral Nutrition and Physical Activity.* Jun 21;10:79. doi: 10.1186/1479-5868-10-79

Lepp, A., Jacob E., Barkley, A., & Karpinski, C. (2014). The relationship between cell phone use, academic performance, anxiety, and satisfaction with life in college students. *Computers in Human Behavior, 31*: 343. doi:10.1016/j.chb.2013.10.049

Li, C., Chang, H-Y., Hsu, C-C., Lu, J. & Fang, H-L. (2013). Joint predictability of health-related quality of life and leisure-time physical activity on mortality risk in people with diabetes. *BMC Public Health, 13,* 67.

Luncheon, C., & Zack, M. (2011). Health-related quality of life and the physical activity levels of middle-age women, California Health Interview Survey, 2005. *Prevention of Chronic Disease, 8,* A36. Epub.

Maher, J. P., Doerksen, S. E., Elavsky, S., & Conroy, D. E. (2014). Daily satisfaction with life is regulated by both physical activity and sedentary behavior. *Journal of Sport and Exercise Psychology, 36,* 166–178.

Maher, J. P., Doerksen, S. E., Elavsky, S., Hyde, A. L., Pincus, A. L., Ram, N., & Conroy, D. E. (2013). A daily analysis of physical activity and satisfaction with life in emerging adults. *Health Psychology, 6,* 647–656.

Martin Luther King, Jr. (n.d.). BrainyQuote.com. Retrieved September 13, 2015, from BrainyQuote. com. http://www.brainyquote.com/quotes/quotes/m/martinluth297515.html

Matheson, G. (2014). Changing level of physical activity and changing degree of happiness. *Clinical Journal of Sport Medicine, 24,* 162–163.

McAuley, E., Doerksen, S., Morris, K., Motl, R., Hu, L., Wojciki, T. R.,… Rosengren, K. R. (2008). Pathways from physical activity to quality of life in older women. *Annals of Behavioral Medicine, 36,* 13–20.

McEwen, L. N., Kim, C., Haan, M. N., Ghosh, D., Lantz, P. M., Thompson, T. J., & Herman, W. H. (2009). Are health-related quality of life and self-rated health associated with mortality? Insights from translating research into action for diabetes (TRIAD). *Primary Care in Diabetes, 3,* 37–42.

Mishra, S I., Scherer, R. W., Geigle, P. M., Berlanstein, D. R., Topaloglu, O., Gotay, C. C., & Snyder, C. (2012a). Exercise interventions on health-related quality of life for cancer survivors. *Cochrane Database Systematic Review,* Aug 15;*8*:CD007566. doi:10.1002/14651858.CD007566.pub2

Mishra, S. I., Scherer, R. W., Snyder, C., Geigle, P. M., Berlanstein, D. R., & Topaloglu, O. (2012b). Exercise interventions on health-related quality of life for people with cancer during active treatment. *Cochrane Database Systematic Review* Aug 15;*8*:CD008465. doi:10.1002/14651858.CD008465.pub2

Motl, R. W., & McAuley, E. (2010). Physical activity, disability, and quality of life in older adults. *Physical Medicine and Rehabilitation Clinics in North America, 21,* 299–308.

National Center for Chronic Disease Prevention and Health Promotion. (2011). *HRQOL tables and maps.* Retrieved March 7, 2014, from http://www.cdc.gov/hrqol/data.htm

Penedo, F. J., & Dahn, J. R. (2005). Exercise and well-being: A review of mental and physical health benefits associated with physical activity. *Current Opinions in Psychiatry, 18,* 189–193.

Puetz, T. W., Beasman, K. M., & O'Connor, P. J. (2006). The effect of cardiac rehabilitation exercise programs on feelings of energy and fatigue: A meta-analysis of research from 1945 to 2005. *European Journal of Cardiovascular Prevention and Rehabilitation, 13,* 886–893.

Puetz, T. W., Flowers, S. S., & O'Connor, P. J. (2008). A randomized controlled trial of the effect of aerobic exercise training on feelings of energy and fatigue in sedentary young adults with persistent fatigue. *Psychotherapy and Psychosomatics, 77,* 167–174.

Puetz, T. W., O'Connor, P. J., & Dishman, R. K. (2006b). Effects of chronic exercise on feelings of energy and fatigue: A quantitative synthesis. *Psychological Bulletin, 132,* 866–876.

Reed, J., & Ones, D. S. (2006). The effect of acute aerobic exercise on positive activated affect: A meta-analysis *Psychology of Sport and Exercise, 7,* 477–514.

Rendi, M., Szabo, A., Szabo, T., Velenczei, A., & Kovacs, A. (2008). Acute psychological benefits of aerobic exercise: A field study into the effects of exercise characteristics. *Psychology, Health, and Medicine, 13,* 180–184.

Richards, J., Jiang, X., Kelly, P., Chau, J., Bauman, A., & Ding, D. (2015). Don't worry, be happy: Cross-sectional associations between physical activity and happiness in 15 European countries. *BMC Public Health, 15,* 53. doi:10.1186/s12889-015-1391-4

Schmitz, K.H., Courneya, K. S., Matthews, C., Demark-Wahnefried, W., Galvao, D. A.,... American College of Sports Medicine. (2010). American College of Sports Medicine roundtable on exercise guidelines for cancer survivors. *Medicine and Science in Sports & Exercise, 42,* 1409–1426.

Schwerdtfeger, A., Eberhardt, R., & Chmitorz, A. (2008). Gibt es einen Zusammenhang zwischen Bewegungsaktivität und psychischem Befinden im Alltag? [Is there a correlation between everyday-life physical activity and psychological well-being?]. *Zeitschrift für Gesundheitspsychologie, 16,* 2–11.

Seligman, M. E., & Csikszentmihalyi, M. (2000). Positive psychology. An introduction. *The American Psychologist, 55,* 5–14.

Seligman, M. E., Steen, T. A., Park, N., & Peterson, C. (2005). Positive psychology progress: Empirical validation of interventions. *The American Psychologist, 60,* 410–421.

Standage, M., Gillison, F. B., Ntoumanis, N., & Treasure, D. C. (2012). Predicting students' physical activity and health-related well-being: A prospective cross-domain investigation of motivation across school physical education and exercise setting. *Journal of Sport and Exercise Psychology, 34,* 37–60.

Stone, A. A., Shiffman, S., Atienza, A. A., & Nebeling, L. (2007). *The science of real-time data capture: Self-reports in health research.* New York: Oxford University Press.

Szabo, A., & Abraham, J. (2013). The psychological benefits of recreational running: A field study. *Psychology, Health, and Medicine, 18,* 251–261.

Wang, F., Orpanan, H. M., Morrison, H., de Groh, M., Dai, S., & Luo, W. (2012). Long-term association between leisure-time physical activity and changes in happiness: Analysis of the Prospective National Population Health Survey. *American Journal of Epidemiology, 176,* 1085–1100.

Ware, J. E., & Sherbourne, C. D. (1992). The MOS 36-item Short-Form Health Survey (SF-36): I. Conceptual framework and item selection. *Medical Care, 30,* 473–483.

Wipfli, B. M., Rethorst, C. D., & Landers, D. M. (2009). The anxiolytic effects of exercise: A meta-analysis of randomized trials and dose-response analysis. *Journal of Sport and Exercise Psychology, 30,* 392–410.

World Health Organization. (1948). WHO definition of health. Retrieved April 14, 2014, from http://www.who.int/about/definition/en/print.html

World Health Organization. (1997). WHOQOL. Measuring quality of life. Retrieved March 15, 2015, from http://www.who.int/mental_health/media/68.pdf

World Health Organization. (2012). GLOBOCAN 2012: Estimated cancer incidence, mortality, and prevalence worldwide in 2012. Retrieved April 8, 2014, from http://globocan.iarc.fr/Pages/fact_sheets_cancer.aspx

World Health Organization. (2014). Aging and life course. Retrieved April 16, 2014, from http://www.who.int/ageing/en/

Zack, M. M. (2013). Health-related quality of life—United States, 2006 and 2010. *MMWR, 62,* 105–111.

Zack, M. M., Moriarty, D. G., Stroup, D. F., Ford, E. S., & Mokdad, A. H. (2004). Worsening trends in adult health-related quality of life and self-rated health-United States, 1993–2001. *Public Health Reports, 119,* 493–506.

Zhang, X., Norris, S. L., Chowdhury, F. M., Gregg, E. W., & Zhang, P. (2007). The effects of interventions on health-related quality of life among persons with diabetes: A systematic review. *Medical Care, 45,* 820–834.

Exercise-Related Disorders

Vignette: Katie

It began when I was living with 14 other girls at a residential facility in Connecticut, designed to provide support to emotionally troubled teens. In the 45 minutes a day I was permitted privacy in my own room, I spun through 100 repetitions of lunges, squats, jumping jacks, crunches, and as many pushups as I could manage. All in the hopes of proving to myself, to my body, that I had control over something: that I could make myself smaller.

I'd arrived at the residential facility following a 9-week stay at a boot camp program in Naples, Idaho, that my parents believed might put an end to my pot smoking, my self-harm, and my promiscuity. I was barely 13. Their confusion and concern and their own painful divorce added up to me being too much for either of them to handle. So they sent me away.

Since middle school, I saw my body as defective. I was the last girl in my grade to develop breasts, and the first to be excluded from popular lunch tables and after-school gatherings buzzing with queen bees. I intuited something was inherently wrong with me. And that belief took root in my nascent identity, growing over time into a lifelong self-loathing, fueled by a hypervigilance toward how big or how loud or how unattractive I might, at any moment, suddenly become. I did not believe I could let my guard down. Ever. I felt I always had to be doing something to make myself better. Relaxation and pleasure quickly became enemies.

LEARNING OBJECTIVES

After completing this chapter, you will be able to

- Describe the criteria for a diagnosis of exercise dependence, anorexia nervosa, bulimia nervosa, and muscle dysmorphia.
- Describe the relationship between physical activity and eating disorders.
- Outline the psychological effects of muscle dysmorphia.
- Understand the difference between primary and secondary exercise dependence.

The first culprit was my face. In sixth grade, I'd hide in the bathroom with a turtleneck sweater pulled up over my lips and my nose, refusing to return to class for fear I was too ugly to be seen. The second culprit was my legs—too chicken-like, I thought. I wanted a round backside. Thicker thighs, like my female classmates who got to bask in male attention. I thought if I looked more like them, I wouldn't be as inferior—so unloveable.

Ironically, I strove toward putting on weight at first, hoping to be softer around my edges like the girls at the top of the social totem pole. Then, as time went on and I learned what society deemed attractive—heard the praise heaped on those who could keep their figures in check—my drive to grow larger reversed course. Minimization—reaching my smallest possible size—took precedence above all other goals.

I grew up in Manhattan, a city stuffed to the brim with conspicuous thinness. Women were lauded for svelte physiques and shamed for even the slightest suggestions of corpulence. My father chastised my mother for how high the numbers got on our bathroom scale after she gave birth to me.

"I just stopped finding her attractive," he would say to me over phone calls after he'd moved out.

And when I reached for a box of cookies in his new apartment, he looked at me coldly and said, "You don't want to look like your mother, do you?"

After I left the residential facility and returned to high school—sober now, and hell-bent on getting perfect grades so as to disprove my teachers' assumptions that I would be some kind of failure—I discovered the gym. Here was another tool to aid me in manipulating my body—in pummeling myself into something tighter, smaller, more productively controlled. Even better, I could use "having to work out" as an excuse to escape the social anxiety I felt whenever asked to "hang out" with friends.

The gym organized me. It gave me a schedule. It justified and dictated whatever I ate. Carbs were permissible if used as fuel. Protein and fat, for recovery. Several months into a regular routine, I began to find satisfaction in what I saw in the mirror. To like my own reflection was intoxicating enough to keep me coming back. I was not used to taking pride in my body. And I clung to this new transient confidence, terrified to return to its absence. This meant hitting the gym constantly. Daily. Avoiding stillness at all costs.

Working out wove itself into the fabric of who I was. "Gym rat." "Yoga freak." "Exercise addict," people would call me. All compliments to my stubborn prioritization of burning calories over developing meaningful relationships or spending any modicum of extended time with my family.

By the time I entered college, my world revolved around the gym. No sooner would I finish a class than I'd dash off to the campus fitness center. I'd dabbled in treatment at an outpatient eating disorder clinic prior to my freshman year, but I was unsatisfied by their focus on food. Sure, I had issues surrounding what I ate. But my main problem was my compulsive zeal for physical activity. I had to get to the gym or else anxiety, depression, self-hatred, and a crumbling sense of helplessness would consume me. No matter how tired or sick or stressed or busy I was, I would go. Getting on that elliptical machine, going for that run, lifting those weights, or cycling through that yoga routine was nonnegotiable. Few treatment professionals I met with seemed to understand this and approach it as its own unique disorder.

By the time I graduated college, 99 pounds gripping my 5-foot, 6-inch frame, I could count on two hands the number of friendships and career opportunities I'd lost due to being barely available outside my exercise schedule.

Injuries ensued. By 26 I'd weathered two herniated discs in my spine, a stress fracture in my left foot, and a persistent exhaustion that, no matter how much sleep I got in between gym sessions, never abated. Though I would seek treatment for exercise addiction time and again, my obsession with burning calories and lifting weights would creep back into my life, leaking around the edges of whatever job or hobby or interest outside physical activity I managed to take hold of.

Though I have been able to find love and connection, my ability to participate in relationships is severely limited by my obsession with working out. I feel lucky to have a life partner who tries his best not to take my compulsions personally, and squeezes himself into the narrow time slots left around my hours spent exercising.

Traveling is incredibly difficult for me. My obsessiveness surrounding my routines has grown so thick that even most hotel gym equipment won't suffice. I crave the specificities of my home gym's setup. So enmeshed have I become in my routine that I am terrified to face change, to be uprooted from that which I know offers me a respite from anxiety— over my appearance, at the prospect of losing control, or the overwhelming nature of any given day's tasks. I am equally addicted to the familiarity of my rituals surrounding physical activity as I am to its physiological effects. I know that the behavior has more control over me than I have over it. Yet it is so much of who I am that I can't unravel myself from the transient solace that comes after each daily exercise session.

I want to believe there will be a day when I can sit still in my skin. When I won't wake up dreading the 2-hour workouts I can't seem to say no to, despite the havoc they wreak on my schedule, my mental stability, and my connections to other people. But I know from over 25 years of being in this body, being trapped in this cycle, that it's going to take years to undo the habitual self-abuse that is my daily routine. And the saddest part of all of this to me is that no matter how haggard I look at the gym, or how sick I feel myself to be, there is always someone—a fellow gym-goer, a trainer—who waits for me to come out of a handstand or demount an elliptical machine to tell me, "whatever you're doing, keep it up—it's great."

Introduction

Since the "fitness boom" of the 1970s, much has been written about the benefits of exercise. Everywhere we turn, we hear that we should be more physically active, and with good reason given all of the physiological, psychological, and social benefits of being physically active. Does an activity associated with so many benefits have the potential to be harmful? The answer seems to be, it depends. The following quote by Carl Gustav Jung, the founder of **analytical psychology**, held the belief that any type of addiction is negative. According to Jung (1957), "Every form of addiction is bad, no matter whether the narcotic be alcohol, morphine, or idealism." Although he did not specifically address addiction to physical activity, presumably he would view it as negative.

Many people become physically active to become healthy and to look and feel better. But physical activity may become addictive for a small number of people. It is important to emphasize that while exercise may represent an addictive behavior for a small number of people who engage in it to an extreme and unhealthy level, habitual exercise is not inherently abusive. This chapter focuses on the following three exercise-related disorders that are all associated with excessive physical activity: (1) exercise dependence, (2) eating disorders, and (3) muscle dsymorphia. In this chapter, we will define each of these three exercise-related disorders, describe their significance, and examine the role that exercise plays in each.

Exercise Dependence

Does Exercise Have Negative Health Effects?

Current exercise guidelines identify the minimum amount of exercise needed to experience health benefits. For the general adult population, the guidelines call for at least 150 minutes per week of moderate physical activity or 75 minutes per week of vigorous physical activity (Haskell et al., 2007). These guidelines also note that an increased amount of exercise is associated with additional benefits (U.S. Department of Health and Human Services, 2008). Although increased amounts of exercise above the minimum guidelines are encouraged, no cutoff exists for "how much is too much." Furthermore, although the guidelines also caution that high-intensity exercise increases the risk of musculoskeletal injuries and adverse cardiovascular events, it is unknown at which point increased exercise may become detrimental to one's health (La Gerche, Robberect, & Kuiperi, 2010).

Recent research is beginning to shed a bit of light on the notion that there may be a point at which too much exercise may have detrimental physical health effects. We know that a routine of regular exercise is highly effective for preventing and treating many common chronic diseases and improving cardiovascular health and longevity. However, long-term excessive endurance exercise may induce cardiovascular health issues such as pathological structural remodeling of the heart and large arteries (O'Keefe, Patil, & McCullough, 2012). Emerging data suggest that chronic training for and competing in extreme endurance events such as marathons, **ultramarathons**, **ironman triathlons**, and very long distance bicycle races can cause short-term negative cardiovascular effects. For example, among a group of patients diagnosed with coronary artery disease, those who exercised beyond the recommended 60-minute maximum saw decreases in their antioxidant levels as well as stiffening of their blood vessels (Michaelides et al., 2011). In comparison, those patients who exerted themselves within a more reasonable range saw a reduction in free radicals and improved circulation.

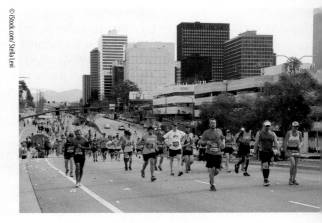

In a large-scale study, researchers found that an upper limit of exercise exists in which the longevity benefits of exercise level off but do not decrease (Arem et al., 2015). Researchers compared the mortality rates with the physical activity levels among 661,137 men and women over a 14-year period in an effort to understand the dose–response relationship between exercise and mortality. In support of the exercise guidelines, they found that adhering to the 2008 Physical Activity Guidelines for Americans of 75 minutes a week of vigorous-intensity or 150 minutes a week of moderate-intensity physical activity significantly reduced mortality. More specifically, they found that adults who either met or engaged in twice the guideline recommendations (i.e., 7.5 to 14.9 METs per week) lowered their risk of mortality by 31%. In comparison, adults who exceeded the recommendations by two to three times (i.e., 15 METs to 22.4 METs per week) saw a 37% decrease in their risk of mortality. An upper threshold for mortality benefit occurred at three to five times the physical activity recommendations. However, compared with the recommended minimum, the additional benefit was modest (i.e., 31% vs. 39%). Of interest, there was no evidence that engaging in 10 or more times the recommended minimum amount of physical activity for health benefits resulted in negative health effects. The researchers concluded that the additional benefit of increased activity was modest, such that meeting the recommended physical activity guidelines was associated with nearly the maximum longevity benefit. While spending large amounts of time engaging in physical activity did not necessarily translate into increased longevity, the researchers found no support for the opposite hypothesis—that there is an upper limit to physical activity beyond which increased activity negatively impacts mortality.

Another study found a very high rate of myocardial fibrosis among lifelong endurance athletes (Wilson et al., 2011). Specifically, the researchers found that 50% of athletes who underwent cardiac magnetic resonance imaging (MRI) displayed signs of the difficult to detect hardening of cardiac cells. This hardening of cardiac cells may play a role in precipitating sudden cardiac arrest or, at the very least, induce an irregular heartbeat (Wilson et al., 2011). And although runners who logged between 0.15 and 15 miles per week (a wide range, indeed) benefited from an estimated 19% reduction in mortality rates, those who consistently surpassed 25 weekly miles had a risk of death comparable to those who did not exercise. Although this preliminary research found that for some individuals long-term excessive endurance exercise can cause adverse health issues, additional research is warranted to determine if a cutoff exists for how much exercise is too much.

CRITICAL THINKING ACTIVITY 14-1

© ecco/Shutterstock, Inc.

Do you think there is a point at which one can engage in too much exercise? In other words, is there a point at which increased exercise duration frequency or intensity may have negative health outcomes?

We do know, however, that for a very small number of people physical activity goes into overdrive. Rather than exercise enhancing their lives, it ends up assuming a life of its own (Cook & Hausenblas, 2012). These people continue to exercise despite injuries, mental health issues, and physical exhaustion. They may even watch their careers crumble and their family and friends drift away. This perspective is illustrated in the following two quotes:

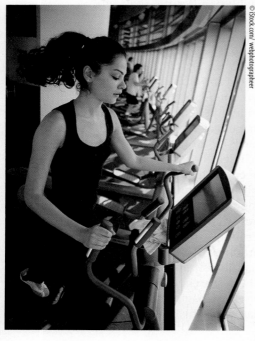

© iStock.com/ webphotographeer

I have learned there is no need for haste, no need to worry, no need to agonize over the future … The world will wait. Job, family, friends will wait; in fact, they must wait on the outcome. And that outcome depends upon the lifetime that is in every day of running … Can anything have a higher priority than running? It defines me, adds to me, makes me whole. I have a job and a family and friends that can attest to that.

(Quote from avid runner, Dr. George Sheehan, in Waters, 1981, p. 51)

As the years went on, I inevitably developed those aches and pains brought about by refusing to rest and pushing through discomfort… Against my doctor's orders, I stuck to my rigorous, daily workouts of 2 (or more) hours a day. The vast majority of that time was spent hunched over an elliptical machine, pursing my lips and wincing through pain. I refused to have surgery, as was clinically recommended, because it would mean too much time off from the gym.

(Schreiber & Hausenblas, 2015, p. 81)

The term often used to describe this compulsive behavior is *exercise dependence*. Other terms used to describe exercise dependence include *exercise addiction*, *compulsive exercise*, and *obligatory exercise*. In this section, we discuss exercise dependence with regard to how it is defined, what researchers have to say about it, and how it might be treated.

Exercise Dependence Defined

Descriptions of exercise dependence have focused on the following: (1) behavioral correlates, including physical activity duration, intensity, frequency, or history; (2) psychological correlates, such as a pathological commitment to physical activity; or (3) a combination of both behavioral and psychological correlates. However, just because someone runs 6 days a week for 45 minutes a session or has been regularly weight lifting for 3 years does not mean that he or she is exercise dependent. In fact, there are thousands of people who can be physically active 5, 6, or even 7 days a week who *should not and could not* be classified as exercise dependent. Dependence is indicated not only by the behavior, but also by the psychological reasons underlying that behavior.

Current exercise guidelines identify the minimum amount of exercise needed to experience health benefits (see **TABLE 14-1**). The guidelines also recommend that an increased amount of exercise is associated with additional benefits (USDHHS, 2008). For example, exercising for more than 300 minutes a week at a moderate intensity is associated with additional health benefits. Although increases above the minimum guidelines are encouraged, no cutoff exists for "how much is too much." Researchers have attempted to determine if there is an upper limit of activity above which there are no additional health benefits.

Recent research has shed some preliminary insight into the question of "how much is too much" from a mental health perspective. Research conducted with adolescents aged 16 to 20 years and adults revealed that very high levels of exercise results in decreased well-being (Kim et al., 2012; Merglen, Flatz, Belanger, Michaud, & Suris, 2014). Further research is needed to clearly determine, however, at which point physical activity may become detrimental to one's health in varying populations.

TABLE 14-1 Adult Guidelines by Physical Activity Level and Health Benefit		
Physical Activity Level	**Moderate-Intensity Minutes per Week**	**Health Benefit**
Inactive	None	None
Low	< 150	Some
Medium	150–300	Substantial
High	> 300	Additional

Determining when "regular exercise" becomes excessive, and thus detrimental to an individual's physical and psychological health, is often referred to as exercise dependence (Berczik et al., 2012). Simply stated, **exercise dependence** is a craving for leisure-time physical activity that results in uncontrollably excessive exercise behavior that manifests itself in physiological (e.g., tolerance) and/or psychological (e.g., withdrawal) symptoms (Hausenblas & Symons Downs, 2002a). Characteris-

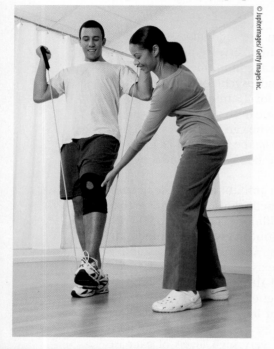

tics of exercise dependence include exercising despite either injury or illness; experiencing withdrawal effects; and giving up social, occupational, and family obligations to exercise (Hausenblas & Symons Downs, 2002a). Exercise dependence may also play a pivotal role in explaining the function of exercise behavior in the development and maintenance of body image disturbance and eating disorders.

The operational definition that has received the most recognition was presented by David DeCoverely Veale (1987, 1995). He advocated the adoption of a set of standards for diagnosing exercise dependence that are based on the American Psychiatric Association's *Diagnostic and Statistical Manual for Mental Disorders, Fourth Edition* (DSM-IV) criteria for substance dependence (APA, 2013). The DSM provides a classification system for mental disorders.

Expanding upon Veale's suggestion, Hausenblas and Symons Downs (2002a) stated that exercise dependence can be defined as a multidimensional maladaptive pattern of physical activity, leading to significant impairment or distress, as manifested

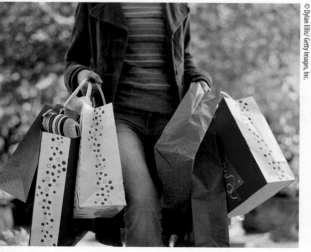

by *three or more* criteria from a list of seven (APA, 2000). The seven criteria for exercise dependence are listed in **TABLE 14-2** . For example, if a person reports feelings of anxiety and depression when unable to exercise, spends little to no time with family or friends because of physical activity involvement, and continues to run despite a doctor's advice to allow an overuse injury to heal, he or she could potentially be classified as exercise dependent.

It is important to note that exercise dependence (or exercise addiction, as it is also commonly referred to) is not included in the DSM-5 (APA, 2013) as a mental disorder. The substance-related disorders section of the DSM-5 includes only gambling as a form of

TABLE 14-2 Exercise Dependence Criteria

Criteria	Description	Example
Tolerance	Need for increased exercise levels to achieve the desired effect, or diminished effects experienced from the same exercise level.	Running 5 miles no longer results in improved mood.
Withdrawal	Negative symptoms are evidenced with cessation of exercise, or exercise is used to relieve or forestall the onset of these symptoms.	Anxiety, depression, and/or fatigue experienced when unable to exercise.
Intention	Exercise is undertaken with greater intensity, frequency, or duration than was intended.	Intended to run for 5 miles, but ran for 7 miles instead.
Lack of control	Exercise is maintained despite a persistent desire to cut down or control it.	Ran during lunch break despite trying to not exercise during work hours.
Time	Considerable time is spent in activities essential to exercise maintenance.	Vacations are exercise related, such as skiing or hiking.
Reduction in other activities	Social, occupational, or recreational pursuits are reduced or dropped because of exercise.	Running rather than going out with friends for dinner.
Continuance	Exercise is maintained despite the awareness of a persistent physical or psychological problem.	Running despite shin splints.

addiction that does not involve ingestion of a substance, reflecting evidence that this repetitive behavior activates the brain's reward system similar to that seen with drugs of abuse. According to the American Psychiatric Association, all other potentially addictive behaviors—not just exercise, but also sex, Internet browsing, and shopping—require further research before unequivocally being denoted as uniquely diagnosable pathologies. In other words, more research is need before exercise addiction/dependence is considered a mental disorder in the DSM.

CRITICAL THINKING ACTIVITY 14-2

© ecco/Shutterstock, Inc.

Do you think that exercise addiction should be included in the DSM as a behavioral addiction?

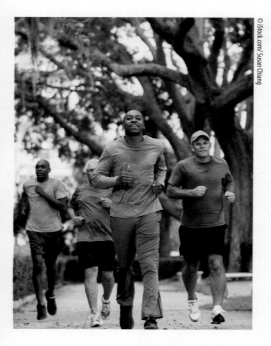

© iStock.com/ Susan Chiang

Origins of Research on Exercise Dependence

Exercise dependence was first identified by "accident" by Frederick Baekeland over 45 years ago. He wanted to study the common belief that exercise promotes sound or deep sleep by conducting a 1-month longitudinal study on the effects of exercise deprivation (i.e., no physical activity) on sleep. Two key study findings led him to the conclusion that some people may become addicted to physical activity. First, he encountered great difficulty recruiting habitual male exercisers (i.e., individuals who exercised 5 to 6 days a week) who were willing to abstain from physical activity for 1 month. In fact, no amount of money was sufficient to persuade these habitual runners to participate in the study. He finally was able to recruit men who regularly exercised 3 to 4 days a week. Second, during the 1-month deprivation period, participants reported decreased psychological well-being.

Baekeland (1970) realized the importance of these complaints and designed a self-report questionnaire to assess the participants' distress sensations. He found that the participants retrospectively reported that their exercise deprivation of 1 month caused increased anxiety, nocturnal awakening and arousal, and decreased sexual drive. In short, he found that habitual runners refused to abstain from physical activity for a 1-month period, whereas regular runners reported withdrawal symptoms during physical activity deprivation.

Subsequent early researchers debated the differences between positive versus negative addiction and whether excessive physical activity could be harmful (Glasser, 1976; Morgan, 1979). William Glasser (1976) argued that excessive physical activity is a positive addiction because of its many beneficial effects on self-esteem, mood, and anxiety. He also claimed that running is "the hardest but surest way to positive addiction" (p. 100).

In contrast, William Morgan (1979) pointed to the increasing number of overuse injuries and the social and occupational problems present in individuals who ran "excessively." As a consequence, he concluded that, for some runners, the benefits of physical activity may be offset by a negative addiction. The common belief held today is that exercise dependence represents a negative addiction.

Subsequently, exercise addiction has been replaced by a variety of terms such as *exercise dependence*, *obligatory exercise*, *compulsive exercise*, *committed exercisers*, *morbid exercise*, *exercise abuse*, *habitual exercise*, and *chronic exercise*. **TABLE 14-3** lists the most commonly applied terms that attempt to define exercise dependence (Hausenblas & Symons Downs, 2002a). Typically, the terms indicate pathological

TABLE 14-3	Terms Used to Describe Exercise Dependence		
Addiction	**Commitment**	**Exercise**	**Running**
Bodybuilder addiction	Attitudinal commitment	Exercise dependence	Compulsive running
Exercise addiction	Exercise commitment	Excessive exercise	Chronic jogging
Negative addiction	Running commitment	Fitness fanaticism	Habitual running
Running addiction	Obsessive commitment	Obligatory exercise	High-intensity running
			Running dependence
			Obligatory running

attitudes and excessive amounts of exercise in the context of addiction, commitment, problems related to exercise in general, and running-specific factors. It is not always apparent whether the various terms represent the same phenomenon because operational definitions are often not provided. This has resulted in a body of literature with no consensus regarding the causes, consequences, and correlates of exercise dependence.

Despite a slow and controversial beginning, in recent years increased interest in exercise dependence has been observed. In general, the exercise dependence research is characterized by four general approaches: (1) comparing exercisers to eating disorder patients (this literature is discussed in a subsequent section in this chapter), (2) determining the prevalence of exercise dependence, (3) examining correlates of exercise dependence, and (4) examining the effects of exercise deprivation on mood (Hausenblas & Symons Downs, 2002a). Each of these research areas will be discussed in more detail in this chapter.

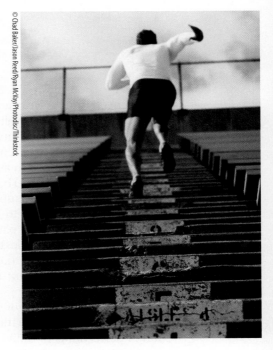

© Chad Baker/Jason Reed/Ryan McVay/Photodisc/Thinkstock

Prevalence of Exercise Dependence

Prevalence represents the proportion of a population found to have a condition. Researchers have been interested in trying to determine how many people are exercise dependent. Several studies have attempted to answer this question, but inconsistent results have emerged largely because of the measures used and the small sample size of the target population participating in either a specific sport

TABLE 14-4	Sample Items from the Exercise Dependence Scale
Subscale	**Item**
Tolerance	I continually increase my exercise duration to achieve the desired effects/benefits.
Withdrawal effects	I exercise to avoid feeling tense.
Continuance	I exercise despite persistent physical problems.
Lack of control	I am unable to reduce how intense I exercise.
Reduction in other activities	I choose to exercise so that I can get out of spending time with family/friends.
Time	A great deal of my time is spent exercising.
Intention effects	I exercise longer than I plan.

Data from Hausenblas, H. A., & Symons Downs, D. (2002b). How much is too much? The development and validation of the Exercise Dependence Scale. *Psychology and Health: An International Journal, 17*, 387–404.

or activity (Berczik et al., 2012). In an attempt to overcome limitations of past prevalence studies, Heather Hausenblas and Danielle Symons Downs (2002b) examined exercise dependence symptoms in over 2,300 exercisers who varied in their physical activity involvement using a standardized exercise dependence measures. The Exercise Dependence Scale (see ▆TABLE 14-4▆ for sample items from this measure) was used to assess the prevalence of exercise dependence in a physically active population. This scale operationalizes exercise dependence based on the DSM-IV criteria for substance dependence. When completing the scale, the participants were asked to refer to their current exercise beliefs and behaviors that had occurred in the past 3 months. The researchers found that about 7% of the exercisers could be classified as at risk for exercise dependence, 61% as nondependent-symptomatic (i.e., displayed some exercise dependence symptoms), and 32% as nondependent-asymptomatic (i.e., displayed no exercise dependence symptoms).

Hausenblas and Symons Downs (2002b) also found a hierarchy of responses for the degree of participation in vigorous exercise, self-efficacy, and the disposition of perfectionism. Individuals classified as at risk for being exercise dependent scored higher on self-efficacy and perfectionism and engaged in more vigorous exercise than those classified as nondependent-symptomatic, and individuals classified as nondependent-symptomatic scored higher than the individuals classified as nondependent-asymptomatic. The study was based exclusively on self-report measures and was correlational in design. Therefore, cause–effect conclusions are not possible. It is not possible to say, for example, that being perfectionistic causes an individual to be exercise dependent.

Brian Cook and his colleagues (2013) examined exercise dependence prevalence in a large sample of 2,660 long-distance runners. They found that the overall prevalence of exercise dependence was only 1.5%. They also found that runners who ran longer distances were more at risk for exercise dependence, in that those individuals who ran longer distance races (i.e., half marathon and marathon) reported higher exercise dependence symptoms than those who ran shorter races (i.e., 10K and 5K distances).

The largest prevalence study to date was conducted with a national representative sample of 2,710 Hungarian adults between the ages of 18 and 64 years (Monok et al., 2012). Of this total sample, the 474 people who reported exercising at least once a week were asked to complete exercise dependence and addiction questionnaires. Based on their responses to the Exercise Dependence Scale, the researchers found that 0.3% of the people could be identified as being at risk for exercise dependence. These research-based estimates are in concordance with the argument that exercise addiction is relatively rare, especially when compared to other addictions (Sussman, Lisha, & Griffiths, 2011). Nevertheless, given the severity of the problem, even a tenth of positive diagnoses among the at-risk cases may be large. In other words, a prevalence of 0.3% translates into 30 cases of exercise dependence for every 10,000 people.

Researchers have also sought to determine the prevalence of exercise dependence with other types of addictions. In other words, do people who are addicted to exercise also have a higher chance of being addicted to other behaviors (e.g., shopping, Internet use, gambling, smartphone use) or substances (e.g., nicotine, alcohol)? Emerging research is revealing that there may be a high co-occurrence of exercise addiction with other types of addictions (Di Nicola et al., 2015).

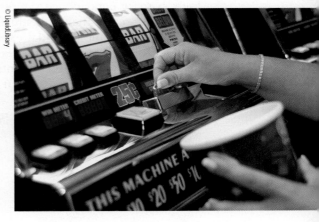
© LiquidLibrary

In a sample of 125 members of a fitness club in Paris, Michael Lejoyeux and his colleagues (Lejoyeux, Avril, Embouazza, & Nivoli, 2008) found that exercise addiction was associated with compulsive buying. And in a sample of 2,853 Italian high school students, Villella and colleagues (2011) found that exercise addiction, compulsive buying, Internet addiction, and work addiction were significantly correlated. The authors concluded that the strong relationship among these different addictions is in line with the hypothesis of a common psychopathological dimension underlying them.

CRITICAL THINKING ACTIVITY 14-3

© ecco/Shutterstock, Inc.

Do you think that being addicted to a behavior, such as exercise, puts a person at risk for other types of addictions? Why or why not?

Correlates of Exercise Dependence

Researchers have been interested in examining correlates or variables that will help identify if someone may be more at risk for exercise dependence. Several demographic and psychological correlates of exercise dependence have been identified. These correlates of exercise dependence are described in more detail in the following discussion and summarized in **TABLE 14-5** .

Personality

Researchers have found that exercise dependence symptoms are associated with certain personality characteristics. For example, Grandi and his colleagues (Grandi, Clementi, Guidi, Benassi, & Tossani, 2011) found that people reporting exercise dependence had more anxiety, hostility, and harm-avoidance behaviors than nonexercise-dependent adults. In another study, Hausenblas and Giacobbi (2004) had 390 American university students complete the Exercise Dependence Scale and the NEO Big Five personality measure. They found positive relationships between exercise dependence symptoms and extraversion and neuroticism and a negative relationship between exercise dependence symptoms and agreeableness. These study findings have been supported by Cecilie Andereassen and colleagues' (2013) research with Norwegian undergraduate students. They also found a positive relationship between exercise dependence and extraversion and neuroticism and a negative relationship with agreeableness. In other words, people reporting high exercise dependence symptoms may be more extraverted, more neurotic, and less agreeable than individuals low in exercise dependence symptoms.

What are some potential explanations for why agreeableness, extraversion, and neuroticism are related to exercise dependence symptoms? Highly neurotic people have limited impulse control, cope poorly with stress, and are often irrational (Costa & McCrae, 1990). It is plausible that people reporting high exercise

TABLE 14-5	Correlates of Exercise Dependence Symptoms	
Category	**Correlate**	**Relationship**
Demographic	Age	Younger adults report more EDS than older adults.
	Gender	Men are more at risk for primary EDS than women.
Psychological	Extraversion	Positive relationship
	Neuroticism	Positive relationship
	Agreeableness	Negative relationship
	Perfectionism	Positive relationship
	Self-esteem	Negative relationship

EDS = exercise dependence symptoms

dependent symptoms may be using exercise as a maladaptive coping strategy for their stress. People who display high neuroticism scores may be prone to excessive worry or concern over their appearance or their health. Therefore, in an effort to reduce these concerns, neurotic individuals may use excessive exercise as a maladaptive coping strategy to either avoid or relieve their withdrawal symptoms.

People with high extraversion are characterized as assertive, energetic, active, upbeat, and as liking excitement. Because a behavioral component of exercise dependence is excessive exercise, it may not be surprising that these individuals report being more energetic, active, and upbeat. Finally, people low in agreeableness tend to be egocentric, skeptical of others' intentions, and competitive (Costa & McCrae, 1992). These people may also view flattery or deception as a necessary social skill. Thus, less sympathetic, altruistic, and cooperative people tend to have more exercise addiction symptoms.

Age

Regarding the relationship between age and exercise dependence, most studies have examined college students. Depending on the sample size and the degree of sophistication of the research design, this can produce valuable information and insights regarding exercise dependence in general. However, the focus on college students and the absence of cross-sectional analyses from different age groups of exercisers makes it difficult to explore risk factors for exercise dependence prevalence by age. Szabo (2000) stated that the prevalence for exercise dependence should decline with age as older exercisers develop a more balanced lifestyle. Furthermore, because of the negative linear relationship between exercise and age, it is likely that a negative relationship also exists between exercise dependence and age, with older adults being less at risk for exercise dependence than their younger counterparts (Sussman et al., 2011).

In support of this, Edmunds and colleagues (2006) found that younger participants (aged 34 years and younger) had higher exercise dependence scores than those 35 years of age and older. As well, Sebastiano Costa and his colleagues (Costa, Hausenblas, Oliva, Cuzzocrea, & Larcan, 2013) found that exercise dependence symptoms declined with age, with the "middle-age adults" (aged 45 to 64 years) reporting lower exercise dependence scores than the "adults" (25 to 44 years) and the "young adults" (18 to 24 years). This may be due to the fact that physical activity levels decrease gradually with age and that older adults may be able to regulate their emotions better than younger adults, thus reducing their risk of exercise dependence.

Limited research, however, has examined exercise dependence in younger populations. One exception is a research study conducted by Danielle Symons Downs and her colleagues (Symons Downs, Savage, & DiNallo, 2013) that examined exercise dependence symptoms in 805 adolescent boys and girls. They found that the boys scored higher than the girls on exercise dependence symptoms, exercise behavior, and exercise motivation. Using **self-determination theory** as a framework, they also found that **integrated regulation** and **introjected regulation** were important determinants of exercise dependence.

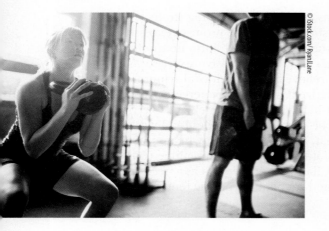
©iStock.com/ RyanJLane

Gender

Male populations display more primary exercise dependence symptoms than female populations (Villella et al., 2011). For example, Danielle Symons Downs and her colleagues (2013) found that adolescent boys display more exercise dependence symptoms than adolescent girls. As well, men displayed more exercise dependence symptoms than women (Costa et al., 2013; Edmunds, Ntoumanis, & Duda, 2006). Although the prevalence of primary exercise dependence tends to be lower among women, the severity of their symptoms is comparable to that seen in men.

CRITICAL THINKING ACTIVITY 14-4

© ecco/Shutterstock, Inc.

What are some plausible explanations for why males are more at risk for exercise dependence than females?

Perfectionism

Perfectionism is a personality trait characterized by a person's striving for flawlessness and setting excessively high performance standards, accompanied by overly critical self-evaluations and concerns regarding others' evaluations (Stoeber et al., 2010). Researchers have found a positive relationship between exercise dependence symptoms and perfectionism (Hagan & Hausenblas, 2003; Hausenblas & Symons Downs, 2002b). Individuals classified as at risk for exercise dependence scored higher on perfectionism than those classified as nondependent-symptomatic, whereas the latter scored higher than individuals classified as nondependent-asymptomatic on perfectionism.

Exercise Identity

Exercise identity is the extent that exercise is descriptive of one's self-concept. Someone who has high exercise identity would most likely strongly agree to the following statement: "When I describe myself to other people, I usually include my involvement in physical exercise" (Anderson & Cychosz, 1994). Not surprisingly, exercise identity has been identified as an important determinant of regular exercise behavior and exercise dependence symptoms. Researchers have found that a stronger exercise identity is associated with greater odds of experiencing exercise dependence symptoms (Lu et al., 2012; Murray, McKensizie, Newman, & Brown, 2013).

Self-Esteem

People scoring high on exercise dependence symptoms also report lower self-esteem (Bruno et al., 2014). Thus, there is a negative relationship between self-esteem and exercise dependence. This is in contrast to regular exercisers who report higher self-esteem than nonexercisers.

Attention-Deficit Hyperactivity Disorder

Attention-deficit hyperactivity disorder (ADHD) is one of the most common childhood disorders and can continue through adolescence and into adulthood. Symptoms include difficulty staying focused and paying attention, difficulty controlling behavior, and hyperactivity (also known as *overactivity*). The symptoms of ADHD usually cause functional impairment in social, occupational, and academic activities.

Using a retrospective design, Nikolas Berger and his colleagues (Berger, Muller, Brahler, Philipsen, & Zwaan, 2014) examined the associations of ADHD with exercise dependence symptoms in 1,615 German adults. The adults completed a retrospective assessment of childhood ADHD and adult ADHD. Their exercise dependence symptoms were assessment via the Exercise Dependence Scale. Adults with childhood-only ADHD had a significantly higher frequency of exercise dependence symptoms than adults without ADHD. More specifically, 9% of the adults with childhood-only ADHD displayed exercise dependence symptoms, compared to only 2.7% of adults without childhood ADHD. These results reveal that excessive exercising is overrepresented in people in which ADHD symptoms in childhood have not persisted into adulthood. It is plausible that some adults may suppress ADHD symptoms by excessive exercise.

Exercise Deprivation

Exercise deprivation sensations (also referred to as *exercise withdrawal symptoms*) are the cardinal identifying components of exercise dependence (Szabo, 1995). These sensations represent the psychological and physiological effects that occur during periods of no physical activity. The individual may either experience withdrawal symptoms, such as anxiety and fatigue, because of a lack of exercise, or engage in exercise to either relieve or avoid the onset of the withdrawal symptoms (APA, 2000).

It is assumed that exercise deprivation symptoms arise for the same reason that regular exercise results in positive psychological states. That is, it is assumed that the onset of physical activity leads to the onset of positive psychological states, whereas the cessation of regular physical activity leads to the onset of negative psychological states or reductions in the positive psychological states. Research has generally supported this assumption that for regular exercisers, exercise withdrawal is associated with negative mood (Glass et al., 2004; Hausenblas, Gauvin, Symons Downs, & Duley, 2008; Weinstein, Deuster, & Kop, 2007). The

TABLE 14-6	Exercise Deprivation Symptoms		
Affective	**Cognitive**	**Physiological**	**Social**
Anxiety	Confusion	Muscle soreness	Increased need for
Depression	Impaired concentration	Disturbed sleep	social interaction
Irritability		Lethargy	
Hostility		Fatigue	
Anger		Increased galvanic skin	
Tension		response	
Guilt		Gastrointestinal problems	
Frustration		Decreased vigor	
Sexual tension		Increased pain	
Decreased self-esteem			

most frequently reported feelings resulting from exercise deprivation are guilt, depression, irritability, restlessness, tension, stress, anxiety, confusion, anger, and sluggishness (Poole, Hamer, Wawrzyniak, & Steptoe, 2011; Szabo, Frenkl, & Caputo, 1997). **TABLE 14-6** lists the withdrawal symptoms commonly reported during exercise deprivation studies. It is important to emphasize that exercise deprivation sensations could be experienced by both nondependent and dependent exercisers, but the former would experience less profound effects than the latter (Szabo, 1995).

One noteworthy study of exercise deprivation was undertaken by Gregory Mondin and his colleagues (1996) at the University of Madison-Wisconsin. They examined the effects of 3 days of exercise deprivation on mood states and anxiety in 10 male and female "habitual" runners. Participants had to run at least 6 to 7 days a week for a minimum duration of 45 minutes per session to be classified as a "habitual" runner.

The study design required that the runners complete their regular workout on the Monday, refrain from physical activity on the Tuesday, Wednesday, and Thursday, and then resume their regular physical activity on the Friday. Also, on the no-exercising days the participants were also asked to limit their lifestyle physical activity. For example, they were asked to take the bus instead of biking to work, park close to buildings to minimize walking, and take the elevator instead of the stairs. Mood and state anxiety were assessed on the Monday and Friday following the workout, as well as on the 3 days of physical activity deprivation. They found that the participants displayed increases in mood disturbance and anxiety during the no-exercise days. When physical

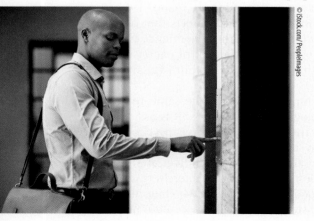

© iStock.com/PeopleImages

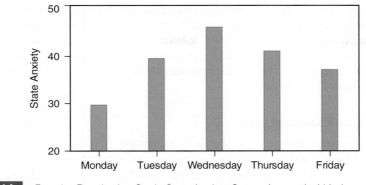

FIGURE 14-1   Exercise Deprivation Study: State Anxiety Scores Across the Week

Data from Mondin, G. W., Morgan, W. P., Piering, P. N., Stegner, A. J., Stotesbery, C. L., Trine, M. R., & Wu, M. (1996). Psychological consequences of exercise deprivation in habitual exercisers. *Medicine and Science in Sports and Exercise*, 28, 1199–1203.

activity was resumed on the Friday, participants showed improvements in mood and anxiety. See   FIGURE 14-1   for a graphical display of the anxiety results. Thus, the researchers concluded that a brief period of physical activity deprivation in habitual exercisers results in mood disturbance within 24 hours.

Explanations of Exercise Dependence

Potential explanations of exercise dependence can be classified into the psychological (i.e., personality traits and affective regulation), physiological (e.g., β-endorphin and sympathetic arousal hypotheses), and psychobiological (i.e., general theory of addiction) domains. Each of these explanations is described below.

Psychological Explanations

The *personality traits* explanation is based on the belief that exercise-dependent people have specific personality characteristics, such as perfectionism, obsessive-compulsiveness, neuroticism, low self-esteem, and high trait anxiety. In support of the personality traits explanation, researchers have usually found a positive relationship between exercise dependence symptoms and perfectionism (Hagan & Hausenblas, 2003), obsessive-compulsiveness (Davis et al., 1995), trait anxiety (Coen & Ogles, 1993), and extraversion (Hausenblas & Giacobbi, 2004). A negative relationship has been evidenced between exercise dependence symptoms and self-esteem, neuroticism, and agreeableness (Hausenblas & Giacobbi, 2004).

The *affective regulation* explanation states that physical activity leads to positive psychological states, whereas the cessation of exercise results in negative psychological states. For example, acute and chronic bouts of exercise are associated with reductions in depression and anxiety and increases in positive mood states in clinical and nonclinical populations. An exercise-dependent individual may use exercise for affective regulation, such as engaging in physical activity to either avoid or reduce his or her anxiety levels. Research support for the affective regulation explanation is found in exercise deprivation studies. In general, researchers have found that exercise deprivation results in increased mood disturbance in habitual exercisers (Szabo, 1995).

Physiological Explanations

The *β-endorphin* explanation is based on the premise that β-endorphin levels in the blood rise with exercise due to an increased need for blood to be transported to the working muscles (Crossman, Jamieson, & Henderson, 1987). β-endorphins are endogenous compounds that decrease people's sensitivity to pain, resulting in a euphoric effect; they also produce addictive behavioral tendencies. Thus, it has been suggested that exercisers may become dependent upon β-endorphins because they make them feel better and mask pain.

Pierce and his colleagues (Pierce, Eastman, Tripathi, Olson, & Dewey, 1993) conducted a study examining the plausibility of the β-endorphin explanation for exercise dependence. They examined the relationship between β-endorphin levels after an acute bout of exercise in eight females who engaged in a minimum of three aerobics classes a week. Blood samples of the participants were taken before and following a 45-minute high-intensity aerobic session. Although their β-endorphin levels were elevated following the exercise session, no relationship was found between the β-endorphins levels and exercise dependence symptoms. It is important to note that the participants did not report high levels of exercise dependence, as their scores on the Negative Addiction Scale (Hailey & Bailey, 1982) ranged from 2 to 6 (mean score = 4) out of a possible maximum score of 14, which indicates high dependence. Thus, additional research is needed to examine the β-endorphin explanation in individuals who report high levels of exercise dependence.

Thompson and Blanton (1987) suggested a *sympathetic arousal* explanation of exercise dependence. According to this explanation, excessive exercise produces an increase in people's fitness level and in their efficiency of energy use. This increased efficiency is a result of lowered sympathetic output that is reflected in a decreased metabolic rate. Because of the lowered sympathetic output, the individual experiences lethargy, fatigue, and low arousal. Thus, regular exercisers must engage in higher intensities and durations of physical activity to produce the same level of physiological arousal during and following an exercise bout. However, no studies have examined the plausibility of the sympathetic arousal hypothesis as an explanation of exercise dependence.

Psychobiological Explanations

In the general theory of addictions, physiological and psychological factors are suggested to interact to produce a predisposition for people to exhibit dependent behaviors (Jacobs, 1986). Jacobs (1986) stated that the two major factors for developing a dependency are: (1) subjective aversion, which is an excessively depressed or excited resting physiological state, and (2) a psychological state characterized by feelings of inadequacy and rejection based on experiences in childhood and early adolescence. Because both factors must be present to develop a dependency, only a limited number of people will be predisposed to dependent behaviors. Furthermore, the dependency remains latent unless at-risk individuals come into contact with a situation that is associated with the alteration of the physiological state to a level that reduces the aversiveness of the existing state.

In a study examining the applicability of the general theory of addiction to exercise behavior, Helen Beh, Sarah Mathers, and John Holden (1996) recorded the electroencephalographic (EEG) readings of three groups of university students who differed in their degree of dependency (i.e., high dependent, low dependent, and nondependent). EEG measures the level of physiological activity, with low EEG frequencies being associated with depression and high frequencies being related to excitation. Thus, in this study, depressed and excited states were defined by EEG parameters. The participants' EEG recordings were assessed before and after a 45-minute exercise session. It was found that the high-dependent group had higher EEG frequencies (i.e., excitation) than the low-dependent group. The authors concluded that their results provided partial support for Jacob's (1986) general theory of addiction with regard to exercise dependence.

■ Eating Disorders

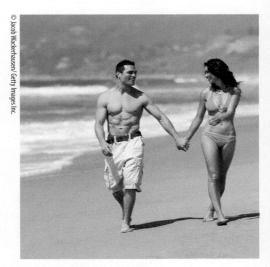

© Jacob Wackerhausen/ Getty Images Inc.

Although physical activity is often part of a safe and healthy program to control weight, individuals may have unrealistic expectations. We are bombarded with images from advertisers of the ideal body. For women, the ideal body that is often seen in the media is that of a thin and toned female (i.e., low percent body fat and physically fit). For men, the ideal physique that is usually portrayed is a lean and muscular body (i.e., low percent body fat and muscular, especially upper body muscularity). To try to achieve these unreasonable body ideals, some individuals turn to dieting, which, when taken to the extreme, can develop into the eating disorders of either anorexia nervosa or bulimia nervosa.

Prevalence rates indicate that 43.5% of people with a lifetime diagnosis of either anorexia or bulimia engage in excessive exercise (Shroff et al., 2006). The cardinal feature of anorexia nervosa is an extreme pursuit of thinness. The primary criteria for bulimia nervosa are eating binges followed by inappropriate compensatory methods to prevent weight gain (APA, 2000). Excessive physical activity has been described as one of the symptoms of an eating disorder. Unfortunately, there is no consensus on how to define and conceptualize excessive amounts of exercise with regard to eating disorders. In this section, we describe these two eating disorders in more detail and the role that excessive exercise plays in their development and maintenance.

Anorexia Nervosa

The criteria for **anorexia nervosa** includes an intense and unrealistic fear of becoming fat and engaging in behaviors intended to produce distinct weight loss (see **TABLE 14-7**). The disturbance of self-evaluation and consequential denial of the severity of one's low weight are defined as maintaining a weight that is less than 85% of what is considered an ideal body weight for that person. Although anorexia nervosa can affect men and women of any age, race, and socioeconomic and cultural background, anorexia nervosa is 10 times more common in females than males (Bennett, 2008).

Bulimia Nervosa

The criteria for **bulimia nervosa** are similar to that of anorexia nervosa in that they also outline an intense fear of becoming fat, but bulimia nervosa differentiates itself by including the requirements of powerful urges to overeat and subsequent binges that are followed by engaging in some sort of purging or compensatory behavior in an attempt to avoid the fattening effects of the excessive caloric intake

TABLE 14-7 Diagnostic Criteria for Anorexia Nervosa and Bulimia Nervosa	
Anorexia Nervosa	**Bulimia Nervosa**
Persistent restriction of energy intake leading to significantly low body weight (in context of what is minimally expected for age, sex, developmental trajectory, and physical health).	Recurrent episodes of binge eating.
Either an intense fear of gaining weight or of becoming fat or persistent behavior that interferes with weight gain (even though significantly low weight).	Recurrent inappropriate compensatory behavior in order to prevent weight gain (e.g., self-induced vomiting, excessive exercise).
Disturbance in the way one's body weight or shape is experienced, undue influence of body shape and weight on self-evaluation, or persistent lack of recognition of the seriousness of the current low body weight.	Binge eating and inappropriate compensatory behaviors both occur, on average, at least once a week for 3 months.
	Body image disturbance.

(see Table 14-7). Similar to anorexia nervosa, the fear experienced by people suffering with bulimia nervosa is in regard to self-evaluation resulting in compensatory behaviors in an attempt to avoid weight gain. The paradox is the presence of **binge eating**, which is defined as uncontrollable urges to overeat. These binges must occur within 2 hours and include an amount of food that is definitely larger than most people would consume in a similar time and setting and a sense of lack of control during the binge (APA, 2013). Compensatory behaviors are separated into *purging type* (i.e., self-induced vomiting; use of laxatives, diuretics, or enemas; or medication abuse) and *nonpurging type* (i.e., other compensatory behaviors, such as fasting or excessively exercising). Unlike anorexia nervosa, there is no criterion defining maintenance of body weight or presence of amenorrhea.

Bulimia nervosa is considered to be less life threatening than anorexia nervosa; however, the occurrence of bulimia nervosa is higher (Manning & Murphy, 2003). Bulimia nervosa is nine times more likely to occur in women than men. The vast majority of those with bulimia nervosa are at normal weight. Antidepressants are widely used in the treatment of bulimia nervosa. Patients who have bulimia nervosa are often linked with having impulsive behaviors involving overspending and sexual behaviors, as well as having family histories of alcohol and substance abuse and mood and eating disorders (Yager, 1991).

Eating Disorders and Exercise

The relationship between exercise and eating disorders is far from clear. Some researchers state that there is no relationship between physical activity and eating disorders, whereas other experts feel strongly that physical activity and eating disorders are related, with exercise dependence playing a key role (see O'Connor & Smith, 1999). With regard to the latter, a distinction has been made between primary exercise dependence and secondary exercise dependence.

Primary exercise dependence is defined as meeting the criteria for exercise dependence and continually exercising solely for the psychological gratification resulting from the exercise behavior itself. **Secondary exercise dependence** is defined as meeting the criteria for exercise dependence, but using excessive exercise to accomplish some other end (e.g., weight loss or body composition changes) that is related to the eating disorder. Thus, for secondary exercise dependence, the excessive exercise is secondary to an eating disorder and the main motivation for physical activity is the control and manipulation of body composition.

CRITICAL THINKING ACTIVITY 14-5

© ecco/Shutterstock, Inc.

What is the difference between primary and secondary exercise dependence? Why is it important from a treatment standpoint to differentiate between the two types of exercise dependence?

David DeCoverely Veale (1987, 1995) suggested that a diagnostic hierarchy must occur to validly identify exercise dependence. He argued that the diagnosis of an eating disorder (i.e., secondary dependence) must first be excluded before a diagnosis of primary exercise dependence can be made; that is, primary exercise dependence can be differentiated from an eating disorder by clarifying the ultimate objective of the exerciser.

Despite a lack of compelling empirical evidence, a misconception exists that excessive exercise leads to the development of an eating disorder. In a review of the literature, Patrick O'Connor and J. Carson Smith (1999) stated that "logic and empirical evidence dictate that excessive exercise cannot be a sole cause of anorexia nervosa" (p. 1010). To illustrate their point, O'Connor and Smith pointed out that about 12% of the adult population participates in regular vigorous physical activity; however, the overwhelming majority of these people never develop anorexia nervosa. Also, increased exercise with anorexia nervosa is paradoxical because starvation results in reduced physical activity and fatigue. Finally, emerging research is revealing that regular exercise may be a viable treatment for eating disorders (Hausenblas, Cook, & Chittester, 2008).

In an attempt to understand the relationship between exercise and eating disorders, Heather Hausenblas and her colleagues (2008) developed the *exercise and eating disorders model* (see FIGURE 14-2). The exercise and eating disorders model states that regular exercise is associated with improvements in several physiological measures (i.e., cardiovascular health, metabolism, adiposity, and bone density), psychological measures (i.e., body image, depression, anxiety, stress reactivity, and self-esteem), and social benefits that are risk and maintenance factors for eating disorders. Hence, the exercise and eating disorders model has consolidated and supported several narrative and meta-analytic reviews that have shown the ability of exercise to impart positive improvements on eating disorder risk, development, and maintenance factors.

The model also extends our current understanding of the relationship between exercise and health status by including exercise dependence. Exercise dependence may explain why the development of eating disorders may supersede the expected benefits of exercise. Simply stated, this model posits that in the absence of pathological psychological factors such as exercise dependence, the benefits conveyed by regular exercise (e.g., improvements in depression, anxiety, stress reactivity, self-esteem, and body composition) may counteract the risk factors for eating disorders (e.g., body dissatisfaction, depression, anxiety, increased body mass).

Researchers have found initial support for the exercise and eating disorder model. For example, Brian Cook and his colleagues (Cook, Hausenblas, Tuccito, & Giacobbi, 2011) had 539 university students complete self-report measures of physical and psychological quality of life, exercise behavior, eating disorder risk, and exercise dependence symptoms. Structural equation modeling analysis found support for the mediation effect of exercise dependence on eating disorders, as well as the effect of psychological well-being on eating disorders. Together, exercise behavior, psychological well-being, and exercise dependence symptoms

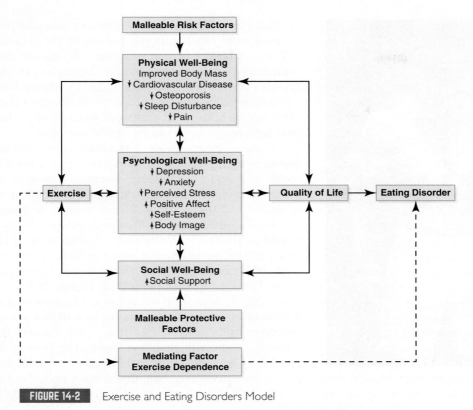

FIGURE 14-2 Exercise and Eating Disorders Model

Reproduced from Hausenblas, H. A., Cook, B. J., & Chittester, N. I. (2008). Can exercise treat eating disorders? *Exercise and Sport Sciences Reviews, 36,* 43–47.

predicted 22.9% of the variation in eating disorders. Thus, these results indicated that the psychological health benefits conveyed by exercise reduced eating disorder risk (Cook et al., 2011). These results were replicated in a more diverse sample of college students (Cook & Hausenblas, 2011).

Initial tests of the exercise and eating disorders model suggest that the model may combine two divergent lines of research (Cook, Hausenblas, Crosby, Cao, & Wonderlich, 2015); that is, exercise may play a role in the development of eating disorders when exercise dependence is simultaneously present. Similarly, the psychological health benefits of exercise may also reduce eating disorder risk for individuals without exercise dependence.

■ Muscle Dysmorphia

Muscle dysmorphia represents the pathological pursuit of muscularity and is characterized by a distressing preoccupation that a person is of insufficient muscularity (despite, in many cases, having well-developed muscles) coupled with

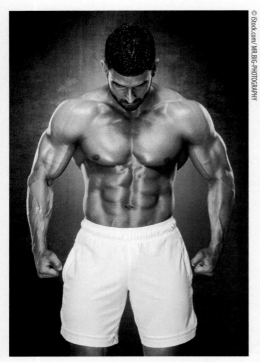

© iStock.com/MR.BIG-PHOTOGRAPHY

excessive exercise and dietary practices that take precedence over other important areas of life (Murray & Touyz, 2013). A person suffering with muscle dysmorphia will most likely perceive themselves to lack muscles despite being very muscular. In other words, a person with muscle dysmorphia will interpret their body size as both small and weak even though they may look normal or even be highly muscular.

Muscle dysmorphia has been conceptually linked to eating disorders, obsessive-compulsive disorder, and body dysmorphic disorder; however, its precise nosology remains unclear (Foster, Shorter, & Griffiths, 2014; Murray, Rieger, Karlov, & Touyz, 2013). The prevalence of muscle dysmophia is estimated at about 2% of the general population (Liao et al., 2010); however, due to the negative connotations often associated with the disorder, many suffering from it remain undetected (Leone, Sedory, & Gray, 2005). Muscle dysmorphia is often viewed as a form of body image disturbance in which a person perceives him- or herself as unacceptably small. For example, some weight lifters, no matter how muscular they become, still see themselves as small and unmuscular. Muscle dysmorphia is perceived as a male-dominated, body image–related psychological condition (Griffiths, Mond, Murray, & Touyz, 2014; Suffolk, Dovey, Goodwin, & Meyer, 2013).

Harrison Pope and his colleagues (Pope, Gruber, Choi, Olivardia, & Phillips, 1997), in their discussion of muscle dysmorphia, provided the following example:

> All of his waking hours are consumed with preoccupations of getting bigger. He tries to resist these thoughts, but reports success only half of the time. He weighs himself 2–3 times daily and checks mirrors 10–12 times a day to monitor his physique. He wears baggy sweatshirts and long pants even in the heat of summer to disguise his perceived smallness.
>
> (p. 554)

A large variety of terms have been used to describe muscle dysmorphia, including *bodybuilding anorexia*, *inverse anorexia*, *reverse anorexia*, *megorexia nervosa*, *bigameraria*, and *vigorexia*.

Harrison Pope and his colleagues (Pope et al., 1997; Pope & Katz, 1994; Pope, Katz, & Hudson, 1993) were among the first researchers to examine muscle dysmorphia. Based on their research, they proposed that persons with muscle dysmorphia are: (1) pathologically preoccupied with the appearance of the whole body; (2) concerned that they are not sufficiently large or muscular; and (3) are consumed by weightlifting, dieting, and steroid abuse. As a consequence, these people experience profound distress about having their bodies seen in public, exhibit impaired social and occupational functioning, and abuse anabolic steroids and other drugs.

Correlates of Muscle Dsymorphia

In recent years, researchers have become interested in examining the correlates or determinants of muscle dsymorphia. Researchers have found a positive relationship between muscle dysmorphia and **drive for muscularity**, social physique anxiety (Ebbeck, Watkins, Concepcion, Cardinal, & Hammermeister, 2009; Grieve, Jackson, Reece, Marklin, & Delaney, 2008), depression (Ebbeck et al., 2009), perfectionism (Kuennen & Waldren, 2007; Murray et al., 2013), and mood intolerance (Murray et al., 2013). In comparison, researchers have found a negative relationship between muscle dysmorphia and perceived body attractiveness (Ebbeck et al., 2009) and self-esteem (Murray et al., 2013). As well, the severity of muscle dsymorphia is greatest in competing bodybuilders compared to noncompeting bodybuilders (Santarneccchi & Derrore, 2012).

Roberto Olivardia and his colleagues (Olivardia, Pope, & Hudson, 2000) conducted interviews with 24 young men with muscle dysmorphia and 30 normal -comparison weight lifters. They found that the muscle dysmorphic men had higher body dissatisfaction, disordered eating, anabolic steroid abuse, and lifetime prevalence of mood and anxiety disorders compared to the normal weightlifters. The researchers also found that the men with muscle dysmorphia frequently reported shame, embarrassment, and impairment of social and occupational functioning in association with their condition. In contrast, the normal weight lifters reported little pathology. More recent research has confirmed the relationship between muscle dysmorphia with steroid use and eating disorder characteristics (Babusa & Tury, 2012).

Exercise is a main focus for individuals with muscle dysmorphia. In particular, resistance exercise (i.e., weightlifting and bodybuilding) is typically undertaken to attain increased muscle mass and decreased fat mass. Ironically, exercise amounts and intensities are often increased despite the fact that people with muscle dysmorphia often possess a large muscular physique that actually meets or exceeds the cultural ideal. Because the preoccupation with one's body is pathological, reaching a level of satisfaction with one's body is not attained despite a muscular appearance. Moreover, Chittester and Hausenblas (2008) found that drive for muscularity is predicted by weightlifting, supplement use, and exercise dependence.

The resulting increases in musculature from increased amounts of exercise often plateau, thus further contributing to body dissatisfaction. Consequently, physically active individuals with muscle dysmorphia often follow a diet of high-protein and low-fat foods along with dietary and **ergogenic supplements** to reduce body fat (Contesini et al., 2013). In particular, dietary supplements and anabolic steroids are often used in an attempt to promote increase muscle

TABLE 14-8	Examples of Muscle Dysmorphia Measure Items
Scale	**Sample Items**
Drive for Muscularity Attitudes Questionnaire (Morrison & Morrison, 2004) Measured on a Likert-type scale (1 "strongly disagree" to 5 "strongly agree").	Being muscular gives me confidence. I would like to be more muscular in the future. I feel less of a man when I have small muscles than when I have large muscles. I think I need to gain a few pounds of "bulk" (muscle mass).
Drive for Muscularity Scale (McCreary & Sasse, 2000) Measured on a Likert-type scale (1 "always" to 6 "never").	I wish that I were more muscular. I lift weights to build up muscle. I use protein or energy supplements. I think about taking anabolic steroids. I think that my legs are not muscular enough.

mass, decrease fat mass, and satisfy the individual's subjective sense of becoming sufficiently big enough (Varnado-Sullivan, Horton, & Savoy, 2006). However, it should be noted that supplements are generally expensive, typically show little impact on muscle mass, and may promote dependence (Kanayama, Pope, & Hudson, 2001). Steroids, however, are efficacious in producing muscle mass gains (Cox, 2012), but they are associated with significant health risks, such as hypertension, disturbed lipid profiles, increased irritability, increased aggression, body image disturbance, and mood disturbances (Hartgens & Kuipers, 2004).

Muscle Dysmorphia Measures

As with other psychological issues, muscle dysmorphia is often measured with self-report measures. **TABLE 14-8** provides sample items from commonly used measures of muscle dysmorphia and drive for muscularity.

■ Summary

This chapter examined some potential negative effects of exercise: exercise dependence, eating disorders, and muscle dysmorphia. For some people, exercise may represent a negative behavior when it becomes excessive, and it can be associated with pathological behaviors such as binging, purging, extreme body dissatisfaction, and steroid use. It is important to emphasize, however, that exercise is largely a positive behavior—a behavior that few adults engage in on a regular basis.

KEY TERMS

analytical psychology
anorexia nervosa
binge eating
bulimia nervosa
drive for muscularity
exercise dependence
exercise deprivation sensations
exercise identity
ergogenic supplements
exercise identity

integrated regulation
introjected regulation
ironman triathlon
muscle dysmorphia
perfectionism
prevalence
primary exercise dependence
secondary exercise dependence
self-determination theory
ultramarathon

REVIEW QUESTIONS

1. Define *exercise dependence*. What are the seven criteria for a diagnosis of exercise dependence?

2. What is the relationship between personality and exercise dependence?

3. Describe exercise deprivation and the symptoms that exercise-dependent individuals may experience when deprived of exercise.

4. Describe the three domains that have been advanced for potential explanations of exercise dependence.

5. Describe the diagnostic criteria for anorexia nervosa and bulimia nervosa.

6. What is the difference between primary and secondary exercise dependence?

7. Describe the exercise and eating disorder model developed by Hausenblas and colleagues. What does the research tell us about this model?

8. Define *muscle dysmorphia*. What other terms are used to describe muscle dysmorphia?

APPLYING THE CONCEPTS

1. Do you think that Katherine exhibits primary or secondary exercise dependence? What aspects of her behavior indicate one over the other?

2. What criteria of exercise dependence does Katherine exhibit?

REFERENCES

American Psychiatric Association. (2000). Diagnostic and statistical manual of mental disorders (4th ed., text rev.). Washington, DC: Author.

American Psychiatric Association. (2013). *Diagnostic and Statistical Manual of Mental Disorders*, Fifth Edition. Washington, DC: Author.

Anderson, D. F., & Cychosz, C. M. (1994). Development of an exercise identity scale. *Perceptual and Motor Skills, 78*, 747–751.

Andreassen, C. S., Griffiths, M. D., Gjertsen, S. R., Krossbakken, E., Kvam, S., & Pallesen, S. (2013). The relationship between behavioral addictions and the five-factor model of personality. *Journal of Behavioral Addictions, 2*, 90–99.

Arem, H., Moore, S. C., Patel, A., Harge, P., Berrington de Gonzalez, A., Visvanathan, K., … Matthews, C. E. (2015). Leisure time physical activity and mortality: A detailed pooled analysis of the dose-response relationship. *JAMA Internal Medicine, 175*, 959–967.

Babusa, B., & Tury, F. (2012). Muscle dysmorphia in Hungarian non-competitive male bodybuilders. *Eating and Weight Disorders, 17*, e49–e53.

Baekeland, F. (1970). Exercise deprivation. Sleep and psychological reactions. *Archives of General Psychiatry, 22*, 365–369.

Beh, H. C., Mathers, S., & Holden, J. (1996). EEG correlates of exercise dependency. *International Journal of Psychophysiology, 23*, 121–128.

Bennett, J. (2008). It's not just white girls. Anorexics can be male, old, Latino, black, or pregnant. A new book undercuts old stereotypes. *Newsweek, 152*, 96.

Berczik, K., Szabó, A., Griffiths, M. D., Kurimay, T., Kun, B., Urbán, R., & Demetrovics, Z. (2012). Exercise addiction: Symptoms, diagnosis, epidemiology, and etiology. *Substance Use and Misuse, 47*, 403–417.

Berger, N., Muller, A., Brahler, E., Philipsen, A., & de Zwaan, M. (2014). Association of symptoms of attention-deficit/hyperactivity disorder with symptoms of excessive exercising in an adult general population sample. *BMC Psychiatry.* Sep 12;*14*:250. doi:10.1186/s12888-014-0250-7

Bruno, A., Quattrone, D., Scimeca, G., Cicciarelli, C., Romeo, V. M., Pandolfo, G., … Muscatello, M. R. A. (2014). Unraveling exercise addiction: The role of narcissism and self-esteem. *Journal of Addiction,* Oct 28, epub. doi:10.1155/2014/987841

Chittester, N. I., & Hausenblas, H. A. (2009). Correlates of drive for muscularity: The role of anthropometric measures and psychological factors. *Journal of Health Psychology, 14*, 872–877.

Contesini, N., Adami, F., Blake, Md., Monterio, C. B., Abreu, L. C., Valenti, L. C., ... Schlickmann, D. E. (2013). Nutritional strategies of physically active subjects with muscle dysmorphia. *International Archives of Medicine*, 26;25. doi:10.1186/1755-7682-6-25

Cook, B. J., & Hausenblas, H. A. (2011). Eating disorder specific health-related quality of life and exercise in college females. *Quality of Life Research*, 20, 1385–1390.

Cook, B. J., Hausenblas, H. A., Crosby, R. D., Cao, L., & Wonderlich, S. A. (2015). Exercise dependence as a mediator of the exercise and eating disorders relationship: A pilot study. *Eating Behaviors*, 16, 9–12.

Cook, B. J., Hausenblas, H. A., Tuccitto, D., & Giacobbi, P. (2011). Eating disorders and exercise: A structural equation modeling analysis of a conceptual model. *European Eating Disorders Review*, 19, 216–225.

Cook, B. J., Karr, T. M., Zunker, C., Mitchell, J. E., Thompson, R., Sherman, R., ... Wonderlich, S. A. (2013). Primary and secondary exercise dependence in a community-based sample of road race runners. *Journal of Sport & Exercise Psychology*, 35, 464–469.

Costa, P. T. Jr., & McCrae, R. R. (1992). *The NEO PI-R: Professional manual*. Odessa, FL: Psychological Assessment Resources.

Costa, P. T. Jr., & McCrae, R. R. (1990). Personality: Another "hidden factor" in stress research. *Psychological Inquiry*, 1, 22–24.

Costa, S., Hausenblas, H. A., Oliva, P., Cuzzocrea, F., & Larcan, R. (2013). The role of age, gender, mood states, and exercise frequency on exercise dependence. *Journal of Behavioral Addictions*, 2, 216–223.

Cox, R. H. (2012). *Sports psychology*. (7th ed.). New York, NY: McGraw-Hill.

Crossman, J., Jamieson, J., & Henderson, L. (1987). Responses of competitive athletes to lay-offs in training: Exercise addiction of psychological relief? *Journal of Sport Behavior*, 10, 28–38.

Davis, C., Kennedy, S. H., Ralevski, E., Dionne, M., Brewer, H., Neitzert, C., & Ratusny, D. (1995). Obsessive compulsiveness and physical activity in anorexia nervosa and high-level exercising. *Journal of Psychosomatic Research*, 39, 967–976.

Di Nicola, M., Tedeschi, D., De Risio, L., Pettorrusa, M., Martinotti, G., Ruggeri, F., ... Janiri, L. (2015). Co-occurrence of alcohol use disorder and behavioral addictions: Relevance of impulsivity and craving. *Drug and Alcohol Dependence*, 148, 118–125.

Ebbeck, E., Watkins, P. L., Concepcion, R. Y., Cardinal, B. J., & Hammermeister, J. (2009). Muscle dysmorphia symptoms and their relationship to self-concept and negative affect among college recreational exercisers. *Journal of Applied Sport Psychology*, 21, 262–275.

Edmunds, J., Ntoumanis, N., & Duda, J. L. (2006). Examining exercise dependence symptomatology from a self-determination perspective. *Journal of Health Psychology*, 11, 887–903.

Foster, A. C., Shorter, G. W., & Griffiths, M. D. (2014). Muscle dysmorphia: Could it be classified as an addiction to body image? *Journal of Behavioral Addictions*, 3, 1–5.

Glass, J. M., Lyden, A. K., Petzke, F., Stein, P., Whalen, G., Ambrose, K., ... Clauw, D. J. (2004). The effect of brief exercise cessation on pain, fatigue, and mood symptom development in healthy, fit individuals. *Journal of Psychosomatic Research*, 57, 391–398.

Glasser, W. (1976). *Positive addiction*. New York, NY: Harper & Row.

Grandi, S., Clementi, C., Guidi, J., Benassi, M., & Tossani, E. (2011). Personality characteristics and psychological distress associated with primary exercise dependence: An exploratory study. *Psychiatry Research*, 189, 270–275.

Grieve, F. G. Jackson, L., Reece, T., Marklin, L., & Delaney, A. (2008). Correlates of social physique anxiety in men. *Journal of Sport Behavior*, 31, 329–337.

Griffiths, S., Mond, J. M., Murray, S. B., & Touyz, S. (2014). Young peoples' stigmatizing attitudes and beliefs about anorexia nervosa and muscle dysmorphia. *International Journal of Eating Disorders*, 47, 189–195.

Hagan, A. L., & Hausenblas, H. A. (2003). The relationship between exercise dependence symptoms and perfectionism. *American Journal of Health Studies*, 18, 133–137.

Hailey, B. J., & Bailey, L. A. (1982). Negative addiction in runners: A quantitative approach. *Journal of Sport Behavior, 5,* 150–154.

Hartgens, F., & Kuipers, H. (2004). Effects of androgenic-anabolic steroids in athletes. *Sports Medicine, 34,* 513–554.

Haskell W. L., Lee I. M., Pate R. R., Powell, K. E., Blair, S. N., Franklin, B. A., ... Bauman, A. (2007). Physical activity and public health: Updated recommendation for adults from the American College of Sports Medicine and the American Heart Association. *Circulation, 116,* 1081–1093.

Hausenblas, H. A., Cook, B. J., & Chittester, N. I. (2008). Can exercise treat eating disorders? *Exercise and Sport Sciences Reviews, 36,* 43–47.

Hausenblas, H. A., Gauvin, L., Symons Downs, D., & Duley, A. R. (2008). Effects of abstinence from habitual involvement in regular exercise on feeling states: An ecological momentary assessment study. *British Journal of Health Psychology, 13,* 237–255.

Hausenblas, H. A., & Giacobbi, P. R. Jr. (2004). Relationship between exercise dependence symptoms and personality. *Personality and Individual Differences, 36,* 1265–1273.

Hausenblas, H. A., & Symons Downs, D. (2002a). Exercise dependence: A systematic review. *Psychology of Sport and Exercise, 3,* 89–123.

Hausenblas, H. A., & Symons Downs, D. (2002b). How much is too much? The development and validation of the Exercise Dependence Scale. *Psychology and Health: An International Journal, 17,* 387–404.

Jacobs, D. (1986). A general theory of addictions. A new theoretical model. *Journal of Gambling Behavior, 2,* 15–31.

Jung, C. G. (1957). *Memories, dreams, reflections.* New York, NY: Vintage.

Kanayama, G., Pope, H. G. Jr., & Hudson, J. I. (2001). "Body image" drugs: A growing psychosomatic problem. *Psychotherapy and Psychosomatics, 70,* 61–65.

Kim, Y. S., Park, Y. S., Allegrante, J. P., Marks, R., Ok, H., Ok Cho, K., & Garber, C. E. (2012). Relationship between physical activity and general mental health. *Preventive Medicine, 55,* 458–463.

Kuennen, M. R., & Waldren, J. J. (2007). Relationships between specific personality traits, fat free mass indices, and the Muscle Dysmorphia Inventory. *Journal of Sports Behavior, 30,* 453–470.

Lejoyeux, M., Avril, M., Embouazza, H., & Nivoli, F. (2008). Prevalence of exercise dependence and other behavioral addictions among clients of a Parisian fitness room. *Comprehensive Psychiatry, 49,* 353–358.

La Gerche A., Robberecht C., & Kuiperi C. (2010). Lower than expected desmosomal gene mutation prevalence in endurance athletes with complex ventricular arrhythmias of right ventricular origin. *Heart, 96,* 1268–1274.

Leone, J. E., Sedory, E., & Gray, K. (2005). Recognition and treatment of muscle dysmorphia and related body image disorders. *Journal of Athletic Training, 40,* 352–359.

Liao, Y., Knoesen, N. P., Deng, Y., Tang, J., Castle, D. J., Bookun, R., ... Liu, T. (2010). Body dysmorphic disorder, social anxiety, and depressive symptoms in Chinese medical students. *Social Psychiatry and Psychiatric Epidemiology, 45,* 963–971.

Lu, F. J., Hsu, E. Y., Wang, J. M., Huang, M. Y., Chang, J. N., & Wang, C. H. (2012). Exercisers' identities and exercise dependence: The mediating effect of exercise commitment. *Perceptual and Motor Skills, 115,* 618–631.

Manning, Y., & Murphy, B. (2003). An introduction to anorexia nervosa and bulimia nervosa. *Nursing Standard, 18,* 14–16.

McCreary, D. R., & Sasse, D. K. (2000). An exploration of the drive for muscularity in adolescent boys and girls. *Journal of American College Health, 48,* 297–304.

Merglen, A., Flatz, A., Belanger, R. E., Michaud, P-A., & Suris, J-C. (2014). Weekly sport practice and adolescent well-being. *Archives of Disease in Childhood, 99,* 208–210.

Michaelides, A. P., Soulis, D., Antoniades, C., Antopoulos, A. S., Miliou, A., & Loakeimidis, N. (2011). Exercise duration as a determinant of vascular function and antioxidant balance in patients with coronary artery disease. *Heart, 97,* 832–837.

Mondin, G. W., Morgan, W. P., Piering, P. N., Stegner, A. J., Stotesbery, C. L., Trine, M. R., & Wu, M. (1996). Psychological consequences of exercise deprivation in habitual exercisers. *Medicine and Science in Sports and Exercise, 28,* 1199–1203.

Monok, K., Berczik, K., Urban, R., Szabo, A., Griffiths, M. D., Farkas, J., ... Demetrovics, Z. (2012). Psychometric properties and concurrent validity of two exercise addiction measures: A population wide study. *Psychology of Sport and Exercise, 13,* 387–404.

Morgan, W. P. (1979). Negative addiction in runners. *The Physician and Sportsmedicine, 7,* 57–77.

Morrison, T. G., & Morrison, M. A. (2004). Scale examining drive for muscularity in males. *Psychology of Men and Muscularity, 5,* 1, 30–39.

Murray, A. L., McKensizie, K., Newman, E., & Brown, E. (2013). Exercise identity as a risk factor for exercise dependence. *British Journal of Health Psychology, 18,* 369–382.

Murray, S. B., Rieger, E., Karlow, L., & Touyz, S. W. (2013). An investigation of the transdiagnostic model of eating disorders in the context of muscle dysmorphia. *European Eating Disorders Review, 21,* 160–164.

Murray, S. B., & Touyz, S. W. (2013). Muscle dysmorphia: Toward a diagnostic consensus. *Australian and New Zealand Journal of Psychiatry, 47,* 206–207.

O'Connor, P. J., & Smith, J. C. (1999). *Physical activity and eating disorders.* In J. M. Rippe (Ed.), *Lifestyle medicine* (pp. 1005–1015). Cambridge, MA: Blackwell Science.

O'Keefe, J. H., Patil, H. R., & McCullough, P. A. (2012). Potential adverse cardiovascular effects from excessive endurance exercise. *Mayo Clinic Proceedings, 87,* 704–716.

Olivardia, R., Pope, H. G., & Hudson, J. I. (2000). Muscle dysmorphia in male weight lifters: A case-control study. *American Journal of Psychiatry, 157,* 1291–1296.

Pierce, E. F., Eastman, N. W., Tripathi, H. L., Olson, K. G., & Dewey, W. L. (1993). B-endorphin response to endurance exercise: Relationship to exercise dependence. *Perceptual and Motor Skills, 77,* 767–770.

Poole, L., Hamer, M., Wawrzyniak, A. J., & Steptoe, A. (2011). The effects of exercise withdrawal on mood and inflammatory cytokine responses in humans. *Stress, 14,* 439–447.

Pope, H. G., Gruber, A. J., Choi, P., Olivardia, R., & Phillips, K. A. (1997). Muscle dysmorphia. An underrecognized form of body dysmorphic disorder. *Psychosomatics, 38,* 548–557.

Pope, H. G., & Katz, D. L. (1994). Psychiatric and medical effects of anabolic steroid use. *Archives of General Psychiatry, 51,* 375–382.

Pope, H. G., Katz, D. L., & Hudson, J. I. (1993). Anorexia nervosa and "reverse anorexia" among 108 male bodybuilders. *Comprehensive Psychiatry, 34,* 406–409.

Santarnecchi, E., & Dettore, D. (2012). Muscle dysmorphia in different degrees of bodybuilding activities: Validation of the Italian version of Muscle Dysmophia Disorder Inventory and Bodybuilder Image Grid. *Body Image, 9,* 396–403.

Schrieber, K., & Hausenblas, H. A. (2015). *The truth about exercise addiction: Understanding the dark side of thinspiration.* Rowman & Littlefield.

Shroff, H., Reba, L., Thornton, L.M., Tozzi, F., Klump, K., Berrettini, W. H., ... Bulik, C. M. (2006). Features associated with excessive exercise in women with eating disorders. *International Journal of Eating Disorders, 39,* 454–461.

Stoeber, J., & Childs, J. H. (2010). The assessment of self-oriented and socially prescribed perfectionism: Subscales make a difference. *Journal of Personality Assessment, 92,* 577–585.

Suffolk, M. T., Dovey, T. M., Goodwin, H., & Meyer, S. (2013). Muscle dysmorphia: Methodological issues, implications for research. *Eating Disorders, 21,* 437–457.

Sussman, S., Lisha, N., & Griffiths, M. D. (2011). Prevalence of the addictions: A problem of the majority or the minority? *Evaluation and the Health Professions, 34,* 3–56.

Symons Downs, D., Savage, J. S., & DiNallo, J. M. (2013). Self-determined to exercise? Leisure-time exercise behavior, exercise motivation, and exercise dependence in youth. *Journal of Physical Activity and Health, 10,* 176–184.

Szabo, A. (1995). The impact of exercise deprivation on well-being of habitual exercisers. *The Australian Journal of Science and Medicine in Sport, 27*, 68–75.

Szabo, A. (2000). Physical activity and psychological dysfunction. In Physical Activity and Psychological Well-being (S. J. H. Biddle, K. Fox, & S. Boutcher, Eds) (pp. 130–153). New York: Routledge.

Szabo, A., Frenkl, R., & Caputo, A. (1997). Relationship between addiction to running, commitment, and deprivation from running: A study on the internet. *European Yearbook of Sport Psychology, 1*, 130–147.

Thompson, J. K., & Blanton, P. (1987). Energy conservation and exercise dependence: A sympathetic arousal hypothesis. *Medicine and Science in Sports and Exercise, 19*, 91–99.

U.S. Department of Health and Human Services. (2008). Physical activity guidelines for Americans. Retrieved August 27, 2015, from health.gov/paguidelines/guidelines/default.aspx.

Varnado-Sullivan, P. J., Horton, R., & Savoy, S. (2006). Differences for gender, weight, and exercise in body image disturbance and eating disorder symptoms. *Eating and Weight Disorders, 11*, 118–125.

Veale, D. (1987). Exercise dependence. *British Journal of Addiction, 82*, 735–740.

Veale, D. (1995). Does primary exercise dependence really exist? In J. Annett, B. Cripps, & H. Steinberg (Eds.), *Exercise addiction: Motivation for participation in sport and exercise.* (pp. 1–5). Leicester, UK: British Psychological Society.

Villella, C., Martinotti, G., Di NiCola, M., Cassano, M., La Torre, G., Gliubuzzi, M. D., … Conte, G. (2011). Behavioural addictions in adolescents and young adults: Results from a prevalence study. *Journal of Gambling Studies, 27*, 203–214.

Waters, B. (1981). Defining the runner's personality. *Runner's World, 16*, 48–51.

Weinstein, A. A., Deuster, P. A., & Kop, W. J. (2007). Heart rate variability as a predictor of negative mood symptoms induced by exercise withdrawal. *Medicine and Science in Sports and Exercise, 39*, 735–741.

Wilson, M. G., O'Hanlon, R., Prasad, S., Deighan, A., Macmillan, P., Oxborough, D., … Whyte, G. (2011). Diverse patterns of myocardial fibrosis in lifelong, veteran endurance athletes. *Journal of Applied Physiology, 110*, 1622–1626.

Yager, J. (1991). Bulimia nervosa. *The Western Journal of Medicine, 155*, 523–524.

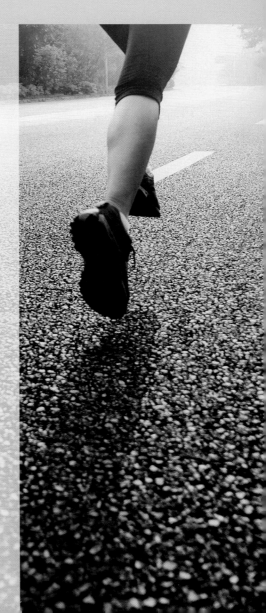

SECTION 4

Environmental Effects of Exercise and Sedentary Behavior

A long-standing dictum in psychology is that behavior is a product of the individual and the situation (i.e., physical and social environment). Thus, it follows directly from this dictum that we need to gain an understanding of the physical and social environment if we hope to understand individual involvement in physical activity. In other words, an important characteristic that helps to define the psychology of exercise and sedentary behavior as a discipline is its focus on the environmental factors that influence individual behavior. Section 4 of the text provides an overview of research that has centered on the individual participant's social and physical environments. Chapter 15 focuses on the social environment (e.g., family, friends, and teammates); Chapter 16 outlines aspects of the physical environment (e.g., neighborhoods, parks, green spaces) that have been found to impact physical activity and sedentary behavior.

15

Social Environment

Runner: © Izf/Shutterstock

Runner: © Izf/Shutterstock

Vignette: Madeline

I'm embarrassed to run outside or on a treadmill. Any time I've tried, I just think of the bright purple track suits my parents would go jogging in around our neighborhood in West Virginia when my older sister and I were kids. They may have been fitter than most parents in our Huntington school district, but they were also the laughingstock of most kids I knew.

My mom was the one who really pushed fitness on our family. She implored my sister and me to join her on jogs, harangued us for watching too much television, and gave us the stink eye when we'd come home with ice cream stains on our clothes or sticky fingers from furtive trips to the bakery after school. My sister had a much harder time with mom's insistence on eating healthy and exercising every day. She went on to develop an eating disorder and had to drop out of college for some time to get treatment.

I, on the other hand, tried to avoid fitness trends, gyms, or involvement in team sports as long as I could hold out. That's not to say I didn't get any physical activity. I took favorably to bike rides outdoors, walks, and the occasional hike. But if ever my activities of choice were associated with willful physical activity—that is, the kind people rely on to "get in

LEARNING OBJECTIVES

After completing this chapter, you will be able to

- Outline the importance of group dynamics to physical activity promotion.
- Differentiate among the four dimensions of group cohesion.
- Describe the relationships between group cohesion, class attendance, and individual-level cognition.
- Explain how the presence of social support influences our involvement in physical activity.
- Understand how parents, peers, and healthcare providers influence our physical activity behaviors.
- Describe how leaders affect physical activity cognitions and behaviors.

shape"—my interests immediately shifted to secluding myself at home or in a library with a thick, heavy book.

Of course, as I've gotten older and settled into the working world I don't have as much time to exercise leisurely as I used to. My fiancé has asked me numerous times to join him in CrossFit, but the intensity of that trend intimidates me. I also don't really see how being able to do 10 pull-ups in a row would benefit me outside of the gym.

One thing that has helped me stay active, however, is the Siberian husky my fiancé and I adopted shortly after we moved in together 6 months ago. I don't consider taking the energetic young pup out two—sometimes more—times a day as formal exercise. But I will say that being dragged around by this tireless fur ball keeps me on my toes. (It also happens to be the closest I'll come to running—ever. At least, I hope.)

Getting the dog has definitely benefitted my social life. My future husband and I are new to Portland, Oregon—where we were both able to secure jobs, buy a sizable house, and still have some savings left over to start our lives together—and I've found it slightly challenging to make friends.

What's more, a lot of employees at the graphic design office where I now work are huge fans of the outdoors. Like me, many of them also eschew the rigidity of most fitness programs marketed by gyms. And so, although I scaled back my time spent moving around when I was first settling in, 9 months into this job I've felt encouraged by my coworkers to get back out there and explore. (Many of them have some great tips for hiking, and I've gone out with a couple of them on some really nice outdoor walks.)

I've been incredibly lucky to escape that lingering sense of shame I felt for not forcing myself to jog or be on some sports team I couldn't care less about. Maybe being thousands of miles away from mom helps. (Though I still worry about my sister, who continues to live at home.)

Part of what keeps me wanting to be active is the social nature of it. Even if I strike out on my own for a bike ride or a hike, I can still share my experience with friends at work who are genuinely interested in my experiences—and have their own to share and compare. And that my dog shows me so much more love when I bring him along for a leisurely outdoor adventure makes me even happier.

Introduction

Humans are social beings. In fact, our need to form and maintain strong social attachments with other people is fundamental to our overall health and well-being (Baumeister & Leary, 1995). C. S. Lewis, a famous novelist, illustrated the importance of our social relations in the following quote: "Those who are enjoying something, or suffering something together, are companions (1945, p. 145)." Indeed, social relationships—whether they are positive or negative—influence our thoughts, emotions, and behavior.

Moreover, the absence of supportive social relationships can have a detrimental impact on our physical and psychological health. A lack of social support is associated with higher morbidity and mortality (Tay, Tan, Diener, & Gonzalez, 2013). For example, divorce (where there is a disruption to social support) leads to an early death. How much earlier than married people? The risk of dying early is 23% greater among divorced adults than married couples. And the health risk associated with divorce is similar to other well-established risk factors, such as smoking up to 15 cigarettes a day, doing insufficient physical activity, being overweight, and drinking alcohol heavily (Sbarra, Law, & Portley, 2011).

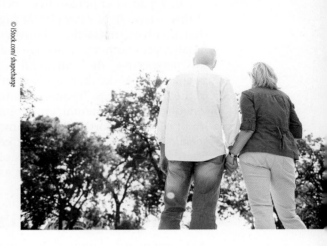

The **social environment** comprises the physical surroundings, social relationships, and cultural milieu within which people function and interact (Barnett & Casper, 2001). The social environment refers to the environment developed by people such as your family, friends, physicians, peers, classmates, neighbors, teachers, and others who you come into contact with regularly. In this chapter, we will examine how our social environment affects physical activity and sedentary behavior by focusing on social support and the group dynamics variables of cohesion and leadership.

■ Social Support

The term **social support** is relatively new in the social sciences. The study of the nature, antecedents, and consequences of social support represents an emerging field of study. As is the case in any emerging field of study, researchers and theoreticians have advanced a variety of perspectives on the nature of social support. The result is that while there is almost universal consensus that social support is important for health and well-being, there is considerable discrepancy in our understanding of what social support actually is and how it should be defined and measured.

Social support is a complex phenomenon. One measure of that complexity is the number of perspectives adopted in an attempt to define it. In one general perspective, the role of *information* is emphasized. Cobb (1976), for example, defined social support as information that leads the individual to feel: (1) cared for; (2) loved, esteemed, and valued; and (3) a sense of belonging to a reciprocal network.

In another similar perspective, the role of *emotion* is emphasized. For example, Cassel (1976) proposed that social support reflects the gratification of an individual's basic needs.

In yet another perspective, social support is viewed as a *process*. As an example of this perspective, Vaux (1992) suggested that social support is a dynamic process that involves transactions between individuals within a specific social context. Finally, yet another perspective draws upon the idea of *networks* of support. From this perspective, the individual is seen as the focus of networks (collection) of people—networks that can vary in structure (e.g., size, number of links), nature of the linkages (e.g., frequency, intensity of interactions), and the function(s) provided (e.g., instrumental, emotional support; Israel, 1982). Perhaps the complexity of social support was best summed up by Alan Vaux (1988) who stated that social support represents a wide cross section of concepts, including "belonging, bonding, and binding; attributes of groups, relationships, and persons; and processes that are social, behavioral, and affective in nature" (p. 33).

Taxonomies for Social Support

A second manifestation of the complexity of social support is the variety of terms that are used interchangeably. In an attempt to distinguish among social support–related concepts, Anton Laireiter and Urs Baumann (1992) proposed a taxonomy. One of the components, **social integration** (also known as *social embeddedness*), represents the degree to which the individual participates and is involved in family life, the social life of the community (e.g., churches, community events), and has access to resources and support systems. Social integration is similar to social networks; it is the extent that the individual has regular contact with friends, neighbors, and family.

A second component, **support networks** (also known as *network resources*), represents the individual's social network from a functional perspective. Who does the individual turn to for assistance or emotional support? Who are the individual's potential supporters? Who are the individual's actual supporters? The people an individual routinely turns to for support represent his or her network resources. As the term implies, support networks represent the pool of support resources available to the individual.

Supportive climates (or *supportive environments*) represent the quality of social relationships and systems. Is the family unit cohesive? To what extent is there frequent conflict in the family? As might be expected, cohesive families, workgroups, and friendship groups are perceived by the individual to be more supportive.

A fourth component of the taxonomy, received and enacted support, represents two aspects of the social support exchange. When social support is viewed as a process, two individuals are involved. One, the provider of social support, represents enacted support; the other individual in the exchange, the recipient, represents received support.

Another component, perceived support, represents the individual's cognitive appraisal. Support received is not synonymous with support perceived. An individual might receive advice, encouragement, and financial assistance from a large network of people, including family, close friends, fellow workers, and health and business professionals. Yet that same individual could perceive that he or she is socially isolated or has been abandoned insofar as access to support is concerned. Thus, social support cannot simply be determined by counting the amount of contacts between a focal person and his or her social network.

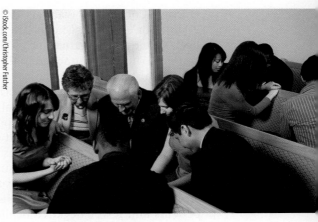

According to Laireiter and Baumann (1992), the complex phenomena in their taxonomy are related to one another in a hierarchical manner. As **FIGURE 15-1** shows, social integration represents the broadest, most fundamental category. Without social integration, there could be no support networks, supportive climates, enacted and received support, and/or perceived support. In turn, support networks are a necessary precondition before questions of supportive climate, received and enacted support, or perceived support can arise. As Figure 15-1 shows, the hierarchy continues until, finally, received and enacted support serve as a precondition for perceived support.

Negative Aspects of Social Support

A third reflection of the complexity of social support is the fact that the implicit assumption that social support is always positive is not true (e.g., Chogahara,

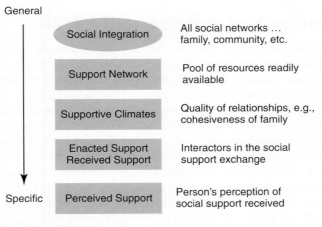

FIGURE 15-1   Hierarchy of Social Support

O'Brien Cousins, & Wankel, 1998; Rafaeli, Cranford, Green, Shrout, & Bolger, 2008). For example, Chogahara and his colleagues (1998) noted that there have been numerous negative social influences identified in fields such as health psychology. The labels attached to those negative social influences include, for example, social hindrance, social rejection, social inhibition, unsupportive behaviors, unhelpful behaviors, negative social ties, social strain, negative social interactions, social pressure, social disapproval, and stereotypes. None of these influences can be considered positive social support, but they all can have an impact on behavior. For example, social pressure and social norms are often cited as reasons for why adolescents begin smoking (Sarason, Mankowski, Peterson, & Dinh, 1992).

Relative to positive social support, negative social support occurs less frequently but likely will have a greater influence on health outcomes (Chogahara et al., 1998). Positive social reactions are associated with more psychological health benefits and fewer negative health symptoms, whereas negative social reactions are associated with increased negative psychological health symptoms (Sylaska & Edwards, 2014). Negative social support also has a stronger immediate impact, and it retains its influence over a longer duration. Thus, a supportive statement from parents to their children such as "you can do it" could positively influence physical activity involvement. However, the negative impact of statements such as "act your age" and "you're too old to ride a bike" would likely carry more weight initially and persist as an influence on activity behavior over a longer period of time.

CRITICAL THINKING ACTIVITY 15-1

© ecco/Shutterstock, Inc.

When might social support have a negative effect on exercise behavior? How can this impact long-term health?

Social Support as a Personality Trait

A final reflection of complexity lies in the fact that although social support is by its very definition a *social* construct, there is also evidence that it is an *individual* construct. In their research, Sarason and colleagues (Sarason, Levine, Basham, & Sarason, 1983; Sarason, Pierce, Sarason, 1990; Sarason et al., 1991; Sarason, Sarason, & Pierce, 1992) observed that perceptions of the availability of social support represent a stable personality trait. We possess an enduring disposition to see ourselves as being supported by others. Some people, of course, may see themselves as the chronic recipients of considerable support from others (even in the presence of evidence to the contrary). Conversely, some people may have the tendency to see themselves as receiving minimal or no support from others (again, even in the presence of evidence to the contrary). The tendency to perceive oneself as being supported is positively related to both self-concept and self-esteem (Sarason, Sarason, & Pierce, 1992).

Measurement of Social Support

Given the complex nature of social support, it is not surprising that a number of approaches have been taken in its measurement. Generally, these different approaches have reflected differences in the specific research question asked. Who gives the person social support? What type(s) of social support does an individual receive? What is the quantity and quality of that social support?

Essentially, the measurement of social support has taken three general approaches (see TABLE 15-1). One approach is concerned with determining an individual's *social network resources* (Vaux, 1982). Throughout the school year, for example, a student might have the need for financial assistance (e.g., money to pay for books and tuition), practical assistance (e.g., for a ride to school), emotional support (e.g., for love, affection), advice or guidance (e.g., in course selection), and positive social interactions (e.g., someone to go to coffee with). Measures of social network resources are concerned with who that student could go to for support. There could be more than one person in any or all of the categories, of course. When social support is assessed through measures of social network resources, the focus is on questions of size and density. The index or measure could be in the form of global estimates (e.g., how many people in total are available to provide support) or domain-specific estimates (e.g., how many people are available to provide financial assistance).

A second approach is concerned with determining an individual's *support appraisal* (Russell & Cutrona, 1984). In this approach, the focus is on satisfaction, sufficiency, or helpfulness of the support. The prototypical student introduced

TABLE 15-1   Typical Approaches in the Measurement of Social Support

Approach	Concept	Example of Possible Measures
Social network resources	Significant others available to provide support	Size of the network Density of the network
Support appraisal	Satisfaction, sufficiency, or helpfulness of support in important domains	Attachment (emotional support) Social integration (network support) Opportunity for nurturance (self-worth from assisting others) Reassurance of worth (esteem support) Reliable alliance (tangible aid) Guidance (information support)
Support behavior	Frequency of occurrence or likelihood of behavior	Financial assistance Practical assistance Emotional support Advice or guidance Positive social interactions

Adapted from Vaux, A. (1992). Assessment of social support. In H. O. F. Veiel & U. Baumann (Eds.), *The meaning and measurement of social support* (pp. 193–216). New York, NY: Hemisphere Publishing.

above can serve as an example to illustrate support appraisal. The student might have a number of individuals available for positive social interactions (e.g., to have coffee with). However, the student's support appraisal—that is, the satisfaction expressed with his or her positive social interactions—could be either moderate or low. The appraisal of support could be "I have support but it's just not very good."

Support appraisal has been examined frequently insofar as its relationship to issues such as self-efficacy for physical activity in elderly populations (e.g., Duncan, Duncan, & McAuley 1993). Generally, the appraisal of social support has centered on six important social needs identified by Weiss (1974). These are *attachment*, which reflects emotional support; *social integration*, which reflects network support; *opportunity for nurturance*, which reflects increased self-worth from assisting others; *reassurance of worth*, which reflects esteem support; sense of *reliable alliance*, which reflects tangible aid; and obtaining of *guidance*, which reflects information support. The relationship of these various forms of social support to exercise and sedentary behavior is discussed later in the chapter.

A third, somewhat related approach is concerned with determining support behavior (Barrera, Sandler, & Ramsay, 1981). In this approach, the focus is on the frequency of occurrence or the likelihood that others will provide the behavior. Again, it might be useful to use the prototypical student to illustrate the approach taken. Although the student might have a large number of individuals available for coffee, he or she might rate the frequency of social interactions to be minimal over a month period.

The three approaches are similar in that they are designed to assess some manifestation of social support. However, it should be apparent that there are subtle differences as well. Thus, the specific approach taken would depend upon the question asked. Is the health professional or researcher interested in whether the person has a large number of people available for social support? If so, social network resources would be assessed. Is the health professional or researcher interested in whether the person's social support is either frequent or infrequent? If so, support behavior would be assessed. Finally, is the interest in whether the social support available to the person is either more or less satisfying? If so, support appraisal would be assessed.

In summary, although there are a variety of instruments used to assess social support, there is no single, "best" measure. This situation may be partially due to the fact that a wide range of different measurement strategies have yielded "scores" that have successfully been related to a variety of health outcomes. Measures range from single items used to assess whether or not types of social support (e.g., emotional, instrumental) are available (using yes/no responses) to more extensive measures that include multiple items asking about various types of social support.

See **TABLE 15-2** for a measure of the functional components of social support developed by Cohen and colleagues (Cohen, Mermelstin, Kamarck, & Hoberman, 1985). This questionnaire has three different subscales designed to measure the

TABLE 15-2   Measuring the Functional Components of Social Support

Instructions: This scale is made up of a list of statements, each of which may or may not be true about you. For each statement circle (4) "definitely true" if you are sure it is true about you and (3) "probably true" if you think it is true but are not absolutely certain. Similarly, you should circle (1) "definitely false" if you are sure the statement is false and (2) "probably false" if you think it is false but are not absolutely certain.

1	2	3	4
definitely false	probably false	probably true	definitely true

1. If I wanted to go on a trip for a day (for example, to the country or mountains), I would have a hard time finding someone to go with me.

2. I feel that there is no one I can share my most private worries and fears with.

3. If I were sick, I could easily find someone to help me with my daily chores.

4. There is someone I can turn to for advice about handling problems with my family.

5. If I decide one afternoon that I would like to go to a movie that evening, I could easily find someone to go with me.

6. When I need suggestions on how to deal with a personal problem, I know someone I can turn to.

7. I don't often get invited to do things with others.

8. If I had to go out of town for a few weeks, it would be difficult to find someone who would look after my house or apartment (the plants, pets, garden, etc.).

9. If I wanted to have lunch with someone, I could easily find someone to join me.

10. If I was stranded 10 miles from home, there is someone I could call who could come and get me.

11. If a family crisis arose, it would be difficult to find someone who could give me good advice about how to handle it.

12. If I needed some help in moving to a new house or apartment, I would have a hard time finding someone to help me.

Scoring:
Items 1, 2, 7, 8, 11, 12 are reverse scored.
Items 2, 4, 6, 11 make up the Appraisal Support subscale.
Items 1, 5, 7, 9 make up the Belonging Support subscale.
Items 3, 8, 10, 12 make up the Tangible Support subscale.

Cohen, A., Mermelstein, R., Kamarck, T., & Hoberman, H. M. (1985). Measuring the functional components of social support. In I. G. Sarason & B. R. Sarason (Eds.), *Social support: Theory, research, and applications*. The Hague, Netherlands: Martinus Niijhoff.

following dimensions of perceived social support: appraisal support, belonging support, and tangible support. Each item is measured by four items on a 4-point scale ranging from "definitely true" to "definitely false."

Social Support, Physical Activity, and Sedentary Behavior

The degree to which people sense that they receive the support of others will influence the development of cognitions associated with their involvement in exercise. Carron, Hausenblas, and Mack (1996) statistically summarized available research on the relationship between social support and intention to be physically active through the use of a meta-analysis. They found that social support from family members has a moderate effect (i.e., ES = .49) on an individual's intention to engage in physical activity. In addition, important others—physicians, work colleagues, for example—also have a moderate effect on intention (i.e., ES = .44), although their influence is slightly lower than that of the family. So, social support has an important role to play in terms of its impact on people's intentions to be physically active.

Social support from important others (e.g., work colleagues) has an even more important role to play than family in terms of the positive affect people develop around physical activity (Carron et al., 1996). Why this is the case is uncertain. Possibly, it is related to the informational and motivational aspects of social reinforcement. Social reinforcement from people who are not intimates can be more motivating because it is generally less frequent and more selective and therefore provides more information to the recipient.

CRITICAL THINKING ACTIVITY 15-2

© ecco/Shutterstock, Inc.

How do you think the social support from a wife could affect a husband's exercise intention and behavior?

TABLE 15-3 provides an overview of the results of the meta-analysis by Carron, Hausenblas, and Mack (1996) that examined the relationship between social support from a variety of sources and adherence to physical activity regimes. The effect of social support on adherence is in the small to moderate range. Nonetheless, social support is an important variable for understanding people's exercise intentions and behaviors.

As Table 15-3 also shows, adherence behavior is more strongly influenced by social support from important others than from family members. As was the case with attitude, the reason for this is unknown. Again, possibly, social support from important others is more motivating because it provides more information.

TABLE 15-3 Results of the Meta-Analysis on the Influence of Social Support on Physical Activity Behavior		
Nature of the Social Support	**Nature of the Behavior**	**Effect Size**
Support from family	Adherence behavior	.36
Support from family	Compliance behavior	.69
Support from important others	Adherence behavior	.44

Data from Carron, A.V., Hausenblas, H., & Mack, D.A. (1996). Social influence and exercise: A meta-analysis. *Journal of Sport and Exercise Psychology, 18,* 1–16.

The difference between adherence and compliance is essentially the difference between maintaining involvement in a self-selected program (i.e., adherence) versus maintaining involvement in a prescribed program (i.e., compliance). Physical activity is often prescribed by physicians and healthcare professionals for a variety of reasons, such as the treatment of obesity and to facilitate recovery after surgery for coronary heart disease. When this is the case, social support from family plays an important role.

Social support is positively and consistently associated with physical activity level across the lifespan (Barber, 2012; Maier & James, 2014; Mendonca, Cheng, Melo, & de Farias Junio, 2014; Oliveira et al., 2011). For example, adolescents who receive more overall social support as well as specific support from both parents and friends have higher levels of physical activity than adolescent who receive less support. As another example, pregnant and postpartum women who perceived greater levels of social support are more likely to exercise than women who perceive they have less social support for exercise during this transitional time into motherhood (McIntyre & Rhodes, 2009).

A large-scale study by Anne Kouvonen and her colleagues (2012) illustrates the complex effects social support can have on physical activity. They conducted a prospective cohort study of 5,395 adults (mean age = 55.7 years) who completed measures of their confiding/emotional support (e.g., wanting to confide, sharing interests) and practical support, as well as exercise behavior at baseline assessment. At the follow-up assessment 5 years later the participants' exercise behavior was reassessed. The researchers found that among the participants who reported the recommended levels of exercise at baseline, those who experienced high confiding/emotional support were more likely to report participating in recommended levels of exercise at follow-up. Among those participants who did not meet the recommended target of exercise at baseline, high confiding/emotional support was not associated with improvement in activity levels. High practical support was associated with both maintaining and improving exercise levels. The researchers concluded that emotional and practical support from those closest to the person may help the individual to maintain the recommended level of exercise. Practical support also predicted a change toward a more active lifestyle.

Parents

Kathryn Hesketh and her colleagues (2014) examined the correlation between objectively measured maternal and preschool-age children's physical activity in a cohort of 554 4-year-olds and their mothers. Physical activity was measured using

accelerometry. The researchers found that mother–child daily activity levels were positively associated at all the activity intensities (i.e., sedentary, light physical activity, moderate to vigorous physical activity). In other words, if a mother spent a large portion of her day being sedentary, it was likely that her child spent a large portion of the day being sedentary also. In short, mothers who were physically active had children who were more physically active. Interestingly, mothers often perceived their young children to be more active than they really were. Almost 90% of mothers of inactive preschool-age children perceive their child to be active (Hesketh et al., 2013).

With regard to sedentary behavior, higher parental television viewing is associated with an increased risk of high levels of television viewing for both boys and girls (Jago, Fox, Page, Brockman, & Thompson, 2010). Researchers have found that children are more likely to watch television with their parents and siblings than to engage in physical activity with them (Tandon et al., 2012).

In another study, Andrew Springer and his colleagues (Springer, Kelder, & Hoelschler, 2006) examined the associations of two types of social support (i.e., social participation in and social encouragement for physical activity) and two social support sources (i.e., family and friends) with self-reported daily minutes of physical activity and sedentary behavior (television/video viewing and computer/video game play) among 718 sixth-grade girls. Students were asked to rate four items that assessed social support. Students were asked to report how often during the past month their (1) family did physical activities with them; (2) family encouraged them to be physically active; (3) friends did physical activities with them; and (4) friends encouraged them to be physically active.

They found that friend physical activity participation and friend and family encouragement were positively related to moderate to vigorous physical activity. Family participation in physical activity had the strongest negative correlation with total minutes of television/video viewing and computer/video game play. The researchers concluded that social support is an important correlate of physical activity among adolescent girls but suggest that the source and type of social support may differ for physical activity and sedentary behaviors.

Peers

While parents are the most important influence early in a child's life, parental influence on the child's day-to-day behavior becomes less evident as the child matures. Children and adolescents spend a significant portion of their time at school with friends and peers. Thus, it is not surprising that their friend's health behaviors influence their individual health behaviors, such as diet. What role do friends play in influencing physical activity and sedentary behavior?

Friendship networks are associated with physical activity among children and adolescents, with some, albeit less, evidence suggesting that friendship networks might also be associated with sedentary behavior (Sawka, McCormack, Nettel-Aquirre, Hawe, & Doyle-Baker, 2013). In fact, children and adolescents who report low social support from family and friends are more likely to be insufficiently active for health benefits compared to those with high levels of social support. As well, children and youth's physical activity is positively associated with encouragement from friends, their friends' own physical activity behavior, and engagement with friends in physical activity (Maturo & Cunningham, 2013).

In other words, youth tend to befriend peers who do similar amounts of physical activity, and subsequently emulate their friends' behaviors. Thus, there is a mutually dependent relationship between adolescent friendship networks and physical activity (de la Haye, Robins, Mohr, & Wilson, 2011). Involvement in physical activity plays an important role in adolescents' friendship choices, with youth showing a preference for friends whose activity levels are similar to their own. Friends also influence changes to physical activity over the course of the school year, evidenced by friends' engagement in leisure-time exercise becoming increasingly similar.

Less research has examined the relationship between sedentary behavior and social support. Existing research has found that playing video games with friends is related to decreased exercise and increased sedentary behavior in children (Marques et al., 2014).

Teasing and Bullying

Teasing and **bullying** reflect negative aspects of social support, and not surprisingly it has a negative effect on young people's physical activity (Roman & Taylor, 2013). Children who are teased during physical activity or physical education class are less likely to participate in exercise a year later (Jensen, Cushing, & Elledge, 2014). The negative impact of teasing during gym class was found in both overweight children as well as those who were of a healthy weight. However, overweight or obese children who experienced

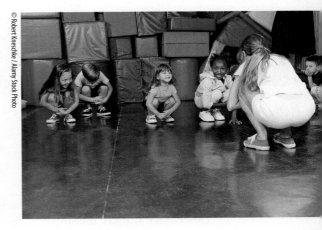
© Robert Kneschke / Alamy Stock Photo

teasing during physical activity had a lower perceived health-related quality of life (referring to physical, social, academic, and emotional functioning) 1 year later. Another study of 7,786 American middle school children found that bullying was associated with fewer days in physical education classes and lower odds of meeting the physical activity guidelines of exercising at least 60 minutes each day (Roman & Taylor, 2013).

What type of perceptions do students and teachers have about bullying in physical education and about both peer and adult support? O'Connor and Graber (2014) used a qualitative interview design to ask these questions of sixth-grade teachers and students. The researchers found that adults acculturate students to support a bullying climate by providing mixed information regarding social interactions, ignoring nonphysical instances of bullying, and promoting inappropriate curricular selections. The students reported that perceived differences such as appearance, body size, physical ability, and personal attire start most episodes of harassment or bullying in their physical education classes. As well, students perceive fear that prevents many of them from following up on important issues, such as reporting instances of bullying to those in authority, assisting bullied friends, and feeling safe in certain physical education locations. Not surprisingly, bullying negatively impacts the students' desire to engage in physical education classes. Children must be encouraged to engage in physical activity at school within a safe and friendly environment (Jensen et al., 2014).

CRITICAL THINKING ACTIVITY 15-3

© ecco/Shutterstock, Inc.

Why do you think bullying can have such a long-term effect on people's exercise behavior?

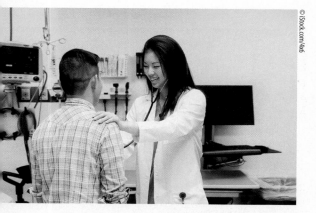
© iStock.com/4x6

Healthcare Providers

Physicians and other healthcare providers have an ethical, and some would even say legal, obligation to assess and prescribe exercise to their patients. Physicians are in a critical position to help patients develop healthy lifestyles by actively counseling them on physical activity (Joy et al., 2013). Research indicates that physicians can influence patients to improve their health through proactive advising on the positive health impacts of physical activity during an office visit (Orrow, Kinmonth, Sanderson, & Sutton, 2012).

Unfortunately, many physicians are not talking to their patients about physical activity and are missing a unique opportunity to raise awareness about its benefits. Physicians report several barriers that make it difficult for them to counsel their patients on exercise. Some of these barriers include time demands, insufficient reimbursement, lack of education on the benefits of physical activity, lack of knowledge on how to write an effective exercise prescription, and limited support systems for patient education (McKenna, Naylor, & McDowell, 1998). One study found that over half of the physicians trained in the United States receive no formal education in physical activity (Cardinal, Park, Kim, & Cardinal, 2014). Lastly, physically active physicians are more likely to counsel patients to be active. Thus, a key message for the healthcare provider community is the importance of serving as a positive physical activity role model.

Dogs

In most developed countries, rates of dog ownership are high. For example, about 40% of Australian and 37% of U.S. households own at least one dog (American Veterinary Medical Association, 2012; Animal Health Alliance, 2013). This high level of dog ownership shows the high level of attachment that exists between people and their dogs. In fact, most dog owners consider their pets to be family members. A common activity for dog owners is to walk their dog.

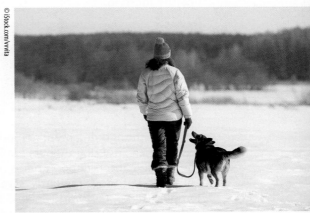

However, is dog ownership related to physical activity? The answer is a clear yes! People who own a dog are more likely to be physically active (Christian, Trapp, et al., 2013; Lentino, Visek, McDonnell, & DiPietro, 2012; Solomon, Rees, Ukoumunne, Metcalf, & Hillsdon, 2013). Dog owners tend to be more physically active than those who do not own a dog (Toohey & Rock, 2011). Just how much more active are dog owners? Hayley Christian and her colleagues (Christian, Westgarth et al., 2013) conducted a review of 29 studies that compared the physical activity levels of dog owners to nondog owners. They found small to moderate effect sizes that showed that dog owners engaged in more walking and physical activity than nondog owners. More specifically, they found that about 60% of dog owners walked their dog with a median duration and frequency of 160 minutes a week and four walks per week. They concluded that while dog walking has significant potential to increase the proportion of people who are physically active, either by encouraging those who do not walk their dog to do so or by increasing the amount of walking owners do with their dog, more high-quality research is needed to further our understanding of the correlates and determinants of dog-walking behavior.

This positive effect of dog ownership on physical activity is evidenced across the lifespan (Shibata et al., 2012). For example, researchers from Australia found that dog ownership was associated with children getting 29 more minutes of walking and 142 more minutes of physical activity per week than nondog owners (Christian, Trapp, et al., 2013). They also found that children with a dog are 49%

more likely to achieve the recommended level of weekly physical activity and 32% more likely to have walked in their neighborhood in the last week, compared with nondog owners. Dog ownership, however, was not associated with screen use.

Interestingly, people who do not own dogs have greater risk of diabetes, hypertension, hypercholesterolemia, and depression compared with people who regularly walked their dogs (Lentino et al., 2012). Because of the health benefits associated with dog walking, it has been suggested that dog walking should be encouraged within communities as a method of promoting and sustaining a healthy lifestyle.

CRITICAL THINKING ACTIVITY 15-4

Do you think that owning other types of pets besides dogs can result in increased exercise for pet owners as opposed to nonowners?

Even though dog owners report more leisure-time walking than nonowners, less than 25% of dog owners walk their dogs regularly (Cutt et al., 2008). Thus, one possible intervention area is to promote dog walking among owners who do not walk their dogs regularly. Ryan Rhodes and his colleagues (Rhodes, Murray, Temple, Tukko, & Wharf Higgins, 2012) examined the viability of dog walking for a physical activity intervention using messages targeting canine exercise. In their study, 58 inactive dog owners completed a baseline questionnaire package and wore a pedometer for 1 week. They were then randomized to either a standard control condition or the intervention condition. The intervention condition consisted of persuasive material about canine health benefits from walking and a calendar to mark walks. The control group participants were instructed to continue with their current dog walking schedule for the study's duration.

Participants in the intervention group were instructed to read and use the materials provided and to add more dog walking to their lifestyle. The materials detailed the benefits of exercise for dogs; dogs' exercise needs; the proper types and amounts of exercise for dogs of different breeds, age, and health; tips for regular dog walking; and a variety of exercises for dogs and their owners. The materials also included safety and health tips for starting a walking routine and motivational quotes from dog owners.

The researchers found that both the control and intervention groups increased physical activity across the 12 weeks of the study. The intervention group, however, had higher increases in step-counts per day as well as minutes of both dog walking and nondog walking per week compared to the control group. **FIGURE 15-2** displays the steps per day for the intervention and control group. As is evidenced in this figure, the intervention group was approaching the 10,000 steps per day needed to be classified as physically active. This pilot study reveals that targeted information might be helpful to increase dog walking. Larger-scale studies are needed to verify these results.

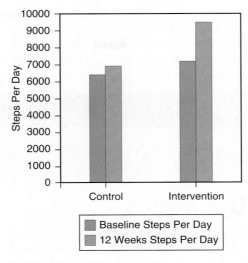

FIGURE 15-2   Steps Taken at Baseline and at 12 Weeks

Data from Rhodes, R. E., Murray, H., Temple, V., Tuokko, H., & Wharf Higgins, J. (2012). Pilot study of a dog walking intervention: Effects of a focus on canine exercise. *Preventive Medicine, 54*, 309–312.

Social Media

Rapid developments in technology have encouraged the use of **social media**, including **mobile applications (apps)**, to help people increase their physical activity. Providing social support via these apps is becoming an increasingly popular technique in attempts to change people's physical activity behavior (Conroy, Yang, & Maher, 2014; Yang, Maher, & Conroy, 2015). These apps typically provide social support, information about others' approval, instructions on how to perform an exercise behavior, demonstrations of the exercise behavior, and feedback on the exercise behavior (Yang et al., 2015). Because many people do not have access to behavior change programs, these apps can help to promote the adoption and maintenance of exercise in a variety of populations. Preliminary research reveals that social support networking via social media (e.g., smartphones, Facebook) may be an effective strategy to encourage physical activity change (Bort-Roig, Gilson, Puig-Ribera, Contrera, & Trost, 2014).

   Researchers examined the efficacy of a Facebook social support group to increase the steps per day in 63 female college freshman (Rote, Klos, Brondino, Harley, & Swartz, 2015). The students were randomized to either a Facebook social support group or a standard walking group for 8 weeks. The women in both groups received weekly step goals, and they tracked their steps per day with a pedometer. Women in the Facebook social support group were also enrolled in a Facebook group and asked to post information about their steps per day and provide feedback to one another. The researchers found that women in both intervention groups significantly increased their steps per day from baseline to the 8-week assessment. Women in the Facebook social support group, however, increased their steps per day significantly more than women in the standard walking intervention. In fact, women in the Facebook social support group increased their walking by about 1.5 miles more per day than the women in the standard walking intervention.

CRITICAL THINKING ACTIVITY 15-5

© ecco/Shutterstock, Inc.

What type of app would you design to increase exercise behavior of high school students?

Group Dynamics

Group dynamics includes the study of the nature of groups, individual relationships within groups, and group members' interactions with each other. **Group dynamics** can be defined as the positive and negative forces at play within a group of people. Within the domain of physical activity, a number of group dynamics variables have been related to sustained behavior (Carron, Hausenblas, & Estabrooks, 1999). In this section, the following two group dynamics topics are examined in more detail: cohesion and leadership.

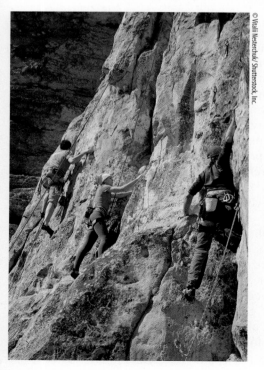
© Vitalii Nesterchuk/Shutterstock, Inc.

Cohesion

The degree to which a group is cohesive determines the individuals' level of success as a group. When examining the forces that bind individuals together, a logical starting point is the cohesive nature of the physical activity group. Physical activity groups, like other action-based groups (e.g., sport, work, or military groups), become bound together based upon the task and social components of the environment. This bond is referred to as group **cohesion**, and it is defined as "a dynamic process that is reflected in the tendency for a group to stick together and remain united in pursuit of its instrumental objectives and/ or for the satisfaction of member affective needs" (Carron, Brawley, & Widmeyer, 1998, p. 213).

Cohesion is often conceptualized as a multidimensional model (Carron, Widmeyer, & Brawley, 1985) that consists of four dimensions distinguished on two levels. The first level is the *individual* versus *group* bases for cohesion. For example, an individual has personal attractions to the group as well as perceptions regarding the collectivity of the group. Simply said, the individual basis for cohesion is exemplified by "I" and "me" statements (e.g., "I like the exercises I do in this class"), whereas the group basis for cohesion is exemplified by "we" and "us" statements (e.g., "We all like the exercises we do in this class").

The second level of group cohesion is based on a distinction between the *task* and *social* aspects of group involvement. For example, both individually and as a group there are social outcomes (e.g., activities related to the development and maintenance of social relations) and task outcomes (e.g., activities related to accomplishing a task, productivity, and performance). A social outcome of physical activity classes could be the development of friendships. A task outcome could be the increased attraction to the exercises done in class.

Based upon these two levels of distinction (i.e., individual versus group and social versus task), the following four dimensions of group cohesion are conceptualized: individual attractions to the group–task, individual attractions to the group–social, group integration–task, and group integration–social (see FIGURE 15-3 ; Carron et al., 1985). Bert Carron and his colleagues hypothesized that people can feel personally attracted to the specific physical activity offered in the class (i.e., individual attractions to the group–task) and to the people who attend the class (i.e., individual attractions to the group–social). People may also perceive that the physical activity group as a whole interacts with one another to get the best work out (i.e., group integration–task) or to socialize (i.e., group integration–social). Within exercise class settings, social cohesion changes over time, whereas task cohesion remains more steady (Dunlop, Falk, & Beauchamp, 2013).

Over the past 20 years, a large body of research has revealed the positive relationship between group cohesion and physical activity adoption and maintenance

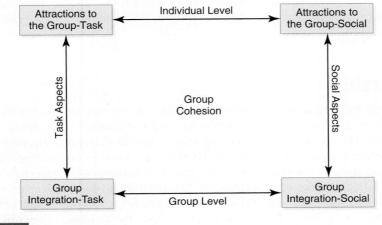

FIGURE 15-3 Group Cohesion

Data from Carron, A. V., Widmeyer, W. N., & Brawley, L. R. (1985). The development of an instrument to assess cohesion in sport teams: The group environment questionnaire. *Journal of Sport Psychology, 7*, 244–266.

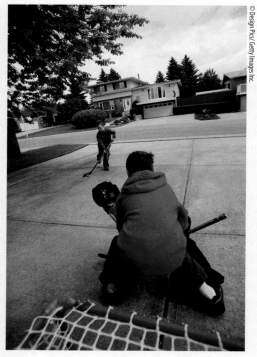

© Design Pics/ Getty Images Inc.

(Burke, Carron, Eys, & Estabrooks, 2006; Estabrooks, 2000; Smith-Ray et al., 2012). More specifically, people who have strong perceptions of group cohesion attend group sessions more often, are late less often, and drop out less frequently. Group cohesion also has a positive relationship with attitudes toward physical activity and enhanced perceptions of self-efficacy and personal control.

As well, neighborhood social cohesion is positively related to exercise participation (Cradock, Kawachi, Colditzm Gortmaker, & Buka, 2009). Parent-reported neighborhood social cohesion is positively associated with weekday and weekend physical activity in youth (Pabayo, Belsky, Gauvin, & Curtis, 2011). This association is most pronounced for boys. Parental perception of neighborhood social environment is also an important source of children's activity levels.

Because cohesion is positively related to exercise adherence, attitudes, and cognitions, it is important to foster it. Researchers, for example, have found that competition is a strong predictor of cohesion (Harden, Estabrooks, Mama, & Lee, 2014). Facilitating a sense of friendly competition may increase physical activity levels in group-based programs by bolstering group cohesion. Friendly competition is a sense of competition that is connected to the overall success of the group and can reflect a generalized sense of intragroup competition as well as intergroup competitions within a single intervention. With friendly competition, people are inspired to compete against each other with the recognition that even if someone else wins it benefits the group as a whole.

Leadership

Researchers and program planners also have been interested in the role that exercise leaders play in participants' attitudes toward and adherence to physical activity programs. Effective physical activity leaders are those whom the participants feel are properly qualified, are able to develop a personal bond with participants, and can use their knowledge about the group to demonstrate collective accomplishments (Estabrooks et al., 2004). It is important to have effective exercise leaders because they influence participant's attitudes, cognitions, and behaviors toward physical activity. Indeed, a meta-analysis by Carron, Hausenblas, and Mack (1996) on social influences in exercise adherence showed that there is a small effect for the influence that exercise leaders have on adherence behavior.

McAuley and Jacobson (1991) examined the relationship between member adherence and instructor influence with formerly sedentary females. Following an 8-week exercise program, participants were asked how they felt the instructor had influenced their adherence to the program. McAuley and Jacobson concluded that participant perceptions of the leader influence did have a small positive association with in-class adherence.

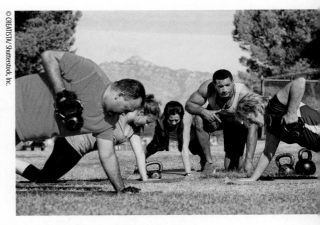

In a similar study, Nancy Gyurcsik and her colleagues (Gyurcsik, Culos, Bray, & DuCharme, 1998) examined the relationship between elements of leadership and the adherence of regular exercisers. After assessing participants' confidence in their activity leader's abilities (a measure referred to as *instructor efficacy*), they monitored attendance for 12 weeks. A small, but significant, relationship was found between instructor efficacy and attendance.

Fox and her collaborators (Fox, Rejeski, & Gauvin, 2000) investigated the impact of leadership style and group dynamics on intention to return to a structured fitness class. Each participant completed a single program session under four conditions in which both leadership style (i.e., an enriched versus a bland leadership style) and group environment (i.e., an enriched versus a bland class environment) were systematically varied. **TABLE 15-4** provides an overview of the approach taken in each instance. The enriched group environment was manipulated with the use of trained confederates.

At the completion of the session, the participants completed assessments of their intention to return to a similar class and enjoyment of the previous session. Interestingly, a positive effect was found for the interaction between the leader style and group environment for enjoyment of the aerobics session. In other words, the participants enjoyed the class more when the environment had both enriched leadership and group dynamics. A positive relationship was also found between the group environment and intention. So, those participants in the enriched group environments intended to return to a similar exercise session, regardless of the style of the leader.

Just as group cohesion is related to other cognitive and affective factors in addition to adherence in the physical activity domain, so, too, is class leadership. Turner, Rejeski, and Brawley (1997) examined the influence of leadership behavior on participants' self-efficacy and the exercise-induced feeling states of revitalization, positive engagement, tranquility, and physical exhaustion. Again, college women were assigned to classes structured to be either socially enriched or socially bland in terms of interactions from the program leader. The participants in the socially enriched classes reported more enhanced mood states from involvement in the exercise than those in the bland classes. Furthermore, the socially

TABLE 15-4	Bland versus Enriched Leadership Styles and Group Environment		
Leadership Style		**Group Environment**	
Socially Enriched	**Bland**	**Socially Enriched**	**Bland**
Use participants' names.	Do not use participants' names.	Introduce themselves to others as soon as they arrive in class.	Do not introduce themselves to others at any time in class.
Engage participants in general conversation before, during, and after class.	Do not engage in general conversation before, during, or after class.	Initiate casual interactions with other members early in each session.	Do not initiate or promote casual interactions with other members at any time in the class.
Provide specific reinforcement for positive behaviors.	No reinforcement or praise for positive behaviors.	Be compliant with the instructor's wishes.	Be compliant but not enthusiastically.
Give encouragement before and after a skill or mistake.	Fail to follow up with praise after a skill or mistake.	Provide encouragement to the group as a whole.	No encouragement to others or the instructor.
Focus on positive comments during instruction.	Focus on negative comments during instruction.	Respond to all questions the leader directs to the group.	Do not respond to questions the leader directs to the group.
Verbal reward of effort and ability immediately after the exercise and ignore mistakes.	Verbally note mistakes and do not reward effort and ability after the exercise.	Make positive and encouraging remarks to the instructor about the class in general.	No remarks to the instructor even if she directed instructions or corrections toward an individual.

Fox, L. D., Rejeski, W. J., & Gauvin, L. (2000). Effects of leadership style and group dynamics on enjoyment of physical activity. *American Journal of Health Promotion, 14,* 277–283.

enriched leadership style had a greater impact on the participant's self-efficacy beliefs.

Caperchione and colleagues (Caperchione, Mummery, & Duncan, 2011) examined the relationship between leader behaviors and group cohesiveness within women's physical activity groups. They had 95 women who were previously involved in a physical activity/walking program assess their group leaders' behavior using items pertaining to enthusiasm, motivation, instruction, and availability, and their groups' cohesiveness using the Physical Activity Group Environment Questionnaire (see TABLE 15-5 for sample items). They found that

TABLE 15-5 Sample Items from the Physical Activity Group Environment Questionnaire

Scale	Sample Item
Individual attractions to the group—task	I like the amount of physical activity I get in this program.
Individual attractions to the group—social	I enjoy my social interactions within this physical activity group.
Group integration—task	Members of our group are satisfied with the intensity of physical activity in this program.
Group integration—social	We spend time socializing with each other before or after our activity sessions.

Data from Burke, S. M., Carron, A. V., Eys, M. A., & Estabrooks, P. A. (2006). Group versus individual approach? A meta-analysis of the effectiveness of interventions to promote physical activity. *Sport and Exercise Psychology Review, 2,* 13–29.

group cohesion was strongly related to leadership behavior. Simply stated, group leaders who were perceived as being highly enthusiastic, having the ability to motivate, being able to provide personal instruction, and who were available outside of the group's regular activities were associated with higher levels of group cohesion.

■ Summary

The definition and measurement of social support is an ongoing source of discussion and debate in the health sciences. What seems to be generally accepted, however, is the belief that social support is essential for human well-being. It influences our emotions, cognitions, and behavior. Thus, not surprisingly, it influences involvement in physical activity. More research is needed examining the effects of social support on sedentary behavior. Among the cognitions and emotions found to be positively associated with social support are intention to be physically active and perceptions of the degree of cohesiveness present in the exercise class. Moreover, social support is also positively associated with both adherence and compliance to activity programs. Finally, the probability of being ill or suffering from a premature death is increased in the absence of social support.

KEY TERMS

bullying
cohesion
group dynamics
mobile application
social environment

social integration
social media
social support
support network
supportive climate

REVIEW QUESTIONS

1. Considerable discrepancy exists in our understanding of what social support actually is and how it should be defined and measured. Provide examples of why social support is a complex phenomenon.

2. What effect does social support have on exercise adherence? Provide research support for your answer.

3. What role do parents play with regard to the physical activity levels of their children? Explain.

4. Do you think that healthcare providers should provide physical activity counseling to their patients? Justify your answer with research support.

5. What type of social support does bullying represent? What role does teasing play for children's physical activity behavior and quality of life?

6. Define the term *cohesion*. How is cohesion related to exercise adherence?

7. Can technology represent a form of social support for physical activity? Explain.

8. Is a dog an effective intervention to increase physical activity levels? Provide research support for your answer.

APPLYING THE CONCEPTS

1. How have Madeline's work colleagues influenced her exercise behavior?

2. Do you think Madeline would be physically active were it not for her work colleagues? Why or why not?

REFERENCES

American Veterinary Medical Association. (2012). *U.S. Pet ownership and demographic sourcebook.* Retrieved June 4, 2014, from https://www.avma.org/KB/Resources/Statistics/Pages/Market-research-statistics-US-pet-ownership.aspx.

Animal Health Alliance. (2013). *Pet ownership in Australia summary.* Retrieved August 28, 2015, from http://kb.rspca.org.au/How-many-pets-are-there-in-Australia_58.html.

Barber, F. D. (2012). Social support and physical activity engagement by cancer survivors. *Clinical Journal of Oncology Nursing, 16*, E84–E98.

Barnett, E., & Casper, M. (2001). A definition of "social environment." *American Journal of Public Health, 91*, 465.

Barrera, M., Jr., Sandler, I. N., & Ramsay, T. B. (1981). Preliminary development of a scale of social support: Studies on college students. *American Journal of Community Psychology, 9*, 435–447.

Baumeister, R. F., & Leary, M. R. (1995). The need to belong: Desire for interpersonal attachments as a fundamental human motivation. *Psychological Bulletin, 117*, 497–529.

Bort-Roig, J., Gilson, N. D., Puig-Ribera, A., Contrera, R. S., & Trost, S. G. (2014). Measuring and influencing physical activity with smartphone technology: A systematic review. *Sports Medicine, 44*, 671–686.

Burke, S. M., Carron, A. V., Eys, M. A., & Estabrooks, P. A. (2006). Group versus individual approach? A meta-analysis of the effectiveness of interventions to promote physical activity. *Sport and Exercise Psychology Review, 2*, 13–29.

Caperchione, C., Mummery, W. K., & Duncan, M. (2011). Investigating the relationship between leader behaviours and group cohesion within women's walking groups. *Journal of Science and Medicine in Sport, 14*, 325–350.

Cardinal, B. J., Park, E. A., Kim, M., & Cardinal M. K. (2014). If Exercise is Medicine®, where is exercise in medicine? Review of U.S. medical education curricula for physical activity-related content. *Journal of Physical Activity and Health*, epub.

Carron, A. V., Brawley, L. R., & Widmeyer, W. N. (1998). The measurement of cohesiveness in sport groups. In J. L. Duda (Ed.), *Advances in sport and exercise psychology measurement* (pp. 213–226). Morgantown, WV: Fitness Information Technology.

Carron, A. V., Hausenblas, H. A., & Estabrooks, P. A. (1999). Social influence and exercise involvement. In S. Bull (Ed.), *Adherence issues in sport and exercise* (pp. 1–17). New York, NY: John Wiley & Sons.

Carron, A.V., Hausenblas, H., & Mack, D.A. (1996). Social influence and exercise: A meta-analysis. *Journal of Sport and Exercise Psychology, 18*, 1–16.

Carron, A. V., Widmeyer, W. N., & Brawley, L. R. (1985). The development of an instrument to assess cohesion in sport teams: The group environment questionnaire. *Journal of Sport Psychology, 7*, 244–266.

Cassel, J. (1976). The contributions of the social environment to host resistance. *American Journal of Epidemiology, 104*, 107–123.

Chogahara, M., O'Brien Cousins, S., & Wankel, L. M. (1998). Social influence on physical activity in older adults: A review. *Journal of Aging and Physical Activity, 6*, 1–17.

Christian, H. E., Trapp, G., Lauritsen, C., Wright, K., & Giles-Corti, B. (2013). Understanding the relationship between dog ownership and children's physical activity and sedentary behaviour. *Pediatric Obesity, 8*, 392–403.

Christian, H. E., Westgarth, C., Bauman, A., Richards, E. A., Rhodes, R. E., Evenson, K. R., ... Thorpe, R. L. (2013). Dog ownership and physical activity: A review of the evidence. *Journal of Physical Activity and Health, 10*, 750–759.

Cobb, S. (1976). Social support as a moderator of life stress. *Psychosomatic Medicine*, *3B*, 300–314.

Cohen, A., Mermelstein, R., Kamarck, T., & Hoberman, H. M. (1985). Measuring the functional components of social support. In I. G. Sarason & B. R. Sarason (Eds.), *Social support: Theory, research, and applications*. The Hague, Netherlands: Martinus Niijhoff.

Conroy, D. E., Yang, C. H., & Maher, J. P. (2014). Behavior change techniques in top-ranked mobile apps for physical activity. *American Journal of Preventive Medicine*, *46*, 649–652.

Cradock, A. L., Kawachi, I., Colditz, G. A., Gortmaker, S. L., & Buka, S. L. (2009). Neighborhood social cohesion and youth participation in physical activity in Chicago. *Social Science and Medicine*, *68*, 427–435.

Cutt, H., Giles-Corti, B., Knuiman, M., Timperio, A., & Bull, F. (2008). Understanding dog owners' increased levels of physical activity: Results from RESIDE. *American Journal of Public Health*, *98*, 66–69.

De la Haye, K., Robins, G., Mohr, P., & Wilson, C. (2011). How physical activity shapes, and is shaped by, adolescent friendships. *Social Science and Medicine*, *73*, 719–728.

Duncan, T. E., Duncan, S. C., & McAuley, E. (1993). The role of domain and gender-specific provisions of social relations in adherence to a prescribed exercise program. *Journal of Sport and Exercise Psychology*, *15*, 220–231.

Dunlop, W. L., Falk, C. F., & Beauchamp, M. R. (2013). How dynamic are exercise group dynamics? Examining changes in cohesion within class-based exercise programs. *Health Psychology*, *32*, 1240–1243.

Estabrooks, P. A. (2000). Sustaining exercise participation through group cohesion. *Exercise and Sport Science Reviews*, *28*, 63–67.

Estabrooks, P. A., Munroe, K. J., Fox, E. H., Gyurcsik, N. C., Hill, J. L., Lyon, R., … Shannon, V. R. (2004). Leadership in physical activity groups for older adults: A qualitative analysis. *Journal of Aging and Physical Activity*, *12*, 232–245.

Fox, L. D., Rejeski, W. J., & Gauvin, L. (2000). Effects of leadership style and group dynamics on enjoyment of physical activity. *American Journal of Health Promotion*, *14*, 277–283.

Gyurcsik, N. C., Culos, S. N., Bray, S. R., & DuCharme, K. A. (1998). Instructor efficacy: Third-party influence of exercise adherence. *Journal of Sport and Exercise Psychology*, *2*, S9.

Harden, S. M., Estabrooks, P. A., Mama, S. L., & Lee, R. E. (2014). Longitudinal analysis of minority women's perceptions of cohesion: The role of cooperation, communication, and competition. *International Journal of Behavioral Nutrition and Physical Activity*, *29*, 57.

Hesketh, K. R., Goodfellow, L., Ekelund, U., McMinn, A. M., Godfrey, K. M., Inskip, H. M., … van Sluijs, E. M. (2014). Activity levels in mothers and their preschool children. *Pediatrics*, *133*, e973–e980.

Hesketh, K. R., McMinn, A. M., Griffin, S. J., Harvey, N. C., Godfrey, K. M., Inskip, H. M., … van Sluijs, E. M. (2013). Maternal awareness of young children's physical activity: Levels and cross-sectional correlates of overestimation. *BMC Public Health*, Oct 3;*13*:924. doi:10.1186/1471-2458-13-924

Israel, B. A. (1982). Social networks and health status: Linking theory, research, and practice. *Patient Counseling and Health Education*, *4*, 65–69.

Jago, R., Fox, K. R., Page, A. S., Brockman, R., & Thompson, J. L. (2010). Parent and child physical activity and sedentary time: Do active parents foster active children. *BMC Public Health*, Apr 15;*10*:194. doi:10.1186/1471-2458-10-194

Jensen, C. D., Cushing, C. C., & Elledge, A. R. (2014). Associations between teasing, quality of life, and physical activity among preadolescent children. *Journal of Pediatric Psychology*, *39*, 65–73.

Joy E. L., Blair, S. N., McBride, P., & Sallis, R. (2013). Physical activity counseling in sports medicine: A call to action. *British Journal of Sports Medicine*, *47*, 49–53.

Kouvonen, A., De Vogli, R., Stafford, M., Shipley, M. J., Marmot, M. G., Cox, T., … Kivimaki, M. (2012). Social support and the likelihood of maintaining and improving levels of physical activity: The Whitehall II study. *European Journal of Public Health*, *22*, 514–518.

Laireiter, A., & Baumann, U. (1992). Network structures and support functions—theoretical and empirical analyses. In H. O. F. Veiel & U. Baumann (Eds.), *The meaning and measurement of social support* (pp. 33–55). New York, NY: Hemisphere Publishing.

Lentino, C., Visek, A. J., McDonnell, K., & DiPietro, L. (2012). Dog walking is associated with a favorable risk profile independent of moderate to high volume of physical activity. *Journal of Physical Activity and Health, 9,* 414–420.

Lewis, C. S. (1945). *That hideous strength.* New York, NY: Scribner.

Maier, K. J., & James, A. E. (2014). Hostility and social support explain physical activity beyond negative affect among young men, but not women, in college. *Behavioral Medicine, 40,* 34–41.

Marques, A., Sallis, J. F., Martins, J., Diniz, J., & Carreiro Da Coasta, F. (2014). Correlates of urban children's leisure-time physical activity and sedentary behaviors during school days. *American Journal of Human Biology, 26,* 407–412.

Maturo, C. C., & Cunningham, S. A. (2013). Influence of friends on children's physical activity: A review. *American Journal of Public Health, 103,* e23–e38.

McAuley, E., & Jacobson, L. (1991). Self-efficacy and exercise participation in sedentary adult females. *American Journal of Health Promotion, 5,* 185–191.

McIntyre, C. A., & Rhodes, R. E. (2009). Correlates of leisure-time physical activity during transitions to motherhood. *Women and Health, 49,* 66–83.

McKenna, J., Naylor, P. J., & McDowell, N. (1998). Barriers to physical activity promotion by general practitioners and practice nurses. *British Journal of Sports Medicine, 32,* 242–247.

Mendonca, G., Cheng, L. A., Melo, E. N., & de Farias Junio, J. S. (2014). Physical activity and social support in adolescents: A systematic review. *Health Education Research, 29,* 822–839.

O'Connor, J. A., & Graber, K. C. (2014). Sixth-grade physical education: An acculturation of bullying and fear. *Research Quarterly in Exercise and Sport, 85,* 398–408.

Oliveira, A. J., Lopes, C. S., de Leon, A. C., Rostila, M., Griep, R. H., Werneck, G. L., & Faerstein, E. (2011). Social support and leisure-time physical activity: Longitudinal evidence from the Brazilian Pro-Saude study. *International Journal of Behavioral Nutrition and Physical Activity,* Jul 26;8:77. doi:10.1186/1479-5868-8-77

Orrow, G., Kinmonth, A. L., Sanderson, S., & Sutton, S. (2012). Effectiveness of physical activity promotion based in primary care: Systematic review and meta-analysis of randomised controlled trials. *BMJ, 344,* e1389.

Pabayo, R., Belsky, J., Gauvin, L., & Curtis, S. (2011). Do area characteristics predict change in moderate-to-vigorous physical activity from ages 11 to 15 years? *Social Science and Medicine, 72,* 430–438.

Rafaeli, E., Cranford, J. A., Green, A. S., Shrout, P. E., & Bolger, N. (2008). The good and bad of relationships: How social hindrance and social support affect relationship feelings in daily life. *Personality and Social Psychology Bulletin, 34,* 1703–1718.

Rhodes, R. E., Murray, H., Temple, V., Tuokko, H., & Wharf Higgins, J. (2012). Pilot study of a dog walking intervention: Effects of a focus on canine exercise. *Preventive Medicine, 54,* 309–312.

Roman, C. G., & Taylor, C. J. (2013). A multilevel assessment of school climate, bullying victimization, and physical activity. *Journal of School Health, 83,* 400–407.

Rote, A., Klos, L. A., Brondino, M. J., Harley, A. E., & Swartz, A. M. (2015). The efficacy of a walking intervention using social media to increase physical activity: A randomized trial. *Journal of Physical Activity and Health, 12*(Suppl 1), S18–S25.

Russell, D., & Cutrona, C. (1984, August). The provisions of social relationships and adaptation to stress. Paper presented at the annual meeting of the American Psychological Association. Toronto, Ontario, Canada.

Sarason, B. R., Pierce, G. R., & Sarason, I. G., (1990). Social support: The sense of acceptance and the role of relationships. In B. R. Sarason, I. G. Sarason, & G. R. Pierce (Eds.), *Social support: An interactional view* (pp. 97–128). New York, NY: Wiley.

Sarason, B. R., Pierce, G. R., Shearin, E. N., Sarason, I. G., Waltz, J. A., & Poppe, L. (1991). Perceived social support and working models of self and actual others. *Journal of Personality and Social Psychology, 60,* 273–287.

Sarason, I. G., Levine, H. M., Basham, R. B., & Sarason, B. R. (1983). Assessing social support: The Social Support Questionnaire. *Journal of Personality and Social Psychology, 44,* 127–139.

Sarason, I. G., Mankowski, E. S., Peterson, A. V. Jr., & Dinh, K. T. (1992). Adolescents' reasons for smoking. *Journal of School Health, 62,* 185–190.

Sarason, I. G., Sarason, B. R., & Pierce, G. R. (1992). Three contexts of social support. In H. O. F. Veiel & U. Baumann (Eds.), *The meaning and measurement of social support* (pp. 143–154). New York, NY: Hemisphere Publishing.

Sawka, K. J., McCormack, G. R., Nettel-Aquirre, A., Hawe, P., & Doyle-Baker, P. K. (2013). Friendship networks and physical activity and sedentary behavior among youth: A systematic review. *International Journal of Behavioral Nutrition and Physical Activity,* Dec. 1;*10*:130. doi:10.1186/1479-5868-10-130

Sbarra, D. A., Law, R. W., & Portley, R. M. (2011). Divorce and death: A meta-analysis and research agenda for clinical, social, and health psychology. *Perspectives on Psychological Science, 6,* 454–474.

Shibata, A., Oka, K., Inoue, S., Christian, H., Kitabatake, Y., & Shimomitsu, T. (2012). Physical activity of Japanese older adults who own and walk dogs. *American Journal of Preventive Medicine, 43,* 429–433.

Smith-Ray, R. L., Mama, S., Reese-Smith, J. Y., Estabrooks, P. A., & Lee, R. E. (2012). Improving participation rates for women of color in health research: The role of group cohesion. *Prevention Science, 13,* 27–35.

Solomon, E., Rees, T., Ukoumunne, O. C., Metcalf, B., & Hillsdon, M. (2013). Personal, social, and environmental correlates of physical activity in adults living in rural south-west England: A cross-sectional analysis. *International Journal of Behavioral Nutrition and Physical Activity,* Nov 21;*10*:129. doi: 10.1186/1479-5868-10-129

Springer, A. E., Kelder, S. H., & Hoelschler, D. M. (2006). Social support, physical activity, and sedentary behavior among 6th-grade girls: A cross-sectional study. *International Journal of Behavioral Nutrition and Physical Activity,* Apr 6;*3*:8.

Sylaska, K. M., & Edwards, K. M. (2014). Disclosure of intimate partner violence to informal social support network members: A review of the literature. *Trauma, Violence, and Abuse, 15,* 3–21.

Tandon, P. S., Zhou, C., Sallis, J. F., Cain, K. L., Frank, L. D., & Saelens, B. E. (2012). Home environment relationships with children's physical activity, sedentary time, and screen time by socioeconomic status. *International Journal of Behavioral Nutrition and Physical Activity,* Jul 26;*9*:88. doi: 10.1186/1479-5868-9-88

Tay, L., Tan, K., Diener, E., & Gonzalez, E. (2013). Social relations, health behaviors, and health outcomes: A survey and synthesis. *Applied Psychology, Health and Well-Being, 5,* 28–78.

Toohey, A. M., & Rock, M. J. (2011). Unleashing their potential: A critical realist scoping review of the influence of dogs on physical activity for dog-owners and non-owners. *International Journal of Behavioral Nutrition and Physical Activity,* May 21;*8*:46. doi:10.1186/1479-5868-8-46

Turner, E. E., Rejeski, W. J., & Brawley, L. R. (1997). Psychological benefits of physical activity are influenced by the social environment. *Journal of Sport and Exercise Psychology, 19,* 119–130.

Vaux, A. (1988). *Social support: Theory, research, and intervention.* New York, NY: Praeger.

Vaux, A. (1992). Assessment of social support. In H. O. F. Veiel & U. Baumann (Eds.), *The meaning and measurement of social support* (pp. 193–216). New York, NY: Hemisphere Publishing.

Weiss, R. S. (1974). The provisions of social relationships. In Z. Rubin (.), *Doing unto others* (pp. 17–26). Englewood Cliffs, NJ: Prentice-Hall.

Yang, C. H., Maher, J. P., & Conroy, D. E. (2015). Implementation of behavior change techniques in mobile applications for physical activity. *American Journal of Preventive Medicine, 48,* 452–455.

CHAPTER 16

Physical Environment

Runner © lzf/Shutterstock

Runner © lzf/Shutterstock

Vignette: Clayton

I played sports in high school and lifted weights in college. But when I graduated from business school, went into finance, got married, and quickly became a dad, my involvement in physical activity all but vanished. I jokingly competed with two work buddies over whose waistband was expanding the fastest.

A few of my colleagues would get up at unreasonably early hours to hit the gym. But most of the fellow junior analysts I worked with came down on the side of preferring a bit more sleep before work hours—not to mention drinks and steak dinners whenever the bulk of us clocked out.

My health wasn't the only thing I wasn't paying attention to. I was pretty absentminded when it came to my home life. My wife wasn't happy with my long hours at work. Nor was she all that approving of my drinking habits. I loved my kids, but I could tell they felt I wasn't there for them as strongly as she was. I kept arguing that I should get cut a bit more slack since I was bringing home most of our income. But I see now that my reasoning was not just selfish but misguided.

She filed for divorce shortly after our youngest boy's third birthday. The stress of dealing with lawyers, the tumult and adjustment of moving into my own studio apartment in midtown Manhattan, and the radical shift in my mood resulted in my putting on even more weight and plowing my body with more alcohol.

LEARNING OBJECTIVES

After completing this chapter, you will be able to

- Outline the importance of the physical and built environment on physical activity and sedentary behaviors.
- Describe how modernization has influenced levels of physical activity and sedentary behavior.
- Describe the influence of the environment on travel patterns.
- Describe environmental prompts that increase physical activity.
- Differentiate between perceived and actual access to physical activity resources.
- Outline physical environmental correlates of physical activity and sedentary behavior.

399

It was only when my habits started affecting my work that I considered making some health-related changes. I was told during an annual physical that I had high blood pressure, high cholesterol, and would be at risk of an imminent heart attack if I didn't alter my habits as soon as possible. When my boss pulled me aside and said he was worried about how my unraveling was impacting the morale of our company, the reality of all I was doing to myself truly hit.

I took 10 days off work, per my boss's recommendation. I booked appointments with a nutritionist and trainer who had each been recommended by one of my college friends. I held out on the mental health component for some time because I was, to be honest, ashamed of needing emotional help of any kind—or admitting I had issues that couldn't be solved with the perfect algorithm on a spreadsheet. But once I returned to work I tentatively started seeing a psychiatrist, who specialized not only in prescribing the right drugs but also in counseling.

I'd say the transition away from whole boxes of pizza, six packs chugged in the dank presence of my dimly lit bachelor pad, and the insidious comfort of my couch and television was quite possibly one of the hardest behavioral adjustments I ever made. I'd put it on par with the actual divorce itself. So ensconced in my own self-destructive routine had I become that I wasn't even aware of how insurmountable it would be to wriggle out of it until I actually tried.

My wife and kids ended up coming over one weekend to help me get my place into shape. She and I were on talking terms and, though there would always be some level of tension and resentment between us, she did care enough about me to ensure I wouldn't fall through any cracks. Together, we single-handedly discarded all junk food in the apartment, as well as all beer, liquor, and wine (despite my pleading with her to not throw out the top-shelf stuff). The kids helped, too. And I have to say that seeing an obvious look of worry in their young faces made me keep at it. It wasn't about doing this just for myself, it was about doing this, also, for my family. Or what was left of it.

As part of my plan with my personal trainer, I started walking to and from work. I used to just take cabs, even though my new apartment was only about 15 blocks from the office. Another change: taking the stairs. I've been at it for about 2 months now and I can make it up about 12 flights before I have to take the elevator the rest of the way up to the 35th floor where my office is. (When I started I could barely do one flight.) My goal by the end of the year is to be able to make it the whole way.

I consider myself lucky to live in such a walkable environment as New York City. It's not as hard as I thought to squeeze more activity into my day. And with access to my company's gym, I can—if time permits—lift weights during those rare extended breaks from work.

A big shift in how much I work out is keeping a pair of sneakers and having several days' worth of gym clothes at my office. If I had to go home to change I'd honestly stay parked on the couch watching television.

What's been the best outcome of my new effort to be healthy is the quality time I now spend with my boys. My coworkers also have kids and they don't give me slack for leaving work early every other Friday to take the boys out for dinner. And while I have yet to spend a Saturday or Sunday without my Blackberry attached to my hip, I'm able to at least run around Central Park with them as they learn to bike ride.

I'm hoping the fact that I can keep up with them might work in my favor as I soon try to get back into the dating world.

■ Introduction

In George Orwell's classic novel *1984*, a dark picture of a futuristic society in fear of the ever-present, watchful eye of the enigmatic dictator called Big Brother is described (Orwell, 1949). In *1984*, members of the "Outer Party" were awakened with a whistle every morning at the same time. Three minutes after the sound of the whistle, a fitness instructor would appear on the telescreen. Outer Party members did not think about having time for exercise, they did not consider if they had the confidence to complete the exercise, nor did they have intentions regarding the frequency, duration, intensity, or type of physical activity. They simply did their morning exercises. Why? Because their environment was structured so that each day they would do what was called the "Physical Jerks." No questions, no options. And, if they did attempt to miss the physical activity, they would be quickly chastised and brought back into behavioral conformity. Unlike the dismal exercise adherence we have in most countries, in Big Brother's world there were no exercise adherence problems—only 100% prevalence, 100% maintenance.

So, did Orwell find the answer to promoting the initiation and maintenance of physical activity? Is it a plausible model for current society? Definitely not. However, some components of Big Brother's world are appealing. For example, in his world there are no motivational problems associated with being physically active. What is clear is that one's physical environment has the potential to be related to behavioral outcomes. In this chapter, we focus on factors within one's physical environment that may be related to either improved or diminished levels of physical activity and sedentary behavior. The **physical environment** includes all of your indoor and outdoor surroundings. Thus, the physical environment includes both designed and natural infrastructures. Designed infrastructures include houses, stores, fitness facilities, and recreational parks. In comparison, examples of natural infrastructures include oceans, lakes, and mountains.

The **built environment** is part of the physical environment, but it refers to only the designed, human-made surroundings. The built environment ranges in scale from infrastructures for walking and cycling, availability of public transit,

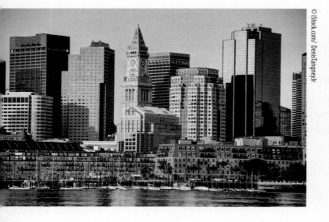

© iStock.com/ DenisTangneyJr

street connectivity, housing density, parks, **green spaces** (i.e., an area of grass, trees, or other vegetation set apart for recreational purposes), and **land use mix** (i.e., diversity or variety of land uses such as residential, commercial, industrial, and agricultural). For example, a diverse land use mix is associated with shorter travel distances between places of interest and activities.

Examining the effect of the physical environment on people's exercise and sedentary behavior is a more recent area of inquiry. The physical environment represents an intense area of study, accounting for about 30% of all exercise psychology research (Rhodes & Nasuti, 2011). When reviewing the literature examining the impact of physical environmental factors on physical activity participation, a pattern of research emerges. Based on this pattern of research, the following components of the physical environment and its relationship to exercise and sedentary behavior are addressed in this chapter: modernization, travel, climate/seasonal variations, point-of-choice prompts, and environmental correlates of exercise and sedentary behavior. To better understand how the physical environment affects our physical activity behavior, let's first take a closer look at how the environment influences young children's ability to delay gratification.

Influences of the Physical Environment on Delayed Gratification

Delayed gratification is the ability to reject immediately available smaller rewards in favor of later larger rewards. For example, can you forgo buying those jeans to save money to buy a car in the next year? People's ability to delay gratification has been linked to many positive outcomes, including academic success, physical health, psychological health, and social competence (Drobetz, Maercker, & Forstmeier, 2012; Moffitt et al., 2011).

For the purposes of this chapter, a functional starting point is with Walter Mischel and his colleagues' research regarding delayed gratification in 4-year-old children (for a review, see Mischel, Shoda, & Rodriguez, 1989). Using primarily laboratory research techniques, the typical protocol involved children being shown toys, marshmallows, or candies. The researcher then explained to the children that they can either have the treat or play with the toy immediately or have additional treats or toys if they wait a few minutes until the researcher returns to the room. In other words, the child could eat the one marshmallow right away or wait 20 minutes for two marshmallows. The researcher would then leave the room and return in 20 minutes. As expected, the children, on average, were not very successful in delaying their gratification. Most would quickly play with the toys or eat the candies. Only about one-third of the children could wait until the researcher returned (Mischel et al., 1989). A longitudinal study of these children found that a child's ability to delay gratification for a longer time as a preschooler was associated with important outcomes such as adolescent academic strength, social competence, and the ability to handle stress as an adult. In some children, it was also associated with higher Scholastic Aptitude Test (SAT) scores and decreased likelihood of illegal drug use in adulthood (Ayduk et al., 2000).

CRITICAL THINKING ACTIVITY 16-1

© ecco/Shutterstock, Inc.

How successful are you at delaying gratification? How has this affected your overall health?

A number of potential explanations were offered for why some children could wait and others could not resist the temptation. It was hypothesized that some children have the skills necessary to wait for gratification. Potentially, these skills could be taught to children, or the temptation of early consumption could be removed from the child's environment. In subsequent studies, Mischel and his colleagues (1989) examined different strategies that could help the child become more successful. Using the typical protocol, the children were assigned to one of three possible environments. In Condition 1, the children were asked to wait while the candy was in plain view on the table. In Condition 2, the children were asked to wait while the candy was in plain view on the table but they had been taught to cope by thinking about fun thoughts while waiting for the researcher to return. In Condition 3, the children were asked to wait while the candy was on the table but under a cover. In other words, in Condition 3 the physical environment was changed.

As expected, the children in Condition 1 typically ate the candy and could not delay gratification. In Condition 2, the children were more successful than those who were not taught the coping strategy from Condition 1; that is, the children who had been taught to cope by thinking about fun thoughts (Condition 2) were more successful than those who were not taught the coping strategy (Condition 1). However, for Condition 3, where the physical environment was changed (i.e., the candy was covered), the children were also more successful in waiting for their reward (Mischel et al., 1989). Based on these findings, it appears that changing the physical environment can change children's ability to delay their gratification—changing their physical environment changed their behavior.

Interestingly, Mischel and his colleagues assessed whether the 4-year-olds' performance on the delayed gratification task would predict their body mass index (BMI) 30 years later. As part of a longitudinal study, a subset ($n = 164$) of the children were followed up on about 30 years later and were asked to self-report their height and weight. The researchers found that children who had a longer delay of gratification at age 4 also had a lower BMI 30 years later (Schlam, Wilson, Shoda, Mischel, & Ayduk, 2013). Potentially identifying children with greater difficulty in delaying gratification could help detect children at risk of becoming either overweight or obese.

How does this relate to exercise behavior? David Dzewaltowski and his colleagues (Dzewaltowski, Johnston, Estabrooks, & Johannes, 2000) suggested the following. First, like waiting for a second candy, the benefits of physical activity participation are sometimes more distal than the acute benefits of sedentary behavior. Second, like waiting for candy, physical activity often requires coping skills to complete. Take, for example, an individual who plans to exercise after work. Before he goes to exercise he decides to stop at home. While at home he turns on the television and finds an entertaining program and in the end does not exercise. It can be concluded from Mischel and colleagues' study that if the television option was removed from the environment, then the individual would not have been tempted and would have followed through on his plans to exercise. So, when an environment is risky (i.e., there is a candy waiting to be eaten or a television show waiting to be watched), it is important to ensure that individuals have appropriate coping skills. However, when the environment is supportive (i.e., no candy, accessible physical activity options), even those people without

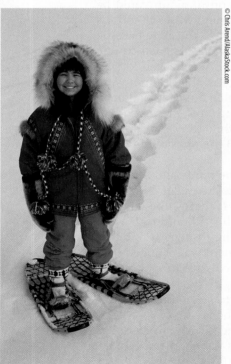

© Chris Arend/AlaskaStock.com

appropriate coping skills can be successful (Dzewaltowski et al., 2000). In short, it is the physical environment that changed the children's behavior regardless of the skills they possessed. Does this generalize to exercise and sedentary behavior? That is, by having a physical environment that makes it easy to be active and stand, will people be more active and stand more? Let's now see what the research says about the role that our physical environment has on our physical activity and sedentary behaviors.

■ Modernization of the Physical Environment: A Comparison of Two Cultures

Modernization refers to the transformation from a rural and agrarian society to an urban and industrial society. To take a look at the effects of modernization of our physical environment on physical activity levels, we can examine the following two very different cultures: (1) the Inuit, who have experienced rapid modernization, and (2) the Old Order Amish, who have resisted modernization. Comparing and contrasting these two cultures has enabled researchers to examine the effects of modernization (or resistance to modernization) on health and physical activity.

The Case of the Inuit

In a landmark series of studies, Andris Rode and Roy Shephard (1993, 1994) examined the effects of a rapidly changing physical environment on the Inuit people living in Igloolik, which is located in the remote northern Canadian territory of Nanavut. Igloolik has a **polar climate**; 9 months of the year the average temperature is below freezing. Historically, the people of Igloolik lived a hunting and trapping lifestyle that required high levels of daily physical activity. However, in the latter half of the 20th century, the people of Igloolik went through a rapid period of acculturation to a sedentary lifestyle. In essence, their hunter-gatherer lifestyle quickly shifted to a more mechanized Western lifestyle.

As shown in **FIGURE 16-1**, the people of Igloolik experience dramatic changes in their physical environment from 1970 to 1990, with significant increases in the ratio of snowmobiles, boats, cars, and all-terrain vehicles to households. Instead of walking, the Inuit could now take a sedentary form of transportation. As well, their outdoor activities declined and were often replaced by sedentary indoor activities such as watching television. Did this dramatic and rapid change in their physical environment affect their health? Yes!

Using a longitudinal study design, Rode and Shephard examined various health outcomes of a sample of Igloolik adults (age range = 20 to 60 years) with surveys and testing that they administered in 1970, 1980, and 1990. In 1970, much of the population continued traditional hunting and fishing activities, and

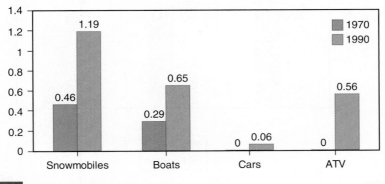

 FIGURE 16-1   Ratio of Vehicles to Households

Adapted from Rode, A., & Shephard, R. J. (1994). Physiological consequences of acculturation: A 20-year study of fitness in an Inuit community. *European Journal of Applied Physiology and Occupational Physiology, 69,* 516–524.

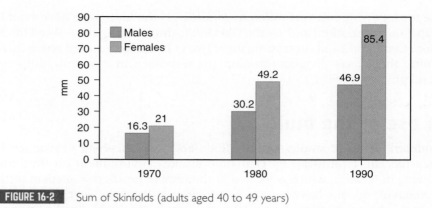

FIGURE 16-2   Sum of Skinfolds (adults aged 40 to 49 years)

Adapted from Rode, A., & Shephard, R. J. (1994). Physiological consequences of acculturation: A 20-year study of fitness in an Inuit community. *European Journal of Applied Physiology and Occupational Physiology, 69,* 516–524.

physical activity levels were high. One of the primary indicators of decreased physical activity was the sum of skinfolds, which assess the amount of subcutaneous body fat. A higher number on this assessment is related to increased adiposity. The 40- to 49-year-old Inuit people assessed in 1970 had a relatively low sum of skinfolds (16.3 mm for men and 21 mm for women). Individuals in the same age category in 1990 had scores four times that of their predecessors (46.9 mm for men and 85.4 mm for women; see **FIGURE 16-2**). Similarly, significant decreases in aerobic power via a step test were found from 1970 to 1990 (see **FIGURE 16-3**). The researchers concluded that changes in the Inuit's physical environment were

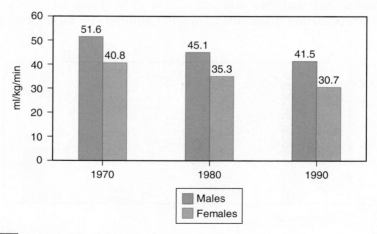

FIGURE 16-3   Changes in Aerobic Power Over a 20-Year Period

Adapted from Rode, A., & Shephard, R. J. (1994). Physiological consequences of acculturation: A 20-year study of fitness in an Inuit community. *European Journal of Applied Physiology and Occupational Physiology, 69,* 516–524.

responsible for the dramatic reduction of lifestyle physical activity, particularly the use of snowmobiles in place of walking through deep snow.

The Case of the Old Order Amish

Another method to assess the impact of modernization on physical activity is to examine the **Old Order Amish** because their lifestyle, in contrast to the Inuit, has not changed much in the last 150 years (Bassett, Schneider, & Huntington, 2004). The Old Order Amish believe in separation from the outside world and a simplistic lifestyle. In their clothing, lifestyle, and religion, the Amish people emphasize humility, nonviolence, and traditional values rather than advancement and technology. They do not drive automobiles, use electrical appliances, or employ other modern conveniences such as dishwashers and washing machines.

They have elected to keep most types of modern technology out of their lives, to live close to the land, and to maintain strong family and community ties. Labor-intensive farming remains the main occupation, whereby the Amish men still till the soil with horses. The Amish people tend to either walk or use horse-drawn carriages for transportation. The Amish women do most of the childcare, cooking, and cleaning. The children are educated in their own schools, and formal education ends after the eighth grade. In short, the Old Order Amish have resisted modernization. Has this resistance to modernization had an effect on their physical activity levels? From the standpoint of physical activity, the Amish people's lifestyle might resemble that of rural residents in North America in the mid-to-late 1800s.

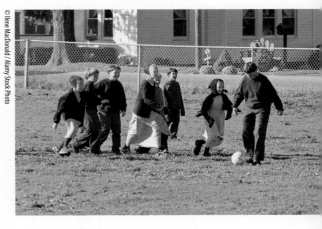

© Ilene MacDonald / Alamy Stock Photo

In a series of studies, David Bassett and his colleagues (2004, 2007; Eslinger et al., 2010; Tremblay, Eslinger, Copeland, Barnes, & Bassett, 2008) examined if resistance to modernization had any effect on physical activity and other health parameters of Old Order Amish children and adults. In one study, the children (aged 6 to 18 years) wore a pedometer for a week and their height and weight were assessed to compute their BMI. The main findings were that the Amish children had higher levels of physical activity (as determined by their pedometer step count), lower rates of sedentary time, and lower rates of overweight and obesity compared to youth living in modern societies.

More specifically, obesity was rare in the Amish children. Only 1.4% of the Amish youth were classified as obese based on their BMI, compared to about 8% of Canadian and American youth at the time the study was conducted. As well, only 7% of Amish youth were overweight, compared with about 25% of Canadian and American youth (see **FIGURE 16-4**).

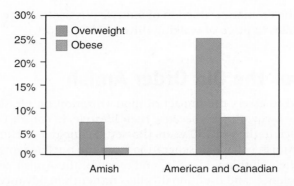

FIGURE 16-4   Percent of Overweight and Obese Amish Children Compared to Their American and Canadian Counterparts

Data from Bassett, D. R. Jr., Tremblay, M. S., Esliger, D. W., Copeland, J. L., Barnes, J. D., & Huntington, G. E. (2007). Physical activity and body mass index of children in an Old Order Amish community. *Medicine and Science in Sports and Exercise, 39,* 410–415.

With regard to physical activity, **FIGURE 16-5** clearly reveals that the Old Order Amish children, on average, took significantly more steps than children in other industrialized countries (age range = 5 to 12 years). As a reasonable rule of thumb, youth should accumulate a minimum of 9,000 steps per day. Of course, more is better for optimal health (Adams, Johnson, & Tudor-Locke, 2013; Tudor-Locke et al., 2011a, 2011b). Based on these values, the Old Order Amish children were very physically active. In fact, the Old Order Amish children took about

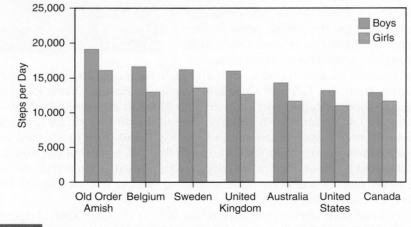

FIGURE 16-5   Average Number of Steps per Day in Elementary School Children in Different Cultures

Adapted from Bassett, D. R. Jr., Pucher, J., Buehler, R., Thompson, D. L., & Crouter, S. E. (2008). Walking, cycling, and obesity rates in Europe, North America, and Australia. *Journal of Physical Activity and Health, 5,* 795–814.

5,000 to 6,000 more steps per day than North American children, and they had significantly lower obesity rates.

Of importance, Old Order Amish youth had higher levels of physical activity than children living in industrialized societies, despite less participation in competitive sports, no fitness facilities, and no physical education classes. Old Order Amish children accumulate steps in a variety of ways throughout the day. For example, they walk to school regardless of the weather, and they perform activity -intense farm and household chores such as feeding and tending to farm animals, harvesting crops, sweeping, cleaning floors on hands and knees, laundry, meal preparation, and childcare. Despite the lack of formal physical education classes, the schoolchildren are given two recesses and a 1-hour lunch each school day, in which most of this time is spent engaged in active play.

Similar results were obtained with Old Order Amish adults, with Amish men accumulating an average of 18,425 steps per day and Amish women accumulating an average of 14,196 steps per day (see **FIGURE 16-6**). These Amish adult daily step values are about two-thirds higher than estimates from other epidemiological pedometer-assessed step values in other American adult populations (Bassett, Wyatt, Thompson, Peters, & Hill, 2010).

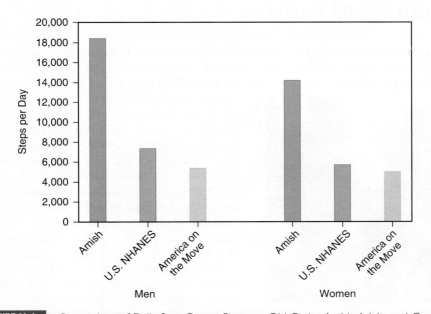

FIGURE 16-6   Comparison of Daily Step Counts Between Old Order Amish Adults and Contemporary U.S. Adults from the "America on the Move" Epidemiological Study

Note: The average number of steps per day taken by Amish men and women were 18,425 steps per day and 14,196 steps per day, respectively. These values are considerably higher than recent estimates for contemporary U.S. adults.

Adapted from Bassett, D. R. Jr., Schneider, P. L., & Huntington, G. E. (2004). Physical activity in an Old Order Amish community. *Medicine and Science in Sports and Exercise, 36,* 79–85.

As well, only 4% of the Amish adults were obese. Of interest, there was no evidence of an age-related decline in physical activity between 6 to 60 years of age for the Old Order Amish. In contrast, American adults take only one-half as many steps as elementary school children in the United States (6,000 vs. 12,000 steps/day; Tudor-Locke et al., 2004). The study of a culture that has resisted modern technology can help us understand the impact of modern technology on people's physical activity and weight status. In short, by examining a culture that refrains from using automobiles, modern labor-saving devices, and screen entertainment, it is possible to estimate how these advances have impacted our lives.

CRITICAL THINKING ACTIVITY 16-2

© ecco/Shutterstock, Inc.

Can you think of other societies that have gone through rapid periods of modernization? How has this affected their health?

■ Travel Patterns

Youth Travel Patterns

Active travel is an approach to transportation that focuses on physical activities such as walking, biking, and skateboarding, as opposed to automobile travel, to get to places like work, school, shops, and parks. Active travel is an important way for youth to get physical activity. School-age children who travel to school by active

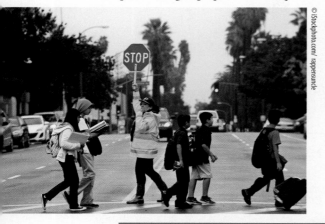

© iStockphoto.com/ rappensunde

means accumulate more exercise and are more physically fit that those who travel by passive means, such as car and bus (Ostergaard, Kolle, Steene-Johannssen, Anderssen, & Anderson, 2013; Pizarro et al., 2013). Unfortunately, there has been a dramatic decline in the number of children who walk, skateboard, or bike to school or engage in active leisure activities in many parts of the world (see Active Healthy Kids Canada, 2013). For example, from 1969 to 1990 the percentage of U.S. children and youth who either walked or biked to school fell from almost 48% to 13% (McDonald, Brown, Marchetti, & Pedroso, 2011).

CRITICAL THINKING ACTIVITY 16-3

© ecco/Shutterstock, Inc.

Did you walk or bike to elementary school? How did this affect your level of daily physical activity as a youth?

The distance from a child's home to school is a strong indicator of active travel. Children living within a quarter mile of their school are 14 times more likely to walk to school than are children living greater than 1 mile away from their school (McDonald et al., 2011). Unfortunately, many students face long trips not possible by active means. The likelihood of children walking or biking to school is positively associated with shorter trips, male gender, higher land use mix, low-density traffic, and presence of street trees (Su et al., 2013). The community and neighborhood environment can facilitate active transportation to school and other nearby locations through the presence of neighborhood schools, sidewalks, bike lanes, and traffic-calming mechanisms such as crosswalks and traffic signals.

In a systematic review of 52 studies, Schoeppe and colleagues (Schoeppe, Duncan, Badland, Oliver, & Curtis, 2013) examined children's (aged 3–18 years) independent mobility and active travel with regard to physical activity, sedentary behavior, and weight status. In children, independent mobility is defined as the freedom to travel around either their own neighborhood or city without adult supervision (Tranter & Whitelegg, 1994). Thus, independent mobility could be for the purposes of either play or travel to places such as school, leisure facilities, parks, and friends' houses. The researchers found that most studies focused on active travel to and/or from school, and that these studies found a positive association with physical activity. In other words, children who walked to school engaged in more physical activity than children who were driven to school. The same relationship was detected for active travel to leisure-related places and independent mobility with physical activity. Unfortunately, few studies have examined whether a correlation exists between active travel to school and self-reported screen time or objectively measured sedentary behavior. The researchers concluded that children who have the freedom to play outdoors and travel actively without adult supervision accumulate more physical activity than those who do not.

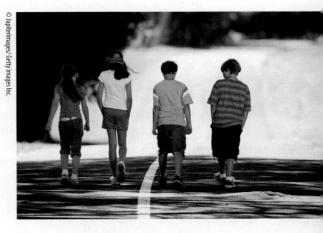

© Jupiterimages/ Getty Images Inc.

Many parents will site safety as a main reason for restricting the independent mobility of their children. In an attempt to bring clarity to this issue, Datar and colleagues (Datar, Nicosia, Shier, 2013) examined the relationship between parent-perceived neighborhood safety and children's physical activity, sedentary behavior, body mass, and obesity status using 9 years of longitudinal data (1999 to 2007) on a cohort of about 19,000 American kindergartners. The children's height and weight measurements and parent perceptions of neighborhood safety were assessed when the children were in kindergarten and in the first, third, fifth, and eighth grades. Dependent variables included age- and gender-specific BMI percentile, obesity status, and parent- or child-reported weekly physical activity and television watching. The researchers found that children whose parents perceived their neighborhoods as unsafe watched more television and participated in less physical activity. No significant association, however, was found between parent-perceived neighborhood safety and children's BMI. Further research is needed to increase our understanding of how crime and pedestrian and traffic safety affect physical activity levels (Bracy et al., 2014).

CRITICAL THINKING ACTIVITY 16-4

© ecco/Shutterstock, Inc.

What types of interventions can be developed to get youth to walk or bike to school more?

Travel in Different Countries

An example of the relationship between physical activity and one's environment can be found in the travel patterns of people from different countries. Bassett and his colleagues (Bassett, Pucher, Buehler, Thompson, & Crouter, 2008) conducted an international examination of the relationship between active transportation (defined as the percentage of trips taken by walking, bicycling, and public transit) and obesity rates in Europe, North America, and Australia. They found that countries with the highest levels of active transportation generally had the lowest obesity rates.

They found that Europeans walked and biked significantly more than Americans. For example, in 2000, European's walked 382 kilometers per person, compared to 140 kilometers per person for Americans. As another example, also in 2000, Europeans bicycled 188 kilometers, compared to Americans biking 40 kilometers per person. The researchers concluded that walking and bicycling are far more common in European countries than in the United States, Australia, and Canada, and that active transportation is inversely related to obesity in these countries.

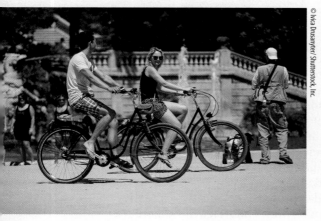

© Ivica Drusany/er/Shutterstock, Inc.

Active travel can also help people meet the recommended levels of physical activity. Buehler and colleagues (Buehler, Pucher, Merom, & Bauman, 2011) conducted a longitudinal study to examine the proportion of walking and cycling trips in Germany and the United States. They found that Germans walk and cycle significantly more than Americans (see **TABLE 16-1**). The researchers concluded that the high prevalence of active travel in Germany shows that daily walking and cycling can help a large proportion of the population meet recommended physical activity levels.

TABLE 16-1 Comparison of Active Travel in the United States and Germany				
	United States		Germany	
	2001/2002	**2008/2009**	**2001/2002**	**2008/2009**
Any walking	18.5%	18.5%	36.5%	42.3%
Any cycling	1.8%	1.8%	12.1%	14.1%
30 minutes of walking a day		7.7%		21.2%
30 minutes of cycling a day		1.0%		7.8%

Note: Between 2001/2002 and 2008/2009, the proportion of "any walking" was stable in the United States (18.5%) but increased in Germany from 36.5% to 42.3%. The proportion of "any cycling" in the United States remained at 1.8% but increased in Germany from 12.1% to 14.1%. In 2008/2009, the proportion of "30 minutes of walking and cycling" in Germany was 21.2% and 7.8%, respectively, compared to 7.7% and 1.0% in the United States.

Data from Buehler, R., Pucher, J., Merom, D., & Bauman, A. (2011). Active travel in Germany and the U.S.: Contributions of daily walking and cycling to physical activity. *American Journal of Preventive Medicine, 41*, 241–250.

People who engage in active travel also have a lower mortality rate. In other words, it appears that people who engage in active travel live longer than those who either drive or take other sedentary forms of travel. For example, Andersen, Schnohr, Schroll, and Hein (2000) observed that cycling to work decreased mortality rates by 40% among Danish men and women. Similarly, a multifaceted cycling demonstration project in Odense, Denmark, reported a 20% increase in cycling levels from 1996 to 2002 and a 5-month increase in life expectancy for men (Pucher et al., 2010). In fact, some evidence suggests that active travel may even have a positive effect on diabetes prevention (Saunders, Green, Petticrew, Steinbach, & Roberts, 2013).

The Case of the Dutch

In the Netherlands, walking and bicycling account for a large proportion of the population's transportation patterns (Pucher & Lefevre, 1996). Researchers found that when the distance to be traveled was 1 kilometer or less, 32% and 60% of the trips were traveled by bicycle and walking, respectively. When the distance to travel was between 1 and 2.5 kilometers, 46% and 21% of the trips were traveled by bicycle and walking, respectively. Transportation by car accounted for only 44% of all trips within urban areas in the Netherlands during the time of the study (Pucher & Lefevre, 1996).

In contrast, North American countries have very low bicycle and walking patterns within urban areas. Canadians bicycle for 1%, walk for 10%, and travel by car for 74% of all trips (travel by public transportation accounts for the remainder). Similarly, Americans travel by car for 84%, bicycle for 1%, and walk for 9% of all urban trips (Pucher & Lefevre, 1996).

One factor that may account for the differences between the three populations compared above is the physical environment of the roadways and the biking infrastructure (Pucher & Lefevre, 1996). In the Netherlands, urban roads and paths are constructed to facilitate cycling and walking. Right-of-way and separate lanes are provided for cyclists. In North America, many urban communities

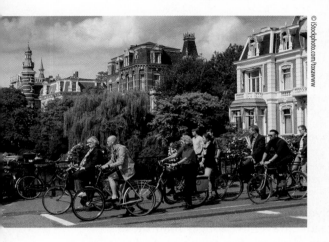

have been developed without sidewalks and with car travel in mind (Pucher & Lefevre, 1996). For many North American homes, the garage is connected to the house, so even walking from the front doorway to the side of the road is eliminated. It could be argued that cultural norms are the primary influence on the travel patterns of populations in the Netherlands, United States, and Canada. Although, cultural norms undoubtedly have some impact on travel patterns, studies in both the United States and Canada have shown that 46% and 70% of respondents, respectively, would cycle to work more often if safe bicycle lanes were provided (Pucher & Lefevre, 1996).

Hence, similar to the research by Mischel and his colleagues (1989), it could be inferred that the environment in the Netherlands is not risky; that is, the environment is free of connected garages and easily accessible and well-developed mass transit roadways. Therefore, the population does not see the attractive "speedy" option of physically inactive modes of travel. As such, coping skills necessary to avoid using one's car for a short trip are not necessary for success. Conversely, the environment is also full of positive environmental factors, such as roads that facilitate more active travel options.

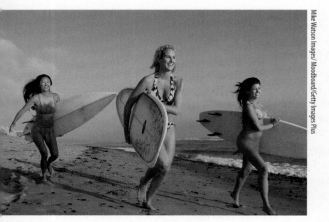

■ Seasonal Variation

A **season** is a division of the year marked by changes in weather, ecology, and hours of daylight. Very hot and humid temperatures, very cold and dry temperatures, high rainfall, strong winds, and snow may reduce the likelihood of people being physically active. Although the meteorological factors associated with the seasons cannot be changed, our ability to identify specific seasons that are associated with low exercise behavior and high sedentary behavior is important for promoting physical activity.

When researchers design studies that focus on physical activity, they typically take great care to assess physical activity at a consistent time of the year across study groups. For example, if an intervention study that targeted increased physical activity completed the baseline measure in the middle of a cold winter and then completed the post assessment in the temperate weather of the spring, chances are that the group would show increased physical activity. This practice highlights the recognition in the scientific community that physical activity varies based upon climatic changes.

Research reveals a relationship between weather and physical activity that is associated with seasonal changes in temperature. For example, in Australia, where the climate is temperate, only swimming varies with the seasons, while every other form of physical activity remains unchanged (Stephens & Caspersen, 1994). In contrast, data collected from Canada and Scotland show wide variations in physical activity across the seasons. For example, walking and cycling are highest in the months of June, July, and August and lowest during November, December, January, and February in these two countries (Stephens & Caspersen, 1994).

Carly Rich and her colleagues (Rich, Griffiths, & Dezateux, 2012) reviewed 16 studies examining seasonal variation in sedentary behavior and physical activity in children aged 2 to 18 years. They only included studies that used accelerometer-determined sedentary behavior and physical activity. Accelerometers are considered the gold standard method to assess physical activity in young populations because self-report or parent proxy reports may overestimate physical activity levels of children. The researchers found seasonal variation in physical activity, particularly for children living in the United Kingdom. Not surprisingly, physical activity levels were highest in the summer and lowest in the winter. The study findings were inconclusive for sedentary behavior, possibly due to the low number of studies examining this relationship. Increasing opportunities for physical activity during poor weather, in particular during winter, may mitigate declines in physical activity.

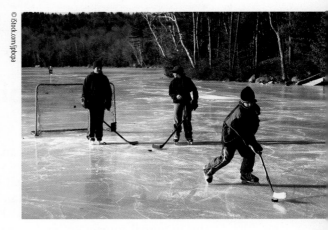
© iStock.com/jpbcpa

A study conducted by Anna Goodman and her colleagues (2014) found that hours of daylight is related to physical activity in children. They examined data on 23,188 children ages 5 to 16 years old from nine different countries. Of this large dataset, 439 of these children were further examined because they contributed data both immediately before and after the clocks changed (i.e., **daylight saving time**). Typically, users of daylight saving time adjust clocks forward 1 hour near the start of spring and then adjust them backward 1 hour in the fall. Although the total number of hours of daylight in the day is fixed, putting the clocks forward in the spring shifts daylight hours from the very early morning to the evening.

Goodman and her colleagues (2014) then examined the correlation between the time of sunset and physical activity levels measured by accelerometers. The date of accelerometer data collection was matched to time of sunset and to weather characteristics such as daily precipitation, humidity, wind speed, and temperature. Adjusting for child (i.e., age and gender) and weather covariates, they found that longer evening daylight was independently related with a small increase in daily physical activity. In other words, a later hour of sunset (i.e., extended evening daylight) was associated with increased daily activity across the full range of time of sunset, and this association was only partly attenuated after adjusting for the weather covariates.

The researchers concluded that their study findings provide evidence that evening daylight plays a casual role in increasing physical activity in the late afternoon and early evening—a time that is important for children's outdoor physical activity. In fact, the researchers calculated that if this proposal would be in effect, British children would have 200 extra waking daylight hours per year. In turn, this would increase the average time children could engage in moderate to vigorous physical activity from 33 to 35 minutes daily. In short, introducing additional daylight hours may positively increase children's evening outdoor play.

CRITICAL THINKING ACTIVITY 16-5

© ecco/Shutterstock, Inc.

Do you think that daylight saving time affects your physical activity level?

■ Point-of-Choice Environmental Prompts

Stair climbing is an activity that can easily be integrated into everyday life and that has positive health effects. **Point-of-choice prompts** (or *point-of-decision prompts*) are informational or motivational signs and messages near stairs and elevators/escalators aimed at increased stair climbing. Kelly Brownell and his colleagues (Brownell, Stunkard, & Albaum, 1980; Study 1) provided the seminal study on the potential impact of one's physical environment on physical activity levels. Their paper outlined the impact of a simple environmental manipulation intended to increase stair use at a shopping mall, a train station, and a bus terminal. In each setting, the stairs and escalator were side by side. Prior to the intervention, the research team documented the naturally occurring activity patterns of individuals confronted with the option of using a set of stairs or an escalator. To ensure that the recorded use rates were reliable, each site was visited on two occasions and stair use was monitored at peak times (i.e., 11 a.m. to 1 p.m. at the mall, 7:30 a.m. to 9:30 a.m. at the train station, and 3:30 p.m. to 5:30 p.m. at the bus terminal). In the initial observations, only about 5% of the people used the stairs.

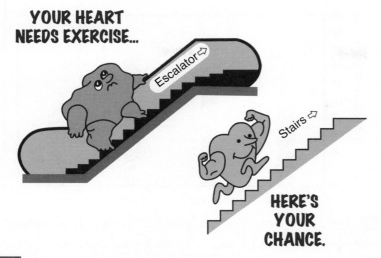

FIGURE 16-7   The Point-of-Choice Prompt to Encourage Stair Use

Reproduced from Brownell, K. D., Stunkard, A. J., & Albaum, J. M. (1980). Evaluation and modification of exercise patterns in the natural environment. *American Journal of Psychiatry, 137*, 1540–1545.

The environmental manipulation introduced was a simple sign placed at the stairs/escalator choice point. The sign—which was 3 × 3 ½ feet in size—depicted a lethargic heavy heart riding up the escalator and a healthy slim heart climbing the stairs (see **FIGURE 16-7**). Over 45,600 observations were made during the baseline and intervention phases of the study. Following the intervention, the percentage of people using the stairs increased to about 16% (Brownell et al., 1980). These results not only demonstrate the usefulness of this paradigm, but also suggest the strength of simple, inexpensive public health interventions to increase people's physical activity.

Interestingly, Brownell and his colleagues found that the impact of the intervention was different for Caucasians and African Americans. Although there were no baseline differences between the groups, African Americans were less likely to use the stairs following the intervention. Furthermore, although men and women differed in their stair use at baseline (7% and 5%, respectively), both increased at the same rate following the intervention (15% and 13%, respectively). Perhaps the most important finding of the study was that the percentage of obese individuals who used the stairs (1.5%) quadrupled (6.7%) during the intervention phase (Brownell et al., 1980).

In a second study, Brownell and his associates (1980; Study 2) examined the lasting impact of their environmental intervention on stair use. To do so, they collected baseline data for a week to determine the typical frequency of stair use at a commuter train station. This time the sign was placed by the set of stairs and escalator for 2 weeks. Average stair use increased from 11% to over 18% during the 2-week intervention period. The sign was then removed and follow-up

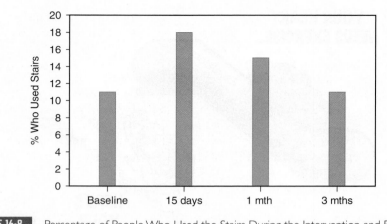

FIGURE 16-8 Percentage of People Who Used the Stairs During the Intervention and Follow-up

Adapted from Brownell, K. D., Stunkard, A. J., & Albaum, J. M. (1980). Evaluation and modification of exercise patterns in the natural environment. *American Journal of Psychiatry, 137*, 1540–1545.

assessments were conducted to examine how long the change would last. After 1 month without the sign, people's stair use had decreased to about 15%; after 3 months, people's stair use had returned to baseline levels (see **FIGURE 16-8**).

More recently, a study conducted in Scotland used a similar point-of-choice design. Using a subway in Glasgow, the researchers placed a sign that read "Stay

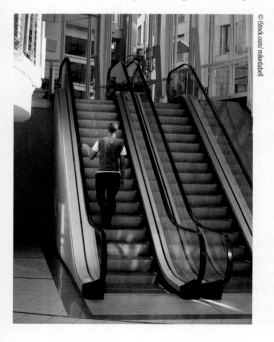

healthy, save time, use the stairs" in close proximity to a set of stairs that was adjacent to an escalator (Blamey, Mutrie, & Aitchison, 1995). Just as in the Brownell studies, stair use improved when the prompt was present. In fact, when the sign was present stair use nearly doubled for men (from 12% to 22%) and almost tripled for women (from 5% to 14%). This study design has been replicated in several other areas (e.g., shopping malls) and countries (Boen, Maurissen, & Opdenacker, 2010).

A recent systematic review of 25 studies assessed the overall effectiveness of point-of-choice prompts for the promotion of stair climbing (Nocon, Muller-Riemenschneider, Nitzschke, & Willich, 2010). The point-of-choice prompts were mostly posters or stair-riser banners in public traffic stations, shopping malls, or office buildings. Only 30% of the results for elevator settings found a significant increase in stair climbing. In comparison, 93% of the results for escalator settings found a significant increase in stair climbing. The authors concluded that point-of-choice prompts are able to increase the rate of stair climbing in escalator settings. However, in elevator settings, point-of-choice prompts are less effective in increasing stair use.

In an interesting study design, Rhian Evans and his colleagues (2012) experimentally examined if point-of-choice prompts could reduce sitting time at work. They examined if point-of-choice prompting software placed on people's computer was able to reduce long uninterrupted sedentary periods and total sedentary time at work. People were randomized to either an education group ($n = 14$) or a point-of-choice prompting group ($n = 14$). The education group received a brief education session on the importance of reducing long sitting periods at work; the point-of-choice group received the same education along with prompting software on their personal computers that reminded them to stand up every 30 minutes. Sitting time was then measured objectively using an activity monitor for 5 workdays at baseline and 5 workdays during the intervention. The number and time spent sitting in events longer than 30 minutes in duration were the main outcome measures.

At baseline, the participants spent almost 6 hours (76%) of their time at work sitting. Of that time, 3.3 hours a day was spent sitting in 3.7 events that lasted longer than 30 minutes. During the intervention, compared with baseline, the point-of-choice prompt group reduced the number and duration of sitting events that were greater than 30 minutes. However, there was no significant difference in total sitting time between groups. The researchers concluded that point-of-choice prompting software on work computers recommending taking a break from sitting plus education is superior to education alone in reducing long, uninterrupted sedentary periods at work.

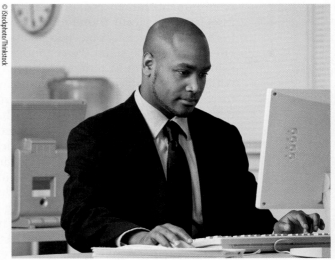

Physical Environment Correlates

Despite the continued effort of health professionals and agencies to encourage people to participate in physical activity, many people are not active enough to achieve optimal health benefits. To develop effective health policies and interventions aimed at increasing people's physical activity levels and reducing their sedentary behaviors, the main correlates and determinants of these behaviors need to be understood. While individual characteristics (e.g., age, gender, and ethnicity) and social characteristics (e.g., parents, peers, teammates) are important correlates of our physical activity and sedentary behavior, so, too, are aspects of the physical environment.

Recently, there has been a growing interest in the relationship between the physical environment in increasing exercise behavior and reducing sedentary behavior. Several reviews have been undertaken in an attempt to examine physical environmental correlates of physical activity, and to a lesser extent sedentary behavior (e.g., Biddle, Petrolini, & Pearson, 2014; Ding, Sallis, Kerr, Lee, & Rosenberg, 2011; Kaushal & Rhodes, 2014; Laxer & Janssen, 2013; Saelens & Handy, 2008; van Loon, Frank, Nettlefold, & Naylor, 2014; Wendel-Vos, Droomers, Kremers, Brug, & van Lenthe, 2007). A major criticism of this research is the reliance on self-report and nonvalidated assessments of both exercise behavior and the physical environment along with a focus on cross-sectional designs (Wendel-Vos et al., 2007). Before strong conclusions can be drawn regarding physical environment correlates of exercise behavior, better quality research is needed in this emerging area of study.

However, with that being said, the existing research reveals that our physical environment influences both our exercise and sedentary behaviors, with larger associations typically found for the perceived versus the actual environment and for self-report versus objective measures. Of importance, the magnitude of the effect tends to be small. Perceptions of one's environment and the actual environment can be quite different. You may perceive a walking path to be quite safe, while your friends may not. Or you may perceive that there are many gyms close to your house, while your neighbors may not. In many cases, personal perceptions are a stronger determinant of behavior than the actual environment. However, there are a number of objective environmental criteria that could influence behavior. Cost is one. For example, the cost of extracurricular physical activities is a main barrier for exercise in disadvantaged neighborhoods (Kottyan, Kottyan, Edwards, & Unaka, 2014). As well, minority women indicate that cost is a main environmental barrier to physical activity (Eyler et al., 1998).

In general, the research examining physical environmental correlates reveals that characteristics such as land use mix, street connectivity, cul-de-sacs, low speed limits, population density, pedestrian infrastructure, aesthetics, and safety are correlated with physical activity (e.g., Ding et al., 2011; Dogra & Stathokostas, 2014; Ferreira et al., 2007; McCormack & Shiell, 2011). For example, access to a mix of local recreational and nonrecreational destinations, such as cafes, grocery stores, food stores, schools, and services, is positively associated with walking. Neighborhoods that have more intersections, such as those with grid-like street patterns, offer direct and alternative routes to destinations supporting walking compared with neighborhoods that have fewer intersections, such as curvilinear street patterns. Higher population densities are positively associated with physical activity. As well, positive associations exist between walking and the quality of pedestrian infrastructure, such as maintained sidewalks, pedestrian lighting, shade, and street furniture. Similarly, associations between walking and neighborhood aesthetics (e.g., greenery, cleanliness), personal safety (e.g., graffiti), and traffic safety (i.e., vehicle volume, speed, crossing aids) have also been evidenced.

TABLE 16-2   Summary of Built Environment Correlates of Physical Activity

Correlate	Relationship to Physical Activity
Cul-de-sacs	Positive
Park space	Positive
Neighborhood walkability (e.g., sidewalks)	Positive
Commercial density	Positive
Residential density	Positive
Distance to school	Negative with youth PA
Recreation sites	Negative with youth PA
Low speed limits	Lower speed limits related to greater PA
Land use mix	Positive
Aesthetics (e.g., greenery, cleanliness)	Positive
Personal safety (e.g., graffiti, incivilities)	Positive
Violence	Negative

See **TABLE 16-2** for a summary of the built environment correlates of physical activity and sedentary behavior.

Urban sprawl is negatively associated with physical activity and health. Urban sprawl (also known as *suburban sprawl*) represents the expansion of auto-oriented, low-density development. In other words, it is the spreading of urban development such as houses and shopping centers on undeveloped land near a city. Characteristics of urban sprawl include increased distances between homes and destinations, lower population densities, and disconnected street patterns.

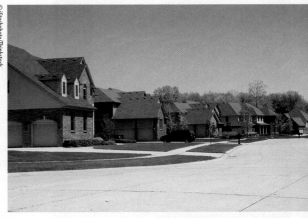
© iStockphoto/Thinkstock

Another physical environmental correlate of physical activity is pollution. Jennifer Roberts and her colleagues (Roberts, Voss, & Knight, 2014) found that increased community level air pollution is associated with reduced exercise, particularly among normal weight individuals. Not surprisingly, air pollution is often perceived as a barrier to exercise in urban areas. Researchers from the University of Copenhagen, however, found that the beneficial effects of exercise are more important for our health than the negative effects of air pollution, as it relates to the risk of premature mortality; that is, the benefits of exercise outweigh the harmful effects of air pollution (Andersen et al., 2015). Despite the adverse effects of air pollution on health, air pollution should be not perceived as a barrier to exercise in urban areas. The researchers concluded that even for those living in the most polluted areas, it is healthier to go for a run, a walk, or to cycle to work than it is to remain inactive.

Home Environment Correlates

It is important to examine if the home environment (also known as the *microenvironment*) is correlated to exercise and sedentary behavior, especially for young children who have limited independent mobility (Kausal et al., 2014; Maitland, Stratton, Foster, Braham, & Rosenberg, 2013). Considering the substantial amount of time children spend at home, there has been little investigation of how the home physical environment either constrains or supports children's exercise and sedentary behavior.

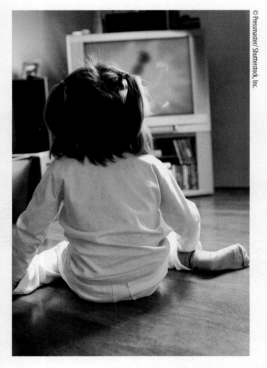

© Pressmaster/ Shutterstock, Inc.

Two reviews of the literature examining the home physical environment on children's physical activity and sedentary behavior have shed some light on this important research area (Kausal & Rhodes, 2014; Maitland et al., 2013). The number of televisions in a home is positively correlated with sedentary behaviors. Interventions that change the home environment by introducing television-limiting devices are effective in reducing sedentary behavior in children. These interventions include such things as television-locking devices, curriculums on media awareness to reduce television watching, setting media use goals, and television-monitoring devices.

In general, home physical activity equipment is unrelated to physical activity behavior, and an inverse relationship exists between physical activity equipment and sedentary behavior. The size of the exercise equipment, however, appears to matter, because large exercise equipment, such as treadmills and prominent exergaming materials (e.g., exergaming bike, dance mats), are more effective than smaller, peripheral devices for increasing physical activity levels. A **peripheral** is a device that is connected to a host computer, but it is not an integral part of the computer. It expands the computer's capabilities, but it does not form part of the core computer architecture.

Socioeconomic status moderates the effects of the home environment on physical activity. For example, children from lower-income households have greater media access in their bedrooms and have more daily screen time compared

TABLE 16-3 Summary of the Home Environment Correlates of Physical Activity	
Correlate	**Relationship**
Media equipment in the home	Positively associated with children's sedentary behavior Inconsistent results for physical activity
Media equipment in the child's bedroom	Positively associated with children's sedentary behavior
Yard space	Positively associated with physical activity
Physical activity equipment	Small positive association with physical activity Inverse relationship with sedentary behavior

to children from higher-income households. As well, children from lower-income households have less access to portable play equipment (e.g., bikes, jump ropes) compared to higher-income children (Tandon et al., 2012). **TABLE 16-3** summarizes the home environment correlates of physical activity.

◼ Summary

George Orwell (1949) described the fictional world of Big Brother where behavior was simply a reaction to environmental cues and stimulants. More scientifically, Walter Mischel and his associates (1989) showed that one's environment has the potential to be related to behavioral outcomes. It was concluded that when an environment is supportive, both individuals with and without appropriate coping skills could be successful.

To examine the generalizability of Mischel's findings this chapter contrasted the Netherlands, a nation with an environment that does not promote physically inactive travel modes (i.e., automobile travel) for urban trips, against Canada and the United States, nations with environments that do promote physically inactive travel modes. Clearly, the population within the Netherlands used physically active travel options with a much higher prevalence than their North American counterparts.

As common sense might predict, climate changes are related to either increased or decreased physical activity. Brownell and associates' (1980) seminal study on the impact of a simple sign to promote the use of stairs rather than escalators provides good support for point-of-choice (i.e., stairs or escalator) environmental influences on physical activity. However, the translation of those findings to more distal physical activity participation within a fitness facility was not supported. Finally, it does seem that individual perceptions of access and actual access to physical activity resources have an impact on physical activity. However, due to the relative infancy of the field, a clear consensus on how best to change environments to promote activity is not available. Some research suggests that the relationship may be influenced by factors such as age. For example, home access may be salient for participation of younger adults, whereas it may be more important for older adults to have access to safe community parks and pathways.

KEY TERMS

active travel
built environment
daylight saving time
delayed gratification
green space
land use mix
modernization
Old Order Amish

peripheral
physical environment
point-of-choice prompt
polar climate
season
street connectivity
urban sprawl

REVIEW QUESTIONS

1. What is the physical environment? What is the built environment? Provide examples of each.

2. Define *delayed gratification*. How is delayed gratification related to participation in physical activity?

3. Define *modernization*. Compare and contrast the Inuit and the Old Order Amish to highlight the effects of modernization (or resistance to modernization) on health and physical activity.

4. Define *active travel*. How is travel related to our physical activity behaviors?

5. How does climate affect our physical activity levels?

6. What are point-of-choice prompts and how to they affect people's behavior with regard to physical activity?

7. Describe some physical environment correlates of physical activity behavior.

APPLYING THE CONCEPTS

1. How did the built environment in which Clayton lived and worked influence his exercise behavior?

2. What changes did Clayton make to his environment (and the way he interacted with it) to increase the likelihood that he would engage in healthy behaviors, such as exercise and dietary changes?

REFERENCES

Active Healthy Kids Canada. (2013). Are we driving our kids to unhealthy habits? Retrieved from http://dvqdas9jty7g6.cloudfront.net/reportcard2013/AHKC-Summary-2013.pdf.

Adams, M. A., Johnson, W. D., & Tudor-Locke, C. (2013). Steps/day translation of the moderate-to-vigorous physical activity guideline for children and adolescents. *International Journal of Behavioral Nutrition and Physical Activity, 2110*:49. doi:10.1186/1479-5868-10-49

Andersen, L. B., Schnohr, P., Schroll, M., & Hein, H. O. (2000). All-cause mortality associated with physical activity during leisure time, work, sports, and cycling to work. *Archives of Internal Medicine, 160*, 1621–1628.

Andersen, N. J., de Nazelle, A., Mendez, M. A., Garcia-Aymerich, J., Hertel, O., Tjonneland, A., ... Nieuwenhuijsen, M. J. (2015). A study of the combined effects of physical activity and air pollution on mortality in elderly urban residents: The Danish Diet, Cancer, and Health cohort. *Environmental Health Perspectives, 123*, 557–563.

Ayduk, O., Mendoza-Denton, R., Mischel, W., Downey, G., Peake, P. K., & Rodriguez M. (2000). Regulating the interpersonal self: Strategic self-regulation for coping with rejection sensitivity. *Journal of Personality and Social Psychology, 79*, 776–792.

Bassett, D. R. Jr., Pucher, J., Buehler, R., Thompson, D. L., & Crouter, S. E. (2008). Walking, cycling, and obesity rates in Europe, North America, and Australia. *Journal of Physical Activity and Health, 5*, 795–814.

Bassett, D. R. Jr., Schneider, P. L., & Huntington, G. E. (2004). Physical activity in an Old Order Amish community. *Medicine and Science in Sports and Exercise, 36*, 79–85.

Bassett, D. R. Jr., Tremblay, M. S., Esliger, D. W., Copeland, J. L., Barnes, J. D., & Huntington, G. E. (2007). Physical activity and body mass index of children in an Old Order Amish community. *Medicine and Science in Sports and Exercise, 39*, 410–415.

Bassett, D. R., Wyatt, H. R., Thompson, H., Peters, J. C., & Hill, J. O. (2010). Pedometer-measured physical activity and health behaviors in U.S. adults. *Medicine and Science in Sport and Exercise, 10*, 1819–1825.

Biddle, S. J., Petrolini, I., & Pearson, N. (2014). Interventions designed to reduce sedentary behaviours in young people: A review of reviews. *British Journal of Sports Medicine, 48*, 182–186.

Blamey, A., Mutrie, N., & Aitchison, T. (1995). Health promotion by encouraged use of stairs. *The British Medical Journal, 311*, 289–290.

Boen, F., Maurissen, K., & Opdenacker, J. (2010). A simple health sign increases stair use in a shopping mall and two train stations in Flanders, Belgium. *Health Promotion International, 25*, 183–191.

Bracy, N. L., Millstein, R. A., Carlson, J. A., Conway, T. L., Sallis, J. F., Saelens, B. E., ... King, A. C. (2014). Is the relationship between the built environment and physical activity moderated by perceptions of crime and safety? *International Journal of Behavioral Nutrition and Physical Activity, 11*(1), 24. doi:10.1186/1479-5868-11-24

Brownell, K. D., Stunkard, A. J., & Albaum, J. M. (1980). Evaluation and modification of exercise patterns in the natural environment. *American Journal of Psychiatry, 137*, 1540–1545.

Buehler, R., Pucher, J., Merom, D., & Bauman, A. (2011). Active travel in Germany and the U.S. Contributions of daily walking and cycling to physical activity. *American Journal of Preventive Medicine, 41*, 241–250.

Datar, A., Nicosia, N., & Shier, V. (2013). Parent perceptions of neighborhood safety and children's physical activity, sedentary behavior, and obesity: Evidence from a national longitudinal study. *American Journal of Epidemiology, 177*, 1065–1073.

Ding, D., Sallis, J. F., Kerr, J., Lee, S., & Ronsenberg, D. E. (2011). Neighborhood environment and physical activity among youth: A review. *American Journal of Preventive Medicine, 41*, 442–455.

Dogra, S., & Stathokostas, L. (2014). Correlates of extended sitting time in older adults: An exploratory cross-sectional analysis on the Canadian Community Health Survey Healthy Aging Cycle. *International Journal of Public Health*. doi: 10.1007/s00038-014-0540-3

Drobetz, R., Maercker, A., & Forstmeier, S. (2012). Delay of gratification in old age: Assessment, age-related effects, and clinical implications. *Aging Clinical and Experimental Research, 24*, 6–14.

Dzewaltowski, D. A., Johnston, J. A., Estabrooks, P. A., & Johannes, E. (2000, October). *Health Places*. Paper presented at the Governors Conference on the Prevention of Child Abuse and Neglect. Topeka, KS.

Eslinger, D. W., Tremblay, M. S., Copeland, J. L., Barnes, J. D., Huntington, G. E., & Bassett D. R. Jr. (2010). Physical activity profile of Old Order Amish, Mennonite, and contemporary children. *Medicine and Science in Sports and Exercise, 42*, 296–303.

Evans, R. E., Fawole, H. O., Sheriff, S. A., Dall, P. M., Grant, P. M., & Ryan, C. G. (2012). Point-of-choice prompts to reduce sitting time at work: A randomized trial. *American Journal of Preventive Medicine, 43*, 293–297.

Eyler, A. A., Baker, E., Cromer, L., King, A. C., Brownson, R. C., & Donatelle, R. J. (1998). Physical activity and minority women: A qualitative study. *Health Education & Behavior, 25*, 640–652.

Ferreira, I., van der Horst, K., Wendel-Vos, W., Kremers, S., van Lenthe, F. J., & Brug, J. (2007). Environmental correlates of physical activity in youth: A review and update. *Obesity Reviews, 8*, 129–154.

Goodman, A., Page, A. S., Cooper, A. R., & International Children's Accelerometry Database (ICAD) Collaborators. (2014). Daylight saving time as a potential public health intervention: An observational study of evening daylight and objectively measured physical activity among 23,000 children from 9 countries. *International Journal of Behavioral Nutritional and Physical Activity*. doi: 10.1186/1479-5868-11-84

Kaushal, N., & Rhodes, R. E. (2014). The home physical environment and its impact of physical activity and sedentary behavior: A systematic review. *Preventive Medicine, 67*, 221–237.

Kottyan, G., Kottyan, L., Edwards, N. M., & Unaka, N. I. (2014). Assessment of active play, inactivity, and perceived barriers in an inner city neighborhood. *Journal of Community Health, 39*, 538–544.

Laxer, R. E., & Janssen, I. (2013). The proportion of youths' physical inactivity attributable to neighbourhood built environment features. *International Journal of Health Geographics*, Jun 18;*12*:31. doi: 10.1186/1476-072X-12-31

Maitland, C., Stratton, G., Foster, S., Braham, R., & Rosenberg, M. (2013). A place for play? The influence of the home physical environment on children's physical activity and sedentary behaviour. *International Journal of Behavioral Nutrition and Physical Activity, 17*. doi:10.1186/1479-5868-10-99

McCormack, G. R., & Shiell, A. (2011). In search of causality: A systematic review of the relationship between the built environment and physical activity among adults. *International Journal of Behavioral Nutrition and Physical Activity*, Nov 13;*8*:125. doi:10.1186/1479-5868-8-125

McDonald, N. C., Brown, A. L., Marchetti, L. M., & Pedroso, M. S. (2011). U.S. school travel, 2009; an assessment of trends. *American Journal of Preventive Medicine, 41*, 146–151.

Mischel, W., Shoda, Y., & Rodriguez, M. L. (1989). Delay of gratification in children. *Science, 244*, 933–938.

Moffitt, T. E., Arseneault, l., Belsky, D., Dickson, N., Hancox, R. J., Harrington, H., … Caspi, A. (2011). A gradient of childhood self-control predicts health, wealth, and public safety. *Proceedings of the National Academy of Sciences of the United States of America, 108*, 2693–2698.

Nocon, M., Muller-Riemenschneider, F., Nitzschke, K., & Willich, S. N. (2010). Review article: Increasing physical activity with point-of-choice prompts: A systematic review. *Scandinavian Journal of Public Health, 38*, 633–638.

Orwell, G. (1949). *1984*. San Diego, CA: Harcourt, Brace, Jovanovich.

Ostergaard, L., Kolle, E., Steene-Johannessen, J., Anderssen, S. A., & Andersen, L. B. (2013). Cross-sectional analysis of the association between mode of school transportation and physical fitness in children and adolescents. *International Journal of Behavioral Nutrition and Physical Activity*, Jul 17;*10*:91. doi:10.1186/1479-5868-10-91

Pizarro, A. N., Ribeiro, J. C., Marques, E. A., Mota, J., & Santos, M. P. (2013). Is walking to school associated with improved metabolic health? *International Journal of Behavioral Nutrition and Physical Activity*. doi: 10.1186/1479-5868-10-12

Pucher, J., & Lefevre, C. (1996). *The urban transportation crisis in Europe and North American*. London: Macmillan.

Pucher, J., Buehler, R., Bassett, D. R., & Dannenbert, A. L. (2010). Walking and cycling to health: A comparative analysis of city, state, and international data. *American Journal of Public Health*, *100*, 1986–1992.

Rhodes, R. E., & Nasuti, G. (2011). Trends and changes in research on the psychology of physical activity across 20 years: A quantitative analysis of 10 journals. *Preventive Medicine*, *53*, 17–23.

Rich, C., Griffiths, L. J., & Dezateux, C. (2012). Seasonal variation in accelerometer-determined sedentary behaviour and physical activity in children: A review. *International Journal of Behavioral Nutritional and Physical Activity*, *30*, 49. doi:10.1186/1479-5868-9-49

Roberts, J. D., Voss, J. D., & Knight, B. (2014). The association of ambient air pollution and physical inactivity in the United States. *PLoS One*. doi:10.1371/journal.pone.0090143

Rode, A., & Shephard, R. J. (1993). Acculturation and loss of fitness in the Inuit: The preventive role of active leisure. *Arctic Medical Research*, *52*, 107–112.

Rode, A., & Shephard, R. J. (1994). Physiological consequences of acculturation: A 20-year study of fitness in an Inuit community. *European Journal of Applied Physiology and Occupational Physiology*, *69*, 516–524.

Saelens, B. E., & Handy, S. L. (2008). Built environment correlates of walking: A review. *Medicine and Science in Sports and Exercise*, *40*, S550–S566.

Saunders, L. E., Green, J. M., Petticrew, M. P., Steinbach, R., & Roberts, H. (2013). What are the health benefits of active travel? A systematic review of trials and cohort studies. *PLoS One*, *15*:e69912.

Schlam, T. R., Wilson, N. L., Shoda, Y., Mischel, W., & Ayduk, O. (2013). Preschoolers' delay of gratification predicts their body mass 30 years later. *Journal of Pediatrics*, *162*, 90–93.

Schoeppe, S., Duncan, M. J., Badland, H., Oliver, M., & Curtis, C. (2013). Association of children's independent mobility and active travel with physical activity, sedentary behavior, and weight status: A systematic review. *Journal of Science and Medicine in Sport*, *16*, 312–319.

Stephens, T., & Caspersen, C. J. (1994). The demography of physical activity. In C. Bouchard & R. J. Shepard (Eds.), *Physical activity, fitness, and health: International proceedings and consensus statement* (pp. 204 – 213). Champaign, IL: Human Kinetics.

Su, J. G., Jerrett, M., McConnell, R., Berhane, K., Dunton, G., Shankardass, K., Reynolds, K., Chang, R., & Wolch, J. (2013). Factors influencing whether children walk to school. *Health Place*. doi: 10.1016/j.healthplace.2013.03.011. Epub 2013 Apr 17.

Tandon, P. S., Zhou, C., Sallis, J. F., Cain, K. L., Frank, L. D., & Saelens, B. E. (2012). Home environment relationships with children's physical activity, sedentary time, and screen time by socioeconomic status. *International Journal of Behavioral Nutritional and Physical Activity*, *26*, 88. doi:10.1186/1479-5868-9-88

Tranter, P., & Whitelegg, J. (1994). Children's travel behaviour in Canberra: Car-dependent lifestyles in a low density city. *Journal of Transport Geography*, *2*, 265–273.

Tremblay, M. S., Esliger, D. W., Copeland, J. L., Barnes, J. D., & Bassett, D. R. (2008). Moving forward by looking back: Lessons learned from long-lost lifestyles. *Applied Physiology, Nutrition, and Metabolism*, *33*, 836–842.

Tudor-Locke, C., Craig, C. L., Beets, M. W., Belton, S., Cardon, G. M., Duncan, S., ... Blair, S. N. (2011a). How many steps/day are enough? For children and adolescents. *International Journal of Behavioral Nutrition and Physical Activity, 28*;78. doi:10.1186/1479-5868-8-78

Tudor-Locke, C., Craig, C. L., Brown, W. J., Clemes, S. A., De Cocker, K., Giles-Corti, B., ... Blair, S. N. (2011b). How many steps/day are enough? For adults. *International Journal of Behavioral Nutritional and Physical Activity, 28*;79. doi:10.1186/1479-5868-8-79

Tudor-Locke, C., Ham, S. A., Macera, C. A., Ainsworth, B. E., Kirkland, K. A., Reis, J. P., & Kimsey, C. D. (2004). Descriptive epidemiology of pedometer-determined physical activity. *Medicine and Science in Sports and Exercise, 36*, 1567–1573.

Van Loon, J., Frank, L. D., Nettlefold, L., & Naylor, P. J. (2014). Youth physical activity and the neighbourhood environment: Examining correlates and the role of neighbourhood definition. *Social Science and Medicine, 104*, 107–115.

Wendel-Vos, W., Droomers, M., Kremers, S., Brug, J., & Van Lenthe, F. (2007). Potential environmental determinants of physical activity in adults: A systematic review. *Obesity Reviews, 8*, 425–440.

Glossary

accelerometer A device that detects and quantifies physical activity and movement via an electronic sensor. Records body acceleration minute to minute, providing detailed information about the frequency, duration, intensity, and pattern of movement. The data provided often are used to estimate energy expenditure.

active travel An approach to travel that focuses on physical activities, such as walking and cycling, as opposed to car travel, to get to work, school, and other destinations.

activity trait A disposition toward a fast lifestyle. Individuals with this trait are high energy, fast talking, and tend to keep busy.

acute pain Sharp, stinging pain that is usually localized in an injured area of the body.

acute physical activity Refers to a single bout of exercise. The exercise activity may take only a few seconds (e.g., lifting a weight or running 50 meters) or many hours (e.g., running a marathon).

affect The broad range of feelings people experience. It encompasses both emotions and moods.

agoraphobia A type of anxiety disorder in which people fear and often avoid places or situations that might cause them to panic and make them feel trapped, helpless, or embarrassed.

agreeableness Tendency to be kind, cooperative, altruistic, trustworthy, and generous.

Alzheimer's disease An irreversible, progressive brain disease that slowly destroys memory and thinking skills, and eventually even the ability to carry out the simplest tasks.

amotivation The absence of motivation toward a behavior.

analytical psychology Branch of psychology that emphasizes the primary importance of the individual psyche and the personal quest for wholeness.

anorexia nervosa An eating disorder characterized by excessive food restriction, an irrational fear of gaining weight, and a distorted body self-perception.

anxiety A negative psychological and physiological state characterized by feelings of nervousness, worry, fatigue, concentration problems, and apprehension and arousal of the body.

apnea Temporary cessation of breathing, especially during sleep.

attention The cognitive process of selectively concentrating on one aspect of the environment while ignoring other things.

attention deficit hyperactivity disorder (ADHD) One of the most common childhood disorders. Symptoms include difficulty staying focused and paying attention, difficulty controlling behavior, and hyperactivity.

attitude An individual's positive or negative evaluation of performing a behavior.

auditory attention The ability to focus on relevant acoustic signals, particularly speech or linguistic stimuli.

bariatric surgery An operation on the stomach and/or intestines that helps patients who are morbidly obese to lose weight. It is an option for people who either cannot lose weight by other means or who suffer from serious health problems related to obesity.

barrier efficacy An individual's beliefs about possessing the capability to overcome obstacles to physical activity.

basal sleep The amount of sleep needed on a regular basis for optimal performance.

behavioral beliefs Perceived consequences of carrying out a specific action and a person's evaluation of each of these consequences.

behavioral medicine An interdisciplinary field of medicine concerned with the development and integration of knowledge in the biological, behavioral, psychological, and social sciences relevant to health and illness.

binge eating Uncontrollable urges to overeat.

biomedical model Health model that excludes psychological and social factors and includes only biological factors in an attempt to understand a person's medical illness or disorder.

biopsychosocial model Health model that states that a combination of biological, psychological, and social factors determines a person's health and illness.

bipolar disorder A condition in which a person has periods of depression and periods of being extremely happy or being cross or irritable.

body image The self-perceptions and attitudes an individual holds with respect to his or her body and physical appearance.

body mass index (BMI) A measure of body fat based on an individual's height and weight.

brain stem The stemlike part of the base of the brain that is connected to the spinal cord. It controls the flow of messages between the brain and the rest of the body, as well as basic body functions such as breathing, swallowing, heart rate, blood pressure, consciousness, and whether one is awake or asleep.

built environment The part of the physical environment that includes the human-made surroundings that provide the setting for human activity.

bulimia nervosa An eating disorder characterized by consuming a large amount of food in a short amount of time, followed by an attempt to rid oneself of the food consumed.

bullying The use of force, threat, or coercion to abuse, intimidate, or aggressively dominate another person.

cancer A broad group of diseases characterized by unregulated cell growth.

cancer survivor A person with cancer of any type who is still living.

cardiometabolic disease An umbrella term used to define the risk relationship between cardiovascular disease and diabetes.

cerebellum A large portion of the brain that serves to coordinate voluntary movements, posture, and balance.

cerebrum The largest part of the brain, which controls thought, feeling, and voluntary movement.

chronic pain Pain that lasts 6 months or longer.

chronic physical activity Prolonged physical activity (i.e., long term).

clinical depression A psychiatric disorder in which feelings of sadness, loss, anger, or frustration interfere with a person's everyday life for weeks, months, or years. Also known as major depression.

cluster randomized controlled trial A type of randomized controlled trial in which groups of subjects (as opposed to individual subjects) are randomized.

cognition The mental processes involved in gaining knowledge and comprehension.

cohesion A dynamic process that is reflected in the tendency for a group to stick together and remain united in pursuit of its instrumental objectives and/or for the satisfaction of member affective needs.

conscientiousness Tendency to be ordered, dutiful, self-disciplined, and achievement oriented.

control beliefs Perceived presence or absence of required resources and opportunities, the anticipated obstacles or impediments to behavior, and the perceived power of a particular control factor to facilitate or inhibit performance of the behavior.

coping appraisal An evaluation of the preventive response of a behavior.

correlate A variable that may be statistically associated with either an increase or decrease (or no relationship) with physical activity. Correlational research assesses only statistical associations; it does not provide evidence of a causal relationship between a factor (e.g., age, gender) and physical activity.

correlational design Research that examines the relationship between two or more nonmanipulated variables. For example, a researcher examining the relationship between height and weight would find a strong positive correlation (i.e., when height increases, weight increases). Neither height nor weight, however, was manipulated by the researcher.

cortisol The body's primary stress hormone. The brain stimulates its release from the adrenal gland into the blood in response to physical or emotional stress.

cross-sectional design Research that involves observation of all of a population, or a representative subset, at one specific point in time.

cues to action Events and strategies that activate a readiness.

daylight saving time Adjustment of the time to achieve longer evening daylight, especially in summer, by setting the clocks an hour ahead of the standard time.

decisional balance The importance that an individual places on the potential advantages, or *pros*, and disadvantages, or *cons*, of a behavior and the subsequent evaluation of these factors.

dehydroepiandrosterone (DHEA) A steroid hormone made from cholesterol by the adrenal glands.

delayed gratification The ability to reject immediately available smaller rewards in favor of later larger rewards.

dementia A serious loss of global cognitive ability in a previously unimpaired person, beyond what might be expected from normal aging.

determinant A variable that has been assessed in a longitudinal observational study and/or experimental design that has a strong causal association with physical activity.

diabetes A group of diseases that affect how the body uses blood glucose.

digital age Refers to an economy based on the digitization of information and widespread use of computers. Also known as the computer age or information age.

digital native A person who was born during or after the general introduction of digital technologies and is therefore familiar with computers and the Internet from an early age.

distress Negative stress; it is the opposite of eustress.

drive for muscularity A desire, typically found in males, to achieve a muscular mesomorphic body.

dysthymia A depressed mood that occurs for most of the day, for more days than not, for at least 2 years (at least 1 year for children and adolescents). Most recently known as persistent depressive disorder.

ecological momentary assessment A category of methods that involve the collection of real-time data about current states (e.g., mood, activity) in the natural environment repeatedly over time.

effect size A standard score used to quantify the difference between two groups.

emotions Intense feelings that are directed at someone or something.

end-stage renal disease Condition where the kidneys stop working well enough to support life; requires dialysis or a transplant.

epidemiology The science that studies the patterns, causes, and effects of health and disease conditions in defined populations.

ergogenic supplements Substances taken in an attempt to enhance performance.

eustress Positive stress that is deemed healthful or that results in feelings of fulfillment.

executive function Cognitive processes that regulate, control, and manage other cognitive processes, such as planning, working, memory, attention, problem solving, and task switching.

exercise Planned, structured, and repetitive activities aimed at improving physical fitness and health.

exercise dependence Craving for leisure-time physical activity that results in uncontrollably excessive exercise behavior that manifests itself in physiological (e.g., tolerance) and/or psychological (e.g., withdrawal) symptoms.

exercise deprivation sensations The psychological and physiological effects that occur during periods of no physical activity (e.g., anxiety, fatigue). Also called exercise withdrawal symptoms.

exercise identity An individual's identification with exercise as an integral part of his or her self-concept.

Exercise-Induced Feeling Inventory A 12-item multidimensional inventory consisting of four 3-item subscales: positive engagement, revitalization, tranquility, and physical exhaustion.

exercise psychology The study of psychological issues and theories related to exercise.

external regulation Engaging in a behavior to receive a reward or to avoid punishment.

extraversion Tendency to be sociable, assertive, energetic, seek excitement, and experience positive affect.

extrinsic motivation Multidimensional concept whereby a person is motivated by external factors, such as rewards or punishments, to accomplish a particular task or engage in a certain behavior.

fibromyalgia A medical condition characterized by chronic widespread pain and a heightened and painful response to pressure.

fight-or-flight response The response of the sympathetic nervous system to a stressful event whereby it prepares the body to fight or flee. It is associated with secretion of epinephrine by the adrenal glands.

fitspiration A message, usually in the form of an image with a quote included, designed to inspire people to attain a fitness goal.

generalized anxiety disorder Long-lasting anxiety that is not focused on any one object or situation. Nonspecific persistent fear and worry and being overly concerned with everyday matters.

green space An area of grass, trees, or other vegetation set apart for recreational or aesthetic purposes in an otherwise urban environment.

group dynamics The positive and negative forces at play within a group of people.

habit The automatic performance of a behavior from consistent cues and practice.

happiness A state of mind or a feeling characterized by contentment, love, satisfaction, pleasure, or joy.

health A state of complete physical, mental, and social well-being, not merely the absence of disease.

health psychology The study of psychological and behavioral processes in health, illness, and health care.

health-related quality of life (HRQoL) An assessment of how an individual's quality of life affects his or her physical, mental, and social health.

hemodialysis A medical procedure performed to remove fluid and waste products from the blood and to correct electrolyte imbalances.

hyperalgesia An increased sensitivity to painful stimuli.

hypoalgesia A decreased sensitivity to painful stimuli.

identified regulation Engaging in a behavior to achieve a personal goal.

inactive behavior Performing insufficient amounts of moderate and/or vigorous physical activity (i.e., not meeting specified physical activity guidelines).

incidental physical activity Unstructured activity taken during the day, such as walking for transport, housework, and activities of daily living.

industriousness-ambition Tendency toward achievement-striving and self-discipline.

insomnia A sleep disorder characterized by long-term difficulties with initiating and maintaining sleep, waking up too early, nonrestorative sleep, and daytime impairment.

integrated regulation Engaging in a behavior because it aligns with other behaviors and choices in one's life.

intelligence quotient (IQ) A score derived from one of several standardized tests designed to assess intelligence.

intention Person's willingness and how much effort he or she is planning to exert to perform a behavior.

intent-to-treat analysis A type of study design where scientists analyze the results based on what the patients were told to do or how they were supposed to be treated rather than what actually happened. For example, if a person in a study is randomized to a medical treatment but ends up getting surgery or no treatment at all, then that person's outcome is still considered as part of the medical treatment group.

intrinsic motivation Engaging in a behavior for its own sake or the pleasure it provides.

introjected regulation Engaging in a behavior to relieve or prevent guilt.

ironman triathlon A long-distance triathlon race consisting of a 2.4-mile (3.86 km) swim, a 112-mile (180.25 km) bicycle ride, and a marathon 26.2-mile (42.2 km) run, raced in that order and without a break.

land use mix The diversity or variety of land uses, such as residential, commercial, industrial, and agricultural. A diverse land use mix is associated with shorter travel distances between places of interest and activities.

mastery experiences Personal experiences with carrying out a task successfully; thought to be the most important cause of self-efficacy beliefs.

maximum oxygen uptake The maximum capacity of an individual's body to transport and use oxygen during incremental exercise, which reflects an individual's physical fitness. Denoted as VO_2 max.

memory The process by which information is encoded, stored, and retrieved in the brain.

mens sana in corpore sano Famous Latin quote that is often translated to mean "a sound mind in a sound body."

meta-analysis A method of reviewing a large body of research evidence that is both systematic and quantitative.

metabolic equivalent (MET) A physiological measure used to express the energy cost of physical activities. It is the ratio of metabolic rate (i.e., the rate of energy consumption) during a specific physical activity to a reference metabolic rate.

mild cognitive impairment An intermediate stage between the expected cognitive decline of normal aging and the more pronounced decline of dementia. It involves problems with memory, language, thinking, and judgment that are greater than typical age-related changes.

mobile application A computer program designed to run on smartphones, tablet computers, and other mobile devices. Often referred to as an app.

moderator variables Variables that directly influence the relationship of an independent variable to a dependent variable.

modernization The transformation of a society from a rural and agrarian society to an urban and industrial one.

mood states A source of self-efficacy beliefs whereby previous successes and failures are stored in memory (and recalled) with associated feelings. Successful experiences are stored in memory with the feelings of joy, elation, vigor, and so on that initially accompanied it. Failures are stored in memory with the feelings of frustration, sorrow, depression, and so on that initially accompanied it. Serves to prime memories of successes or failures, thereby increasing or reducing self-efficacy.

moods Feelings that tend to be less intense than emotions and that usually lack a contextual stimulus.

motor function The ability to use and control muscles and movements.

muscle dysmorphia A form of body image distortion in which the individual perceives him or herself as having unacceptably small muscles.

myocardial ischemia A condition that occurs when there is insufficient blood flow to the heart usually because of a coronary artery obstruction.

neurocognitive function Cognitive functions closely linked to the function of particular areas, neural pathways, or cortical networks in the brain.

neuroticism Tendency to be emotionally unstable, anxious, self-conscious, and vulnerable.

nocioception The process of detecting tissue damage by sensory receptors, which usually causes the perception of pain.

nonclinical depression Transient mental state characterized by feeling unhappy, sad, miserable, down in the dumps, or blue.

noncommunicable diseases Noncommunicable diseases, also known as chronic diseases, are not passed from person to person. They are of long duration and generally slow to progress.

normative beliefs Perceived expectations of important significant others or groups and by the individual's motivation to comply with the expectations of these important significant others.

obstructive sleep apnea A sleep disorder caused by obstruction of the airway during sleep; causes lack of sufficient deep sleep.

Old Order Amish Religious community that emphasizes humility, nonviolence, and traditional values rather than advancement and technology.

100 Marathon Club A primarily British-based club for marathon and ultramarathon runners. Also called the British 100 Marathon Club.

openness to experience/intellect Tendency to be perceptive, creative, and reflective and to appreciate fantasy and aesthetics.

operational definition With regard to data collection, a clear, concise, and detailed definition of a measure.

outcome expectations Expectations an individual has about the outcomes of a particular behavior.

pain An unpleasant sensory and emotional experience associated with actual or potential tissue damage or described in terms of such damage.

pain threshold The point along a curve of increasing perception of a stimulus at which pain begins to be felt. It is an entirely subjective phenomenon.

pain tolerance The maximum level of pain that a person is able to tolerate.

pandemic When a disease is prevalent throughout an entire country or continent or globally.

panic disorder Brief attacks of intense terror and apprehension, often marked by trembling, shaking, confusion, dizziness, nausea, and difficulty breathing.

Parkinson's disease A progressive neurological disorder that leads to shaking (tremors) and difficulty with walking, movement, and coordination.

perceived barriers A person's opinion of the physical and psychological costs of the advised action.

perceived behavioral control Perceived ease or difficulty of performing a behavior.

perceived benefits A person's opinion of the efficacy of the advised action to reduce risk or seriousness of impact.

perceived severity A person's opinion of the seriousness of a condition and its consequences.

perceived susceptibility/vulnerability A person's opinion of his or her chances of getting a particular disease.

perfectionism A personality trait characterized by a person's striving for flawlessness and setting excessively high performance standards. Often accompanied by overly critical self-evaluations and concerns regarding others' evaluations.

peripheral A device that is connected to a host computer but is not an integral part of the computer (e.g., printers).

peripheral artery disease A narrowing of the arteries other than those that supply the heart or the brain.

personality traits Enduring and consistent individual-level differences in tendencies to show consistent patterns of thoughts, feelings, and actions.

physical activity Any body movement produced by skeletal muscles that requires energy expenditure.

physical environment The part of the environment that includes all of a person's indoor and outdoor surroundings, both those that have been designed (e.g., neighborhoods and parks) and those that occur naturally (e.g., oceans and mountains).

physical inactivity The absence of physical activity, usually reflected as the proportion of time not engaged in physical activity of a predetermined intensity.

Physical Self-Perception Profile Assessment tool based on a hierarchical, multidimensional theoretical model of self-esteem in which self-perceptions can be categorized as superordinate, domain, subdomain, facet, subfacet, and state.

physiological state Bodily sensations, such as increased heart rate, increased sweating, and increased respiratory rate, that provide a signal to the individual about his or her current level of self-efficacy.

point-of-choice prompt Informational or motivational signs near stairs and elevators/escalators aimed at increasing stairclimbing.

polar climate Climate characterized by a lack of warm summers. Every month in a polar climate has an average temperature of less than 10°C (50°F).

polysomnography The comprehensive recording of the biophysiological changes that occur during sleep.

population attributable fraction The proportional reduction in population disease or mortality that would occur if exposure to a risk factor were reduced to an alternative ideal exposure scenario.

positive psychology The study of happiness and how people can become happier and more fulfilled.

postpartum depression Moderate to severe depression in a woman after she has given birth.

posttraumatic stress disorder (PTSD) A stress disorder that develops after a traumatic event, such as sexual assault, serious injury, or the threat of death.

prevalence The proportion of a population found to have a condition.

primary exercise dependence Meeting the criteria for exercise dependence and continually exercising solely for the psychological gratification resulting from the exercise behavior itself.

processes of change The behaviors, cognitions, and emotions that people engage in during the course of changing a behavior. In the transtheoretical model, these are proposed as five behavioral and five experiential processes.

processing speed A measure of cognitive efficiency that involves the ability to automatically and fluently perform relatively easy or overlearned cognitive tasks.

prospective cohort study A cohort study that follows over time a group of similar individuals who differ with respect to certain factors in order to determine how the factors affect the occurrence of a particular outcome.

psychoticism Tendency toward risk taking, impulsiveness, irresponsibility, manipulativeness, sensation-seeking, tough-mindedness, and nonpragmatism.

quality of life A broad, multidimensional term that encompasses a person's perceived quality of his or her daily life.

quantitative research The systematic empirical investigation of a phenomena via statistical, mathematical, or numerical data or computational techniques.

quasi-experimental study Type of evaluation that seeks to determine whether a program or intervention has the intended effect on the study participants. Similar to the traditional randomized controlled trial, but specifically lacks the element of random assignment to treatment or control.

reciprocal determinism The interdependency and codetermination of behavior, internal personal factors, and external environmental factors.

recreational screen time Activities such as watching television, playing video games, using the computer, or using other screens during discretionary time (i.e., nonschool or work-based use) that are practiced while sedentary.

recurrent pain Episodes of discomfort interspersed with periods in which the person is relatively pain free for more than 3 months.

restless legs syndrome A neurological disorder characterized by an irresistible urge to move one's body to stop uncomfortable or odd sensations.

scheduling efficacy An individual's beliefs about possessing the capability to schedule physical activity into a daily or weekly routine.

screen time The amount of time people spend in sedentary behaviors such as playing video games, using the computer, watching television, or using mobile devices.

season A division of the year marked by changes in weather, ecology, and hours of daylight.

secondary exercise dependence Meeting the criteria for exercise dependence, but using excessive exercise to accomplish some other end (e.g., weight loss or body composition changes) that is related to a person's eating disorder.

sedentarism Engagement in sedentary behaviors characterized by minimal movement, low energy expenditure, and rest.

sedentary behavior Any waking activity characterized by an energy expenditure of less than or equal to 1.5 metabolic equivalents (METs) and a sitting or reclining posture.

self-concept The multitude of attributes and roles through which a person evaluates him- or herself to establish self-esteem judgments.

self-determination theory Theory that focuses on the degree to which an individual's behavior is self-motivated and self-determined.

self-efficacy Belief in one's capabilities to organize and execute the course of action required to produce a certain outcome.

self-esteem A stable global positive or negative evaluative of a one's own worth.

self-presentation The process by which people attempt to control and monitor how they are perceived and evaluated by others.

separation anxiety disorder Excessive anxiety regarding separation from home or from people to whom the person has a strong emotional attachment, such as a parent, grandparent, or sibling.

sleep A naturally recurring state of rest for the mind and body in which the eyes usually close and consciousness is either completely or partially lost.

sleep debt Accumulated hours of sleep that are lost each night.

sleep disorder A medical disorder of the sleep patterns. Also referred to as somnipathy.

sleep hygiene A variety of different practices that are necessary to have normal, quality nighttime sleep and full daytime alertness.

sleep latency The length of time that it takes to accomplish the transition from full wakefulness to sleep; normally the lightest of the non-REM sleep stages.

social anxiety disorder Intense fear and avoidance of negative public scrutiny, public embarrassment, humiliation, or social interaction.

social environment The part of the environment characterized by human interactions, such as those with family, friends, physicians, peers, classmates, neighbors, teachers, and others a person comes into contact with regularly.

social facilitation The tendency for people to do better on simple tasks when in the presence of others.

social integration The degree to which an individual participates and is involved in family and community social life and has access to resources and support systems. Also known as social embeddedness.

social media Websites and applications that enable users to create and share content or to participate in social networking.

social physique anxiety Anxiety that individuals experience in response to a perception that others will negatively evaluate their physique.

social support The perception and actuality that one is cared for by others, has assistance available from other people, and that one is part of a supportive social network.

specific phobia Fear and anxiety triggered by a specific stimulus or situation.

stages of change Six stages that people pass through in attempting any health behavior change, according to the transtheoretical model: precontemplation, contemplation, preparation, action, maintenance, and termination.

standard of living Refers to the level of wealth, comfort, material goods, and necessities available to a certain socioeconomic class in a certain geographic area.

standard score An individual test score expressed as the deviation from the mean score of the group in units of standard deviation.

state anxiety A state of heightened emotions that develops in response to a fear or danger of a particular situation.

street connectivity How often streets or roadways intersect.

stress The process by which we perceive and respond to events, called stressors, that we appraise as threatening or challenging.

stress hormones Hormones such as cortisol and epinephrine that are released by the body in situations that are interpreted as being potentially dangerous.

stressor Any event or situation that triggers coping adjustments.

subjective norm Perceived social pressure that individuals feel to perform or not perform a particular behavior.

support network The pool of support resources available to an individual.

supportive climate The quality of social relationships and systems.

systematic review A literature review focused on a particular research question that tries to identify, appraise, select, and synthesize all high-quality research evidence relevant to that question.

task efficacy An individual's beliefs about possessing the capability to perform a behavioral act.

temptation The intensity of urges to engage in a specific behavior when in the midst of difficult situations.

theory of planned behavior A theory about the link between beliefs and behavior.

theory of reasoned action A theory about the link between volitional behavior and intention.

threat appraisal An evaluation of the consequences of engaging in an unhealthy behavior (e.g., smoking, sedentary lifestyle).

tomato effect A term James and Jean Goodwin (1984) used to describe a phenomenon whereby highly efficacious therapies are either ignored or rejected.

trait anxiety A preset level of anxiety experienced by an individual who has a tendency to be more anxious (i.e., to react less appropriately to anxiety-provoking stimuli).

type A personality Personality type characterized by a blend of competitiveness and hostility with agitated behavior and continual movement patterns.

ultramarathon Any sporting event involving running and walking farther than the traditional marathon length of 26.21 miles.

urban sprawl The expansion of auto-oriented, low-density development outside of city centers. Also known as suburban sprawl.

verbal persuasion A source of self-efficacy beliefs whereby positive verbal statements ("you can do it") increase self-efficacy. Greatest impact on self-efficacy is found in those individuals who have some reason to believe that they could be successful with a task if they persist.

vicarious experiences Observational learning from the successful or unsuccessful behavior of others used as a comparative standard; thought to be a powerful cause of self-efficacy beliefs.

World Health Organization (WHO) An agency of the United Nations that is concerned with international public health.

Index

Note: Page numbers followed by *f*, or *t* indicate materials in figures, or tables respectively.

A

academic achievement, 169, 169*f*
accelerometers, 53, 168–169
action stage, 143
active stressors, 260, 261*t*
active travel, 116–117, 117*f*, 410, 412
   in United States and Germany,
      comparison of, 413*t*
Activity Limitations Module, 313, 314*t*
activity trait, 222–223
acute exercise, affects of, 294–295
acute pain, 270
acute physical activity, 7, 164
acute *vs.* chronic stress, 262
ADHD. *See* attention deficit
      hyperactivity disorder
adolescents, 195
   exercise and cognition in, 165–172
adults
   guidelines for physical activity, 19, 19*t*
   Old Order Amish, 409–410, 409*f*
   physical activity level and health benefit
      guidelines, 341*t*
   physical inactivity rates, 11, 11*t*
   populations, 172–178, 192–194
   sedentary behavior guidelines for, 45*t*
adverse effects of air pollution, 422
aerobic exercise, 268, 269
Aerobics Center Longitudinal Study, 193
affect, 189–190
   relationship, 190*f*
affective regulation explanation, 353–354
age and exercise dependence, 349
agoraphobia, 205
agreeableness, 218

air pollution, effects of, 421–422
Alzheimer's disease, 174, 176–177
   signs of, 174*t*
American adults reporting, percentage of,
      10, 10*f*
American College of Sports Medicine, 319
American Psychiatric Association's (APA),
      342, 343
American Psychiatric Association's
      Diagnostic and Statistical Manual
      for Mental Disorders, Fourth Edition
      (DSM-IV), 342
amotivation, 100
analytical psychology, 338
anecdotes, 273
anorexia nervosa, 356, 356*t*
antidepressant effects, 302
anxiety
   disorders, 200–201, 201*t*
   physical activity, and sedentary
      behavior, 200–205
   physical fitness, 13
   reduction, 301
APA. *See* American Psychiatric Association's
apnea, 299
apps (mobile applications), 387
attention, 173
attention deficit hyperactivity disorder
      (ADHD), 162, 170–172, 172*f*, 351
   symptoms of, 171*t*
attitude, 113
auditory attention, 176
Australian, physical activity guidelines in
      2012, 22, 22*t*
autonomy, 102

B

Baekeland, Frederick, 344
bariatric surgery, 55
barrier efficacy, 72
barrier self-efficacy, 127
basal sleep, 290
behavior of pain, 272
behavioral beliefs, 113
behavioral medicine, 28
behavioral observation, 124
β-endorphin explanation, 354
Big Brother, 401
binge eating, 357
biomedical model, 26
biopsychosocial model, 26
bipolar disorder, 198–200, 199*f*
Bloom cognitive taxonomy, 164*f*
BMI. *See* body mass index
body image, 234, 241–242, 251–252
    dimensions of, 242*t*
    interventions, 245
    and physical activity, 245–247
    scope and significance of, 243–245
    self-presentational anxiety, 248–251
body mass index (BMI), 9, 10, 22, 168,
        316, 403–404
brain image, 170
brainstem, 163
built environment, 401
    physical activity, correlates of, 421*t*
bulimia nervosa, 356–357, 356*t*
bullying, 383–384

C

Canadian Society for Exercise
        Physiology, 43
cancer, 318
    severity of, 91
cancer populations, 318–319
cancer survivor, 318
cardiometabolic disease, 195
cardiovascular health issues,
        338–339
cell phone use, measure of, 51

Centers for Disease Control and
        Prevention, 170
Centers for Disease Control and
        Prevention's (CDC) HRQoL-14,
        312, 313*t*
cerebellum, 162
cerebral cortex, 162
cerebrum, 162
    functions and four lobes of, 163*f*
children
    with ADHD, 171–172
    exercise and cognition in, 165–172
    independent mobility of, 411
    Old Order Amish, 407–409, 408*f*
    sedentary behavior guidelines for, 44*t*
chronic exercise, affects of, 294–295
chronic pain, 270
chronic physical activity, 7, 164
chronic stress
    acute *vs.*, 262
    cognitive, emotional, physical, and
        behavioral symptoms of, 263*t*
circadian rhythms, 302–303
classroom-based physical activity,
        167–170
classroom-based program, 168
clinical anxiety, 204–205
clinical depression, 191, 196–200
    symptoms of, 192*t*
clinical sleep disorders, 296–301
cluster randomized controlled trial, 168
cognition, 181
    behavior, 179
    definition of, 163–164
    function, 164
    human brain, 162–163
    mechanism of effect, 179–180
    physical activity, and sedentary
        behavior, 164–178
cognitive appraisal, 272
cognitive dimension, 242
cohesion, 388–390
    group, 389*f*, 390
communication intervention, 123

compulsive behavior, 341
conscientiousness, 218
contemplation stage, 142–143
control beliefs, 114
coping appraisal, 95–96
correlates
    definition of, 16
    of exercise, 16–19
    of physical activity, 18, 18t
correlational design, 165–166
cortisol, 267–268
cross-sectional design, 165–166
cues to action, 92

D
daylight saving time, 415
decision-making process, 153
decisional balance, 144–145
dehydroepiandrosterone (DHEA),
        267–268
delayed gratification, 402
dementia, 173
demographic factors, 89
depression, 191–200
determinant, 16
DHEA. *See* dehydroepiandrosterone
diabetes, 319
diabetic populations, 319–320
*Diagnostic and Statistical Manual for
        Mental Disorders, Fourth Edition*
        (DSM-IV) (APA), 342
digital age, 51
digital natives, 51
disease-specific efficacy, 72
dispositional optimism, 222
distress, 263, 264t
dogs, social support, 385–387
dose–response relationship, 42,
        43, 279
drive for muscularity, 361
dropouts, definition of, 94
Dutch, case of, 413–414
Dutch researchers, 176
dysthymia, 198

E
early onset dementia, 174
eating disorders, 355–359
    anorexia nervosa, 356, 356t
    bulimia nervosa, 356–357, 356t
    and exercise, 357–359, 359f
ecological momentary assessment, 323
EEG. *See* electroencephalographic
effect size
    definition of, 14
    interpretation of, 15–16
efficacious therapy, 6–10
electroencephalographic (EEG), 355
embeddedness, 374
emerging research, 42, 49–50
emotion, 189–190
    vs. moods, 190t
    of pain, 272
    relationship, 190f
emotional support, 381
end-of-grade testing, 167
end-stage renal disease, 300
endogenous pain, 273–277
epidemiology, 291
ergogenic supplements, 361
eustress, 262–263, 264t
evening exercise and sleep, 295–296
executive function, 173
exercise, 27, 316–324
    addiction, 341, 344
    aerobic, 268, 269
    eating disorders and, 357–359, 359f
    frequency, 247
    guidelines, 338
    for muscle dysmorphia, 361
    optimal amount of, 205
    relationship with depression, 23, 24f
    restless legs syndrome scores
        in, 301f
    and sedentary behavior, 291–301
        on self-esteem, effects of,
            239–241
    sleep disorders, 296–301
    in special populations, 317–321

exercise dependence, 342
  behavioral component of, 349
  characteristics of, 342
  criteria of, 343*t*
  defined by, 341–343
  exercise deprivation, 351–353
  explanations of, 353–355
  negative health effects, 338–341
  positive vs negative addiction, 344
  prevalence of, 345–347
  primary, 357–358
  research on, origins of, 344–345
  scale, 346, 346*t*
  secondary, 357–358
  symptoms, correlates of,
      348–351, 348*t*
    age, 349
    attention-deficit hyperactivity
      disorder, 351
    exercise identity, 350
    gender, 350
    perfectionism, 350
    personality and, 348–349
    self-esteem, 351
exercise deprivation, 351–353,
      352*t*, 353*f*
  sensations, 351
exercise equipment, 422
exercise identity, 350
Exercise-Induced Feeling Inventory,
      326–328, 327*t*
  definition of, 326
exercise-induced hypoalgesia,
      272–273, 278
exercise programs, 121
exercise psychology, 16
  research topics, 26, 27*t*
exercise-related disorders, 335–362
  eating disorders, 355–359
    exercise dependence. *See* exercise
      dependence
    muscle dysmorphia, 359–362, 362*t*
experimental evidence, 75–79
experimental pain, 275

  and exercise, 279*f*
    stimuli, 278*t*
  experimentally induced pain,
      277–279
  exploratory moderator analyses, 203
  external regulation, 100
  extraversion, 216
  extrinsic motivation, 100–101
    antecedents of, 101–102

F
Facebook, 53
  social support group, 387–388
factor analysis, 216–217
fibromyalgia, 273–274, 277
fibrosis, 23
fight-or-flight response, 261, 268
fitness psychology, 16
fitspiration, 247
FITT. *See* Frequency, Intensity, Time,
      and Thought Process
five-factor model, 219*f*
  vs. personality traits, 220*t*
Frequency, Intensity, Time, and
      Thought Process (FITT), 42*t*
  principle, 28, 28*t*
functional impairments, 270
fundamental lexical hypothesis, 216

G
gender
  exercise dependence symptoms, 350
  self-reported cell phone use by, 53*t*
generalized anxiety disorder, 205
global self-esteem, 235
Goodman, Anna, 415–416
green spaces, 402
group cohesion, 389*f*, 390
group dynamics
  cohesion, 388–390
  definition of, 388
  leadership, 390–393, 392*t*
guidelines for physical activity, 19–25
  upper limit to, 22–25

H

habit, 128–129
happiness, 324–326
  definition of, 324
health, 29, 312
health behavior efficacy. *See* disease-
    specific efficacy
health belief model, 88, 89*f*
  application of, 93–94
  components of, 89–92
  definitions and application of, 90*t*
  limitations of, 98–99
health benefits, adult guidelines
    by, 341*t*
health psychology, 29
health-related quality of life (HRQoL),
    309–315
  definition of, 312
  exercise, and sedentary behavior,
    316–321
  leisure-time physical activity and,
    316, 317*f*
  measurement of, 312–315
    HRQoL-14, 312–313, 313*t*–315*t*
    SF-36 scale, 313–315
  overview of, 309
  in special populations, 317–321
    cancer populations, 318–319
    diabetic populations, 319–320
    older adults, 320–321
healthcare providers, 384–385
healthy days core module, 312, 312*t*
hemodialysis, 300
hierarchical self-esteem, 236*f*
historical developments of physical
    activity psychology, 25–26
Hochbaum, Godrey, 88
home environment, correlates of,
    422–423, 423*t*
household physical activity, 28*f*
HRQoL. *See* health-related quality
    of life
human brain, 162–163, 162*f*
Hutchins, Robert Maynard, 46

hyperalgesia, 272
hypoalgesia, 272
hypoalgesic effects, 272

I

identified regulation, 101
inactive behavior, 39–40
incidental physical activities, 40
industriousness-ambition, 223
information age. *See* digital age
insomnia, 299
instructor efficacy, 391
integrated regulation, 101, 349
intelligence quotient (IQ), 166
intention, 112–113
intention-to-treat analyses, 197
intention–behavior gap, 127–128
International Classification of Sleep
    Disorders, 297
intervention research of
    transtheoretical model,
    151–152
intrinsic motivation, 101
  antecedents of, 101–102
introjected regulation, 100, 349
Inuit physical environment, 405–407,
    405*f*–406*f*
IQ. *See* intelligence quotient
ironman triathlons, 339
isometric exercise, 278–279

K

Kerlinger, Fred, 87–88

L

laboratory stress research, 264–266
land use mix, 402
leadership, 390–393, 392*t*
leisure-time physical activity, 28,
    316, 317*f*
Li, Fuzhong, 103
light physical activity, 39
little brain, 162
lower-order traits, 222–223

M

maintenance stage, 143–144
major depressive disorder, 196–198
marathons, 339
mastery experiences, 68
maximum oxygen uptake, 176
memory, 173
mens sana in corpore sano, 13
mental processes, 163–164
mental states, 74–75
meta-analysis, 13–16, 96, 195
    definition of, 13
    interpretation of effect sizes, 15–16
    research integration, 13–15
metabolic equivalents (METs), 38
METs. *See* metabolic equivalents
microenvironment. *See* home
        environment
mild cognitive impairment, 173–174
mild physical activity, 39
mobile applications (apps), 387
moderator variables, 14
modernization
    definition of, 404
    impact of, 407
    of physical environment, 404–410
        Inuit, case of, 405–407, 405*f*–406*f*
        Old Order Amish, 407–410,
            408*f*–409*f*
mood, 189–190
    disorders, 191
    emotions *vs.*, 190*t*
    relationship, 190*f*
mood states, 70
Morris, Jeremy, 37
motivation, sources of, 100–101
motivational theories of physical
        activity and sedentary
        behavior, 104–105
    health belief model, 88–94
    overview of, 87–88
    protection motivation theory, 94–99
    self-determination theory, 99–104

motor function, 176
MRI scans of brain, 180
multidimensional self-esteem, 236*f*
muscle dysmorphia, 359–362
    correlates of, 361–362
    measures of, 362, 362*t*
muscle pain, 275, 277
musculoskeletal pain, 273
myocardial ischemia, 272

N

National Commission on Sleep
        Disorders Research, 297
National Health and Nutrition
        Examination Survey
        (NHANES), 9
National Sleep Foundation, 293, 296
negative body image, 247
negative health effects, 338–341
negative social support, 376
negative stress, positive *vs.*, 262–263
network resources. *See* support
        networks
networks, 374
neurocognitive function, 173
neurogenesis, 180
neuroticism, 218, 220
neurotransmitters, 180
new media. *See* digital age
NHANES. *See* National Health and
        Nutrition Examination Survey
nociceptors, 271, 272
nocioception, 271
non-exercise activities, 41*f*
nonclinical anxiety, 203–204
nonclinical depression, 191–195
noncommunicable diseases, 20
nonexercisers, 247
    definition of, 97
nonrapid eye movement (NREM), 288
normative beliefs, 113
noxious stimulus, 277
NREM. *See* nonrapid eye movement

O

obligatory exercise, 341
observational studies of
        transtheoretical model, 150
obstructive sleep apnea, 299
occupational physical activity, 28*f*
Old Order Amish, case of, 407–410,
        408*f*–409*f*
older adults, 320–321
    populations, 174–178
100 Marathon Club, 23
openness to experience/intellect, 218
operational definition, 14
opioids, 272
outcome expectations, 66
overactivity, 351

P

PA. *See* physical activity
PAAC. *See* Physical Activity Across
        the Curriculum
pain, 269–271
    acute, 270
    chronic, 270
    components of, 271–272
        behavior, 272
        emotion, 272
        nociception, 271
        perception, 272
    definition of, 270
    endogenous, 273–277
    exercise and sedentary behavior,
        272–273
    experimental, 275
    experimentally induced, effects of,
        277–279
    muscle, 275, 277
    musculoskeletal, 273
    phantom limb, 272
    prevalence of, 271
    recurrent, 270
    stimuli, 277
pain perception threshold, 277–278

pain thresholds, 275, 277, 278
pain tolerance, 276, 277
pandemic, 11
panic disorder, 205
paradox, 357
parents, social support, 382
Parkinson's disease, 177
passive stressors, 260–261, 261*t*
Patient Health Questionnaire, 196, 196*t*
peers, social support, 383
perceived barriers, 92
perceived behavioral control, 113–115
        issues, 126–127
perceived benefits, 91
perceived severity, 91, 95
perceived susceptibility, 90–91
perceived vulnerability, 95
perception of pain, 272
perfectionism, 350
peripheral, 422
peripheral artery disease, 273
personality, in exercise dependence, 348
personality traits, 215–216, 226, 376
    explanation, 353
    five-factor model *vs.*, 220*t*
    and intervention, 224–225
    and physical activity, 219–225
    and sedentary behavior, 225
    structure of, 216–219
phantom limb pain, 272
pharmacotherapy, 197
physical activity (PA), 26–27, 177, 178*f*
    behavior
        effort in, 74
        initiation and maintenance of,
            73–74
    contexts, self-efficacy in, 72–73
    guidelines, 39–40, 124*f*
    incidental, 40
    intensity, 39*t*
    intention, moderator of, 224*f*
    intervention, 97–98
        self-determination theory in,
            103–104

physical activity (*Cont.*)
  model of, 43
  psychology of
    Australian guidelines in 2012,
      22, 22*t*
    benefits of, 8*t*, 12
    correlates of exercise, 16–19
    exercise psychology and research,
      16, 26, 27*t*
    guidelines for, 19–25, 19*t*
    historical developments, 25–26
    meta-analysis, 13–16
    overview, 5–12
    percentage of American adults
      reporting, 10, 10*f*
    related terms of, 26–29, 28*f*
    social ecological framework for,
      17, 17*f*
    and tomato effect, 6–12
    World Health Organization, 21, 21*t*
  therapeutic effect of, 206
Physical Activity Across the
    Curriculum (PAAC), 168
Physical Activity Group Environment
    Questionnaire, 393*t*
physical activity research, 115–118
  examination of, 149–152
    intervention research, 151–152
    observational studies, 150
physical environment
  correlates of, 419–423, 421*t*, 423*t*
  definition of, 401
  on delayed gratification, 402–404
  modernization of, 404–410
    Inuit, case of, 405–407, 405*f*–406*f*
    Old Order Amish, case of,
      407–410, 408*f*–409*f*
  point-of-choice environmental
    prompts, 416–419, 417*f*, 418*f*
  seasonal variation, 414–416
  travel patterns
    in different countries, 412–413
    Dutch, case of, 413–414
    youth travel patterns, 410–412

physical inactivity, 40
physical self-esteem, 236–239, 236*f*
Physical Self-Perception Profile, 236,
    237, 237*f*
  sample items from, 238*t*
  subdomains, 238*t*
physiological explanations of exercise
    dependence, 354
physiological hypotheses, 206
physiological state, 70
planning, 128–129
point-of-choice prompts, 416–419,
    417*f*, 418*f*
point-of-decision prompts. *See*
    point-of-choice prompts
polar climate, 405
polysomnography, 295
population-attributable fraction, 8
positive psychology, 321–328, 321*t*
  definition of, 321
  exercise, and sedentary behavior,
    322–324
  Exercise-Induced Feeling Inventory,
    326–328, 327*t*
  happiness, 324–326
positive social support, 376
positive *vs.* negative stress, 262–263
postpartum depression, 198
posttraumatic stress disorder (PTSD),
    268–269
  symptoms of, 268*t*
potential mechanisms, 206
practical support, 381
precaution strategy, 97
precontemplation stage, 142
preparation stage, 143
prevalence of exercise dependence,
    345–347
primary cognitive processes, 95
primary exercise dependence,
    357–358
processes of change, 145, 146*t*
processing speed, 173
prospective cohort study, 175

protection motivation theory, 94–96, 95f, 98t
  application of, 96–97
  limitations of, 98–99
  and physical activity intervention, 97–98
psychiatric disorder, 191
psychobiological explanations of exercise dependence, 354–355
psychological explanations of exercise dependence, 353–354
psychosocial factors, 89
psychotherapy, 197
psychoticism, 218
PTSD. *See* posttraumatic stress disorder
Public Health Service, 88

Q

quality of life, 309
  integration of, 309, 310f
  World Health Organization (WHO), 309, 310f, 310t
quantitative research, 13
quasi-experimental design, 123

R

rapid eye movement (REM), 288
real-life stress research, 266–267
reciprocal determinism, 67, 68f
recreational physical activity, 28
recreational screen time, 39
recurrent pain, 270
regular exercise, 342
REM. *See* rapid eye movement
research, integration through meta-analysis, 13–15
response efficacy, 95–96
restless legs syndrome, 299

S

SAT. *See* Scholastic Aptitude Test
scheduling efficacy, 72
scheduling self-efficacy, 127
Scholastic Aptitude Test (SAT), 403

screen time, 39
  recreational, 39
SCT. *See* social cognitive theory
season, 414
seasonal variation, 414–416
secondary exercise dependence, 357–358
sedentarism, 39
sedentary behavior, 38, 179, 316–324
  defining, 38–42
  FITT principle to, 42t
  guidelines for, 43–45, 44t–45t
  health significance of, 42–43
  individual correlates of, 50–53, 52t
  measures of, 53–56, 54t, 55f
  overview of, 36–38
  prevalence of, 45–50, 46f, 47f, 49f
  research, 118–119
  social cognitive theory, 78–79
Sedentary Behavior Questionnaire, 53–54, 54t, 55f
self-care physical activity, 28f
self-concept, 235
self-determination theory, 99, 100f, 105, 349
  intrinsic and extrinsic motivation, 101–102
  measurement of, 103
  in physical activity intervention, 103–104
  research of, 102–103
  sources of motivation, 100–101
self-efficacy, 89, 91, 96, 145
  definition of, 65
  enhancement of, 75–79
  and mental states, 74–75
  nature and measurement of, 70–73
  and physical activity behavior, 73–74
  in physical activity contexts, 72–73
  in social cognitive theory, 66–68
  sources of, 68–70, 69f
  strategies for strengthening, 76, 76t

self-esteem, 234–236, 251–252, 351
    effects of exercise and sedentary
        behavior, 239–241
    physical self-esteem, 236–239
self-presentation, 248
    anxiety, 248–251
self-reported cell phone use by
        gender, 53t
separation anxiety disorder, 200–201
Short-Form (SF)-36 scale, 313–315, 315t
Short-Form McGill Pain
        Questionnaire, 276
16PF, 217, 217t
sleep, 287–291
    affects of acute and chronic
        exercise, 294–295
    age group of, 289t
    behaviors improvement with, 292f
    comparison with short and long
        sleepers, 291f
    definition of, 287–288
    evening exercise and, 295–296
    exercise affects sleep, 301–303
        antidepressant effects, 302
        anxiety reduction, 301
        circadian rhythms, 302–303
        thermoregulation, 302
    exercise, and sedentary behavior,
        291–301
    good exercise for, 293f
    stages of, 289t
sleep debt, 290
sleep disorder, 296, 298t
    exercise and clinical, 296–301
sleep hygiene, 296, 297t
sleep latency, 300
social anxiety disorder, 205
social cognitive theory (SCT), 67f
    nature and measurement of
        self-efficacy, 70–73
    overview of, 65–66
    and physical activity behavior, 73–74
    self-efficacy and mental states,
        74–75

self-efficacy enhancement, 75–79
    self-efficacy in, 66–68
    sources of self-efficacy beliefs, 68–70
social ecological framework for
        physical activity, 17, 17f
social embeddedness. See social
        integration
social environment, 371–393
    definition of, 373
    group dynamics, 388–393
    social support. See social support
social facilitation, 25
social integration, 374, 378
social media, 387
social network resources, 377
social physique anxiety, 248, 248t
social reinforcement, 380
social support, 130, 373–374
    appraisal of, 378
    definition of, 373
    functional components of, 379t
    hierarchy of, 375f
    measurement of, 377–380, 377t
    negative aspects of, 375–376
    as personality trait, 376
    physical activity, and sedentary
        behavior, 380–388, 381t
        dogs, 385–387
        healthcare providers, 384–385
        parents, 382
        peers, 383
        social media, 387–388
        teasing and bullying, 383–384
    taxonomies for, 374–375
    types of, 382
specific phobias, 200–201
sport physical activity, 28f
sport psychology, 29
stages of change, 140–144, 141f
    action stage, 143
    contemplation stage, 142–143
    maintenance stage, 143–144
    operational definitions of,
        141, 142t

precontemplation stage, 142
preparation stage, 143
termination stage, 144
STAI. *See* State-Trait Anxiety Inventory
standard of living, 311
standard score, 14
state anxiety, 201–203, 250*f*
    reduction in, 250
State-Trait Anxiety Inventory (STAI),
        202, 203*t*
stimuli, pain, 277
street connectivity, 402
strengthening self-efficacy, strategies
        for, 76, 76*t*
stress, 259–262
    definition of, 260
    disorders and exercise, 268–269
    distress, 263, 264*t*
    effect mechanisms, 267–268
    eustress, 262–263, 264*t*
    exercise and sedentary behavior,
        263–267
    hormones, 267
    laboratory research, 264–266
    real-life research, 266–267
    response, 262
    types of
        acute *vs.* chronic stress, 262
        positive *vs.* negative stress,
            262–263
stressors, 260
    active and passive, 260
    types of, 261*t*
Stroop color-word test, 260, 261
structural factors, 89
subjective norm, 113
    issues, 129–131
substance-related disorders, 342–343
suburban sprawl, 421
support appraisal, 377–378
support networks, 374
supportive climates, 374
supportive environments. *See*
        supportive climates

sympathetic arousal explanation, 354
systematic review, 13

T
talk therapy, 197
task efficacy, 72
teasing, 383–384
temptation, 146
tender points, 274*f*
termination stage, 144
theory for practice, 121,
        123–125
theory of planned behavior
        (TPB), 111–112, 112*f*,
        114*t*, 223
    elicitation studies, 119–121
    for exercise, 114*f*, 116*t*
    limitations of, 125–131
    for pregnant women, 120*t*, 122*t*
    relationship of, 115*f*
    research, 115–119
    for sedentary behavior, 119*t*
    theory for practice, 121, 123–125
    variables, 112–115
theory of reasoned action, 111
thermoregulation, 302
threat appraisal, 95
tomato effect, 6–12
    definition of, 5
TPB. *See* theory of planned behavior
trait anxiety, 201–203
transportation physical activity, 28*f*
transtheoretical model, 137–153
    advantages and limitations of,
        146–149
    constructs of, 140–146
    examination of physical activity
        research, 149–152
    overview of, 139
travel patterns, physical environment
    in different countries, 412–413, 413*t*
    Dutch, case of, 413–414
    youth travel patterns, 410–412
triadic reciprocal determinism, 67

trigger points, 273, 274
Twitter, 53
type A personality, 222

U
ultramarathons, 339
urban sprawl, 421
U.S. Department of Labor, 47

V
variables, 125–126
verbal persuasion, 70
vicarious experiences, 69

W
Wechsler Individual Achievement
        Test-Second Edition, 169
Wheeling Walks, 123
women
    issues for, 243*f*
    report, 245
World Health Organization (WHO), 8
    physical activity guidelines, 21, 21*t*
    quality of life, 309, 310*f*, 310*t*

Y
young populations, 195
youth travel patterns, 410–412